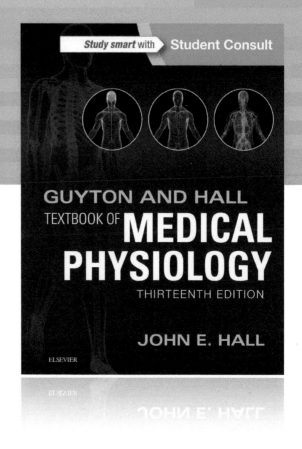
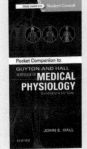
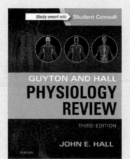

THIRD EDITION

Guyton and Hall
Physiology Review

John E. Hall, PhD

Arthur C. Guyton Professor and Chair
Department of Physiology and Biophysics
Director of the Mississippi Center
for Obesity Research
University of Mississippi Medical Center
Jackson, Mississippi

ELSEVIER

ELSEVIER

1600 John F. Kennedy Blvd.
Ste 1800
Philadelphia, PA 19103-2899

GUYTON AND HALL PHYSIOLOGY REVIEW, THIRD EDITION   ISBN: 978-1-4557-7007-6

Previous editions copyrighted 2011, 2006 by Saunders, an imprint of Elsevier, Inc.

ISBN: 978-1-4557-7007-6

Senior Content Strategist: Elyse O'Grady
Content Development Specialist: Lauren Boyle
Publishing Services Manager: Patricia Tannian
Senior Project Manager: Carrie Stetz
Design Direction: Julia Dummitt

Printed in the United States of America

Last digit is the print number: 9 8 7 6 5 4 3

Working together
to grow libraries in
developing countries

www.elsevier.com • www.bookaid.org

Contributors

Thomas H. Adair, PhD
Professor of Physiology and Biophysics
University of Mississippi Medical Center
Jackson, Mississippi
Units II, IX, X, XI, XII, and XIII

Joey P. Granger, PhD
Billy S. Guyton Distinguished Professor
Professor of Physiology and Medicine
Director of the Cardiovascular-Renal Research Center
Dean of the School of Graduate Studies in the Health
    Sciences
University of Mississippi Medical Center
Jackson, Mississippi
Unit IV

John E. Hall, PhD
Arthur C. Guyton Professor and Chair
Department of Physiology and Biophysics
Director of the Mississippi Center for Obesity Research
University of Mississippi Medical Center
Jackson, Mississippi
Units I, V, and XIII

Robert L. Hester, PhD
Professor of Physiology and Biophysics
Director of the Computer Services, Electronics, and
    Instrumentations Core
University of Mississippi Medical Center
Jackson, Mississippi
Units VII, VIII, and XV

Thomas E. Lohmeier, PhD
Professor Emeritus of Physiology and Biophysics
University of Mississippi Medical Center
Jackson, Mississippi
Unit XIV

R. Davis Manning Jr, PhD
Professor Emeritus of Physiology and Biophysics
University of Mississippi Medical Center
Jackson, Mississippi
Units III and IV

Jane F. Reckelhoff, PhD
Billy S. Guyton Distinguished Professor
Professor of Physiology and Biophysics
Director of the Women's Health Research Center
Director of Research Development
University of Mississippi Medical Center
Jackson, Mississippi
Unit XIV

James G. Wilson, MD
Professor of Physiology and Biophysics
University of Mississippi Medical Center
Jackson, Mississippi
Unit VI

The main goal of this book is the same as in previous editions: to provide students a tool for assessing their mastery of physiology as presented in *Guyton and Hall Textbook of Medical Physiology*.

Self-assessment is an important component of effective learning, especially when studying a subject as complex as medical physiology. *Guyton & Hall Physiology Review* is designed to provide a comprehensive review of medical physiology through multiple-choice questions and explanations of the answers. Medical students preparing for the United States Medical Licensure Examinations (USMLE) will also find this book useful because most of the test questions have been constructed according to the USMLE format.

The questions and answers in this review are based on *Guyton and Hall Textbook of Medical Physiology*, 13th Edition (TMP 13). More than 1000 questions and answers are provided, and each answer is referenced to the *Textbook of Medical Physiology* to facilitate a more complete understanding of the topic. Illustrations are used to reinforce basic concepts. Some of the questions incorporate information from multiple chapters to test your ability to apply and integrate the principles necessary for mastery of medical physiology.

An effective way to use this book is to allow an average of 1 minute for each question in a unit, approximating the time limit for a question in the USMLE examination. As you proceed, indicate your answer next to each question. After finishing the questions and answers, verify your answers and carefully read the explanations provided. Read the additional material referred to in the *Textbook of Medical Physiology*, especially for questions for which incorrect answers were chosen.

Guyton and Hall Physiology Review should not be used as a substitute for the comprehensive information contained in the *Textbook of Medical Physiology*. It is intended mainly as a means of assessing your knowledge of physiology and strengthening your ability to apply and integrate this knowledge.

We have attempted to make this review as accurate as possible, and we hope that it will be a valuable tool for your study of physiology. We invite you to send us your critiques, suggestions for improvement, and notifications of any errors.

I am grateful to each of the contributors for their careful work on this book. I also wish to express my thanks to Lauren Boyle, Rebecca Gruliow, Elyse O'Grady, Carrie Stetz, and the rest of the Elsevier staff for their editorial and production excellence.

John E. Hall

Contents

Guyton and Hall
Physiology Review

Introduction to Physiology: The Cell and General Physiology

1. Which statement about microRNAs (miRNAs) is correct?

   A) miRNAs are formed in the cytoplasm and repress translation or promote degradation of messenger RNA (mRNA) before it can be translated

   B) miRNAs are formed in the nucleus and then processed in the cytoplasm by the dicer enzyme

   C) miRNAs are short (21 to 23 nucleotide) double-stranded RNA fragments that regulate gene expression

   D) miRNAs repress gene transcription

2. Compared with the intracellular fluid, the extracellular fluid has _____ sodium ion concentration, _____ potassium ion concentration, _____ chloride ion concentration, and _____ phosphate ion concentration.

   A) Lower, lower, lower, lower

   B) Lower, higher, lower, lower

   C) Lower, higher, higher, lower

   D) Higher, lower, higher, lower

   E) Higher, higher, lower, higher

   F) Higher, higher, higher, higher

3. In comparing two types of cells from the same person, the variation in the proteins expressed by each cell type reflects which of the following?

   A) Differences in the DNA contained in the nucleus of each cell

   B) Differences in the numbers of specific genes in their genomes

   C) Cell-specific expression and repression of specific genes

   D) Differences in the number of chromosomes in each cell

   E) The age of the cells

4. Which statement about telomeres is incorrect?

   A) Telomeres are repetitive nucleotide sequences at the end of a chromatid

   B) Telomeres serve as protective caps that prevent the chromosome from deterioration during cell division

   C) Telomeres are gradually consumed during repeated cell divisions

   D) In cancer cells, telomerase activity is usually reduced compared with normal cells

5. Which of the following events does not occur during the process of mitosis?

   A) Condensation of the chromosomes

   B) Replication of the genome

   C) Fragmentation of the nuclear envelope

   D) Alignment of the chromatids along the equatorial plate

   E) Separation of the chromatids into two sets of 46 "daughter" chromosomes

6. The term "glycocalyx" refers to what?

   A) The negatively charged carbohydrate chains that protrude into the cytosol from glycolipids and integral glycoproteins

   B) The negatively charged carbohydrate layer on the outer cell surface

   C) The layer of anions aligned on the cytosolic surface of the plasma membrane

   D) The large glycogen stores found in "fast" muscles

   E) A mechanism of cell–cell attachment

7. Which statement is incorrect?

   A) The term "homeostasis" describes the maintenance of nearly constant conditions in the body

   B) In most diseases, homeostatic mechanisms are no longer operating in the body

   C) The body's compensatory mechanisms often lead to deviations from the normal range in some of the body's functions

   D) Disease is generally considered to be a state of disrupted homeostasis

Questions 8–10

   A) Nucleolus

   B) Nucleus

   C) Agranular endoplasmic reticulum

   D) Granular endoplasmic reticulum

   E) Golgi apparatus

   F) Endosomes

   G) Peroxisomes

   H) Lysosomes

   I) Cytosol

   J) Cytoskeleton

   K) Glycocalyx

   L) Microtubules

For each of the scenarios described below, identify the most likely subcellular site listed above for the deficient or mutant protein.

8. The abnormal cleavage of mannose residues during the post-translational processing of glycoproteins results in the development of a lupus-like autoimmune disease in mice. The abnormal cleavage is due to a mutation of the enzyme α-mannosidase II.

9. The observation that abnormal cleavage of mannose residues from glycoproteins causes an autoimmune disease in mice supports the role of this structure in the normal immune response.

10. Studies completed on a 5-year-old boy show an accumulation of cholesteryl esters and triglycerides in his liver, spleen, and intestines and calcification of both adrenal glands. Additional studies indicate the cause to be a deficiency in acid lipase A activity.

Questions 11–13
A) Nucleolus
B) Nucleus
C) Agranular endoplasmic reticulum
D) Granular endoplasmic reticulum
E) Golgi apparatus
F) Endosomes
G) Peroxisomes
H) Lysosomes
I) Cytosol
J) Cytoskeleton
K) Glycocalyx
L) Microtubules

Match the cellular location for each of the steps involved in the synthesis and packaging of a secreted protein listed below with the correct term from the list above.

11. Protein condensation and packaging

12. Initiation of translation

13. Gene transcription

14. Worn-out organelles are transferred to lysosomes by which of the following?

A) Autophagosomes
B) Granular endoplasmic reticulum
C) Agranular endoplasmic reticulum
D) Golgi apparatus
E) Mitochondria

15. Which of the following is not a major function of the endoplasmic reticulum (ER)?

A) Synthesis of lipids
B) Synthesis of proteins
C) Providing enzymes that control glycogen breakdown
D) Providing enzymes that detoxify substances that could damage the cell
E) Secretion of proteins synthesized in the cell

16. Which of the following does not play a direct role in the process of transcription?

A) Helicase
B) RNA polymerase
C) Chain-terminating sequence
D) "Activated" RNA molecules
E) Promoter sequence

17. Which statement is true for *both* pinocytosis and phagocytosis?

A) Involves the recruitment of actin filaments
B) Occurs spontaneously and nonselectively
C) Endocytotic vesicles fuse with ribosomes that release hydrolases into the vesicles
D) Is only observed in macrophages and neutrophils
E) Does not require ATP

18. Which of the following proteins is most likely to be the product of a proto-oncogene?

A) Growth factor receptor
B) Cytoskeletal protein
C) Na$^+$ channel
D) Ca^{++}-ATPase
E) Myosin light chain

19. Which statement is incorrect?

A) Proto-oncogenes are normal genes that code for proteins that control cell growth
B) Proto-oncogenes are normal genes that code for proteins that control cell division
C) Inactivation of anti-oncogenes protects against the development of cancer
D) Several different simultaneously activated oncogenes are often required to cause cancer

20. Which statement about feedback control systems is incorrect?

A) Most control systems of the body act by negative feedback
B) Positive feedback usually promotes stability in a system
C) Generation of nerve actions potentials involves positive feedback
D) Feed-forward control is important in regulating muscle activity

21. Assume that excess blood is transfused into a patient whose arterial baroreceptors are nonfunctional and whose blood pressure increases from 100 to 150 mm Hg. Then, assume that the same volume of blood is infused into the same patient under conditions in which his arterial baroreceptors are functioning normally and blood pressure increases from 100 to 125 mm Hg. What is the approximate feedback "gain" of the arterial baroreceptors in this patient when they are functioning normally?

    A) –1.0
    B) –2.0
    C) 0.0
    D) +1.0
    E) +2.0

22. Which of the following cell organelles is responsible for producing adenosine triphosphate (ATP), the energy currency of the cell?

    A) Endoplasmic reticulum
    B) Mitochondria
    C) Lysosomes
    D) Golgi apparatus
    E) Peroxisomes
    F) Ribosomes

23. Which statement about mRNA is correct?

    A) mRNA carries the genetic code to the cytoplasm
    B) mRNA carries activated amino acids to the ribosomes
    C) mRNA is composed of single-stranded RNA molecules of 21 to 23 nucleotides that can regulate gene transcription
    D) mRNA forms ribosomes

24. "Redundancy" or "degeneration" of the genetic code occurs during which step of protein synthesis?

    A) DNA replication
    B) Transcription
    C) Post-transcriptional modification
    D) Translation
    E) Protein glycosylation

1. A) The miRNAs are formed in the cytoplasm from pre-miRNAs and processed by the enzyme dicer that ultimately assembles RNA-induced silencing complex, which then generates miRNAs. The miRNAs regulate gene expression by binding to the complementary region of the RNA and repressing translation or promoting degradation of messenger RNA before it can be translated by the ribosome.
TMP13 pp. 32-33

2. D) The extracellular fluid has relatively high concentrations of sodium and chloride ions but lower concentrations of potassium and phosphate compared with the intracellular fluid.
TMP13 pp. 3-4

3. C) The variation in proteins expressed by each cell reflects cell-specific expression and repression of specific genes. Each cell contains the same DNA in the nucleus and the same number of genes, and thus differentiation results not from differences in the genes but from selective repression and/or activation of different gene promoters.
TMP13 p. 41

4. D) Telomeres are repetitive nucleotide sequences, located at the end of a chromatid, that serve as protective caps to prevent the chromosome from deterioration during cell division, but they are gradually consumed during cell divisions (see figure below). In cancer cells, the enzyme telomerase is *activated* (not inhibited) and adds bases to the ends of the telomeres so that many more generations of cancer cells can be produced.
TMP13 p. 40

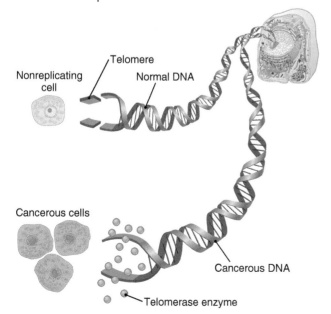

5. B) DNA replication occurs during the S phase of the cell cycle and precedes mitosis. Condensation of the chromosomes occurs during the prophase of mitosis. Fragmentation of the nuclear envelope occurs during the prometaphase of mitosis. The chromatids align at the equatorial plate during metaphase and separate into two complete sets of daughter chromosomes during anaphase.
TMP13 p. 37

6. B) The cell "glycocalyx" is the loose negatively charged carbohydrate coat on the outside of the surface of the cell membrane. The membrane carbohydrates usually occur in combination with proteins or lipids in the form of glycoproteins or glycolipids, and the "glyco" portion of these molecules almost invariably protrudes to the outside of the cell.
TMP13 p. 14

7. B) The term *homeostasis* describes the maintenance of nearly constant conditions in the internal environment of the body, and diseases are generally considered to be states of disrupted homeostasis. However, even in diseases, homeostatic compensatory mechanisms continue to operate in an attempt sustain body functions at levels that permit life to continue. These compensations may result in deviations from the normal level of some body functions as a "trade-off" that is necessary to maintain vital functions of the body.
TMP13 p. 4

8. E) Membrane proteins are glycosylated during their synthesis in the lumen of the rough endoplasmic reticulum. Most post-translational modification of the oligosaccharide chains, however, occurs during the transport of the protein through the layers of the Golgi apparatus matrix, where enzymes such as α-mannosidase II are localized.
TMP13 p. 15

9. K) The oligosaccharide chains that are added to glycoproteins on the luminal side of the rough endoplasmic reticulum, and subsequently modified during their transport through the Golgi apparatus, are attached to the extracellular surface of the cell. This negatively charged layer of carbohydrate moieties is collectively called the *glycocalyx*. It participates in cell–cell interactions, cell–ligand interactions, and the immune response.
TMP13 p. 14; see also Chapter 35

10. **H)** Acid lipases, along with other acid hydrolases, are localized to lysosomes. Fusion of endocytotic and autolytic vesicles with lysosomes initiates the intracellular process that allows cells to digest cellular debris and particles ingested from the extracellular milieu, including bacteria. In the normal acidic environment of the lysosome, acid lipases use hydrogen to convert lipids into fatty acids and glycerol. Other acid lipases include a variety of nucleases, proteases, and polysaccharide-hydrolyzing enzymes.

    TMP13 pp. 15-16

11. **E)** Secreted proteins are condensed, sorted, and packaged into secretory vesicles in the terminal portions of the Golgi apparatus, also known as the trans-Golgi network. It is here that proteins destined for secretion are separated from those destined for intracellular compartments or cellular membranes.

    TMP13 p. 15

12. **I)** Initiation of translation, whether of a cytosolic protein, a membrane-bound protein, or a secreted protein, occurs in the cytosol and involves a common pool of ribosomes. Only after the appearance of the N-terminus of the polypeptide is it identified as a protein destined for secretion. At this point, the ribosome attaches to the cytosolic surface of the rough endoplasmic reticulum. Translation continues, and the new polypeptide is extruded into the matrix of the endoplasmic reticulum.

    TMP13 pp. 33-34

13. **B)** All transcription events occur in the nucleus, regardless of the final destination of the protein product. The resulting messenger RNA molecule is transported through the nuclear pores in the nuclear membrane and translated into either the cytosol or the lumen of the rough endoplasmic reticulum.

    TMP13 pp. 30-31

14. **A)** Autophagy is a housekeeping process by which obsolete organelles and large protein aggregates are degraded and recycled (see figure at right). Worn-out cell organelles are transferred to lysosomes by double membrane structures called autophagosomes that are formed in the cytosol.

    TMP13 p. 20

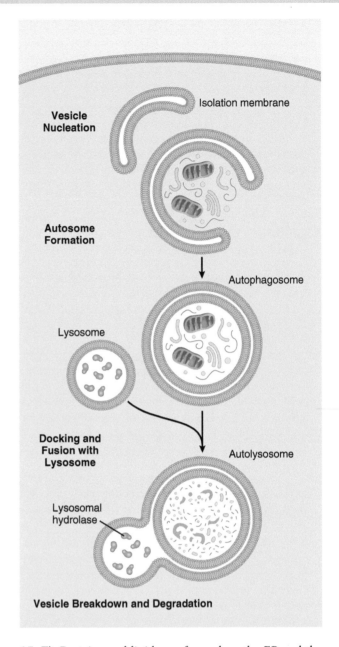

15. **E)** Proteins and lipids are formed on the ER and then passed on to the Golgi apparatus, where they are further processed before being released into the cytoplasm, where they can be used in the cell or secreted. The ER does not secrete proteins and lipids from the cell. The ER also provides enzymes that control glycogen breakdown and help to detoxify substances such as drugs that could damage the cell.

    TMP13 pp. 14-15

16. **A)** Helicase is one of the many proteins involved in the process of DNA replication. It does not play a role in transcription. RNA polymerase binds to the promoter sequence and facilitates the addition of "activated" RNA molecules to the growing RNA molecule until the polymerase reaches the chain-terminating sequence on the template DNA molecule.
    TMP13 pp. 30-31

17. **A)** Both pinocytosis and phagocytosis involve movement of the plasma membrane. Pinocytosis involves invagination of the cell membrane, whereas phagocytosis involves evagination. Both events require the recruitment of actin and other cytoskeleton elements. Phagocytosis is not spontaneous and is selective, being triggered by specific receptor-ligand interactions.
    TMP13 pp. 19-20

18. **A)** An oncogene is a gene that is either abnormally activated or mutated in such a way that its product causes uncontrolled cell growth. A proto-oncogene is simply the "normal" version of an oncogene. By definition, proto-oncogenes are divided into several families of proteins, all of which participate in the control of cell growth. These families include, but are not limited to, growth factors and their receptors, protein kinases, transcription factors, and proteins that regulate cell proliferation.
    TMP13 pp. 41-42

19. **C)** Inactivation of anti-oncogenes, also called tumor suppressor genes, can allow activation of oncogenes that lead to cancer. All the other statements are correct.
    TMP13 pp. 40-41

20. **B)** Positive feedback in a system generally promotes instability, rather than stability, and in some cases even death. For this reason, positive feedback is often called a "vicious cycle." However, in some instances, positive feedback can be useful. One example is the nerve action potential where stimulation of the nerve membrane causes a slight leakage of sodium that causes more opening of sodium channels, more change of potential, and more opening of channels until an explosion of sodium entering the interior of the nerve fiber creates the action potential. Feed-forward control is used to apprise the brain whether a muscle movement is performed correctly. If not, the brain corrects the feed-forward signals that it sends to the muscles the next time the movement is required. This mechanism is often called *adaptive* control.
    TMP13 pp. 8-10

21. **A)** The feedback gain of the control system is calculated as the amount of correction divided by the remaining error of the system. In this example, blood pressure increased from 100 to 150 mm Hg when the baroreceptors were not functioning. When the baroreceptors were functioning, the pressure increased only 25 mm Hg. Therefore, the feedback system caused a "correction" of –25 mm Hg, from 150 to 125 mm Hg. The remaining increase in pressure of +25 mm is called the "error." In this example the correction is therefore –25 mm Hg and the remaining error is +25 mm Hg. Thus, the feedback gain of the baroreceptors in this person is –1, indicating a negative feedback control system.
    TMP13 pp. 8-9

22. **B)** Mitochondria are often called the "powerhouses" of the cell and contain oxidative enzymes that permit oxidation of the nutrients, thereby forming carbon dioxide and water and at the same time releasing energy. The liberated energy is used to synthesize "high-energy" ATP.
    TMP13 pp. 16-17

23. **A)** mRNA molecules are long, single RNA strands that are suspended in the cytoplasm and are composed of several hundred to several thousand RNA nucleotides in unpaired strands. The mRNA carries the genetic code to the cytoplasm for controlling the type of protein formed. The *transfer RNA* transports activated amino acids to the ribosomes. *Ribosomal RNA*, along with about 75 different proteins, forms ribosomes. MiRNAs are single-stranded RNA molecules of 21 to 23 nucleotides that regulate gene transcription and translation.
    TMP13 pp. 31-32

24. **D)** During both replication and transcription, the new nucleic acid molecule is an exact complement of the parent DNA molecule as a result of predictable, specific, one-to-one base pairing. During the process of translation, however, each amino acid in the new polypeptide is encoded by a codon—a series of three consecutive nucleotides. Whereas each codon encodes a specific amino acid, most amino acids can be encoded for by multiple codons. Redundancy results because 60 codons encode a mere 20 amino acids.
    TMP13 pp. 31-32

Membrane Physiology, Nerve, and Muscle

1. Simple diffusion and facilitated diffusion share which of the following characteristics?

   A) Can be blocked by specific inhibitors
   B) Do not require adenosine triphosphate (ATP)
   C) Require transport protein
   D) Saturation kinetics
   E) Transport solute against concentration gradient

2. What is the osmolarity of a solution containing 10 millimolar NaCl, 5 millimolar KCl, and 10 millimolar $CaCl_2$ (in mOsm/L)?

   A) 20
   B) 40
   C) 60
   D) 80
   E) 100

Questions 3–6

Intracellular (mM)	Extracellular (mM)
140 K^+	5 K^+
12 Na^+	145 Na^+
5 Cl^-	125 Cl^-
0.0001 Ca^{++}	5 Ca^{++}

The table above shows the concentrations of four ions across the plasma membrane of a hypothetical cell. Use this table to answer Questions 3–6.

3. Which of the following best describes the equilibrium potential for Cl^- (in millivolts)?

   A) 0
   B) 170
   C) –170
   D) 85
   E) –85

4. Which of the following best describes the equilibrium potential for K^+ (in millivolts)?

   A) 0
   B) 176
   C) –176
   D) 88
   E) –88

5. The net driving force is greatest for which ion when the membrane potential of this cell is –85 millivolts?

   A) Ca^{++}
   B) Cl^-
   C) K^+
   D) Na^+

6. If this cell were permeable only to K^+, what would be the effect of reducing the extracellular K^+ concentration from 5 to 2.5 millimolar?

   A) 19 millivolts depolarization
   B) 19 millivolts hyperpolarization
   C) 38 millivolts depolarization
   D) 38 millivolts hyperpolarization
   E) 29 millivolts depolarization
   F) 29 millivolts hyperpolarization

7. Which of the following best describes the changes in cell volume that will occur when red blood cells (previously equilibrated in a 280-milliosmolar solution of NaCl) are placed in a solution of 140-millimolar NaCl containing 20-millimolar urea, a relatively large but permeant molecule?

   A) Shrink, then swell and lyse
   B) Shrink, then return to original volume
   C) Swell and lyse
   D) Swell, then return to original volume
   E) No change in cell volume

8. A clinical study is conducted to determine the actions of an unknown test solution on red blood cell volume. One milliliter of heparinized human blood is pipetted into 100 milliliters of test solution and mixed. Samples are taken and analyzed immediately before and at 1-second intervals after mixing. The results show that red blood cells placed into the test solution immediately swell and burst. Which of the following best describes the tonicity and osmolarity of the test solution?

   A) Hypertonic; could be hyperosmotic, hypo-osmotic, or iso-osmotic
   B) Hypertonic; must be hyperosmotic or hypo-osmotic
   C) Hypertonic; must be iso-osmotic
   D) Hypotonic; could be hyperosmotic, hypo-osmotic, or iso-osmotic
   E) Hypotonic; must be hyperosmotic or hypo-osmotic
   F) Hypotonic; must be iso-osmotic

9. A single contraction of skeletal muscle is most likely to be terminated by which of the following actions?

   A) Closure of the postsynaptic nicotinic acetylcholine receptor
   B) Removal of acetylcholine from the neuromuscular junction
   C) Removal of Ca^{++} from the terminal of the motor neuron
   D) Removal of sarcoplasmic Ca^{++}
   E) Return of the dihydropyridine receptor to its resting conformation

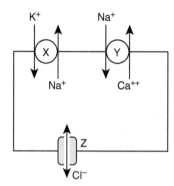

10. A model cell with three different transporters (X, Y, and Z) and a resting membrane potential of −75 millivolts is shown in the above figure. Consider the intracellular and extracellular concentrations of all three ions to be typical of a normal cell. Which of the following best describes transporter Y?

   A) Facilitated diffusion
   B) Primary active transport
   C) Secondary active transport
   D) Simple diffusion

11. Which of the following best describes an attribute of visceral smooth muscle not shared by skeletal muscle?

   A) Contraction is ATP dependent
   B) Contracts in response to stretch
   C) Does not contain actin filaments
   D) High rate of cross-bridge cycling
   E) Low maximal force of contraction

12. The resting potential of a myelinated nerve fiber is primarily dependent on the concentration gradient of which of the following ions?

   A) Ca^{++}
   B) Cl^-
   C) HCO_3^-
   D) K^+
   E) Na^+

13. Calmodulin is most closely related, both structurally and functionally, to which of the following proteins?

   A) G-actin
   B) Myosin light chain
   C) Tropomyosin
   D) Troponin C

14. In the figure below, two compartments (X and Y) are separated by a typical biological membrane (lipid bilayer). The concentrations of glucose in compartments X and Y at time zero are shown. There are no transporters for glucose in the membrane, and the membrane is impermeable to glucose. Which of the figures best represent the volumes of compartments X and Y when the system reaches equilibrium?

   A) A
   B) B
   C) C
   D) D
   E) E

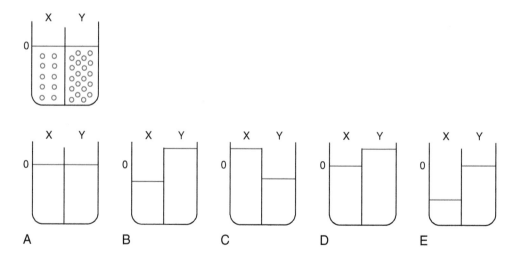

15. During a demonstration for medical students, a neurologist uses magnetic cortical stimulation to trigger firing of the ulnar nerve in a volunteer. At relatively low-amplitude stimulation, action potentials are recorded only from muscle fibers in the index finger. As the amplitude of the stimulation is increased, action potentials are recorded from muscle fibers in both the index finger and the biceps muscle. What is the fundamental principle underlying this amplitude-dependent response?

A) Large motor neurons that innervate large motor units require a larger depolarizing stimulus

B) Recruitment of multiple motor units requires a larger depolarizing stimulus

C) The biceps muscle is innervated by more motor neurons

D) The motor units in the biceps are smaller than those in the muscles of the fingers

E) The muscles in the fingers are innervated only by the ulnar nerve

16. A neurotransmitter activates its receptor on an ion channel of a neuron, which causes the water-filled channel to open. Once the channel is open, ions move through the channel down their respective electrochemical gradients. A change in membrane potential follows. Which of the following best describes the type of channel and mechanism of ion transport?

	Type of Channel	Mechanism of Transport
A)	Ligand gated	Facilitated diffusion
B)	Ligand gated	Simple diffusion
C)	Ligand gated	Secondary active transport
D)	Voltage gated	Facilitated diffusion
E)	Voltage gated	Simple diffusion
F)	Voltage gated	Secondary active transport

17. A 55-year-old woman has a serum potassium of 6.1 mEq/L (normal: 3.5-5.0 mEq/L) and a serum sodium of 150 mEq/L (normal: 135-147 mEq/L). Which of the following sets of changes best describe the K^+ Nernst potential and resting membrane potential in a typical neuron in this woman compared to normal? *(Assume normal intracellular ion concentrations.)*

	K+ Nernst Potential	Resting Membrane Potential
A)	Less negative	Less negative
B)	Less negative	No change
C)	Less negative	More negative
D)	More negative	Less negative
E)	More negative	More negative
F)	More negative	No change
G)	No change	Less negative
H)	No change	More negative
I)	No change	No change

18. Which of the following decreases in length during the contraction of a skeletal muscle fiber?

A) A band of the sarcomere
B) I band of the sarcomere
C) Thick filaments
D) Thin filaments
E) Z disks of the sarcomere

$$E_{Q^-} = -75 \text{ millivolts}$$
$$E_{R^+} = +75 \text{ millivolts}$$
$$E_{S^+} = -85 \text{ millivolts}$$

19. Equilibrium potentials for three unknown ions are shown in the above figure. Note that ions S and R are positively charged and that ion Q is negatively charged. Assume that the cell membrane is permeable to all three ions and that the cell has a resting membrane potential of −90 millivolts. Which of the following best describes the net movement of the various ions across the cell membrane by passive diffusion?

	Q	R	S
A)	Inward	Inward	Inward
B)	Inward	Inward	Outward
C)	Inward	Outward	Inward
D)	Inward	Outward	Outward
E)	Outward	Inward	Inward
F)	Outward	Inward	Outward
G)	Outward	Inward	Outward

20. Tetanic contraction of a skeletal muscle fiber results from a cumulative increase in the intracellular concentration of which of the following?

A) ATP
B) Ca^{++}
C) K^+
D) Na^+
E) Troponin

21. Weight lifting can result in a dramatic increase in skeletal muscle mass. This increase in muscle mass is primarily attributable to which of the following?

A) Fusion of sarcomeres between adjacent myofibrils
B) Hypertrophy of individual muscle fibers
C) Increase in skeletal muscle blood supply
D) Increase in the number of motor neurons
E) Increase in the number of neuromuscular junctions

22. Which of the following transport mechanisms is not rate limited by an intrinsic V_{max}?

    A) Facilitated diffusion via carrier proteins
    B) Primary active transport via carrier proteins
    C) Secondary co-transport
    D) Secondary counter-transport
    E) Simple diffusion through protein channels

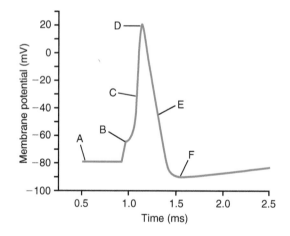

23. Five hypothetical nerve axons are shown in the above figure. Axons A and B are myelinated, whereas axons C, D, and E are non-myelinated. Which axon is most likely to have the fastest conduction velocity for an action potential?

    A) A
    B) B
    C) C
    D) D
    E) E

Questions 24 and 25

The above figure shows the change in membrane potential during an action potential in a giant squid axon. Refer to it when answering Questions 24 and 25.

24. Which of the following is primarily responsible for the change in membrane potential between points B and D?

    A) Inhibition of the Na$^+$, K$^+$-ATPase
    B) Movement of K$^+$ into the cell
    C) Movement of K$^+$ out of the cell
    D) Movement of Na$^+$ into the cell
    E) Movement of Na$^+$ out of the cell

25. Which of the following is primarily responsible for the change in membrane potential between points D and E?

    A) Inhibition of the Na$^+$, K$^+$-ATPase
    B) Movement of K$^+$ into the cell
    C) Movement of K$^+$ out of the cell
    D) Movement of Na$^+$ into the cell
    E) Movement of Na$^+$ out of the cell

26. The axon of a neuron is stimulated experimentally with a 25-millivolt pulse, which initiates an action potential with a velocity of 50 meters per second. The axon is then stimulated with a 100-millivolt pulse. What is the action potential velocity after the 100-millivolt stimulation pulse (in meters per second)?

    A) 25
    B) 50
    C) 100
    D) 150
    E) 200

27. The delayed onset and prolonged duration of smooth muscle contraction, as well as the greater force generated by smooth muscle compared with skeletal muscle, are all consequences of which of the following?

    A) Greater amount of myosin filaments present in smooth muscle
    B) Higher energy requirement of smooth muscle
    C) Physical arrangement of actin and myosin filaments
    D) Slower cycling rate of the smooth muscle myosin cross-bridges
    E) Slower uptake of Ca^{++} ions after contraction

28. An experimental drug is being tested as a potential therapeutic treatment for asthma. Preclinical studies have shown that this drug induces the relaxation of cultured porcine tracheal smooth muscle cells precontracted with acetylcholine. Which of the following mechanisms of action is most likely to induce this effect?

    A) Decreased affinity of troponin C for Ca^{++}
    B) Decreased plasma membrane K$^+$ permeability
    C) Increased plasma membrane Na$^+$ permeability
    D) Inhibition of the sarcoplasmic reticulum Ca^{++}-ATPase
    E) Stimulation of adenylate cyclase

Questions 29 and 30

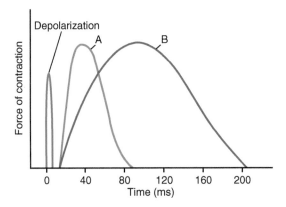

The above figure illustrates the single isometric twitch characteristics of two skeletal muscles, A and B, in response to a depolarizing stimulus. Refer to it when answering Questions 29 and 30.

29. Which of the following best describes muscle B compared with muscle A?

   A) Adapted for rapid contraction
   B) Composed of larger muscle fibers
   C) Fewer mitochondria
   D) Innervated by smaller nerve fibers
   E) Less extensive blood supply

30. The delay between the termination of the transient depolarization of the muscle membrane and the onset of muscle contraction observed in both muscles A and B reflects the time necessary for which of the following events to occur?

   A) ADP to be released from the myosin head
   B) ATP to be synthesized
   C) Ca^{++} to accumulate in the sarcoplasm
   D) G-actin to polymerize into F-actin
   E) Myosin head to complete one cross-bridge cycle

Questions 31–33
A 55-year-old woman visits her physician because of double vision, eyelid droop, difficulty chewing and swallowing, and general weakness in her limbs. All these symptoms worsen with exercise and occur more frequently late in the day. The physician suspects myasthenia gravis and orders a Tensilon test. The test is positive. Use this information when answering Questions 31–33.

31. The increased muscle strength observed during the Tensilon test is due to an increase in which of the following?

   A) Amount of acetylcholine (ACh) released from the motor nerves
   B) Levels of ACh at the muscle end plates
   C) Number of ACh receptors on the muscle end plates
   D) Synthesis of norepinephrine

32. What is the most likely basis for the symptoms described in this patient?

   A) Autoimmune response
   B) Botulinum toxicity
   C) Depletion of voltage-gated Ca^{++} channels in certain motor neurons
   D) Development of macro motor units after recovery from poliomyelitis
   E) Overexertion

33. Which of the following drugs would likely alleviate this patient's symptoms?

   A) Atropine
   B) Botulinum toxin antiserum
   C) Curare
   D) Halothane
   E) Neostigmine

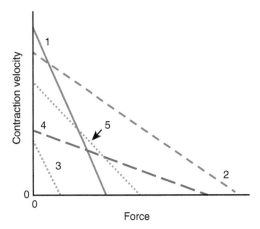

34. The figure above shows a relationship between contraction velocity and force for five different skeletal muscles. Which of the following muscles (A-E) is most likely to correspond to muscle number 1 on the figure shown? *(Assume that all muscles shown are at their normal resting lengths.)*

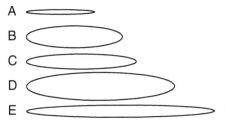

Questions 35–37

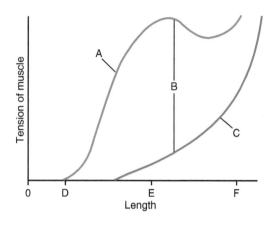

The above figure illustrates the isometric length-tension relationship in a representative intact skeletal muscle. Match the descriptions in Questions 35–37 to one of the points on the figure.

35. So-called "active" or contraction-dependent tension

36. The muscle length at which active tension is maximal

37. The contribution of noncontractile muscle elements to total tension

38. Smooth muscle contraction is terminated by which of the following?

A) Dephosphorylation of myosin kinase
B) Dephosphorylation of myosin light chain
C) Efflux of Ca^{++} ions across the plasma membrane
D) Inhibition of myosin phosphatase
E) Uptake of Ca^{++} ions into the sarcoplasmic reticulum

Questions 39–41
A 56-year-old man sees a neurologist because of weakness in his legs that improves over the course of the day or with exercise. Extracellular electrical recordings from a single skeletal muscle fiber reveal normal miniature end plate potentials. Low-frequency electrical stimulation of the motor neuron, however, elicits an abnormally small depolarization of the muscle fibers. The amplitude of the depolarization is increased after exercise. Use this information to answer Questions 39–41.

39. Based on these findings, which of the following is the most likely cause of this patient's leg weakness?

A) Acetylcholinesterase deficiency
B) Blockade of postsynaptic acetylcholine receptors
C) Impaired presynaptic voltage-sensitive Ca^{++} influx
D) Inhibition of Ca^{++} re-uptake into the sarcoplasmic reticulum
E) Reduced acetylcholine synthesis

40. A preliminary diagnosis is confirmed by the presence of which of the following?

A) Antibodies against the acetylcholine receptor
B) Antibodies against the voltage-sensitive Ca^{++} channel
C) Mutation in the gene that codes for the ryanodine receptor
D) Relatively few vesicles in the presynaptic terminal
E) Residual acetylcholine in the neuromuscular junction

41. The molecular mechanism underlying these symptoms is most similar to which of the following?

A) Acetylcholine
B) Botulinum toxin
C) Curare
D) Neostigmine
E) Tetrodotoxin

Questions 42–44

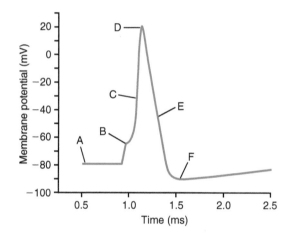

Match each of the descriptions in Questions 42–44 to one of the points of the nerve action potential shown in the above figure.

42. Point at which the membrane potential (V_m) is closest to the Na^+ equilibrium potential

43. Point at which the driving force for Na^+ is the greatest

44. Point at which the ratio of K^+ permeability to Na^+ permeability (P_K/P_{Na}) is the greatest

45. A physiology experiment is conducted in which a motoneuron that normally innervates a predominantly fast type II muscle is anastomosed to a predominantly slow type I muscle. Which of the following is most likely to decrease in the type I muscle after the transinnervation surgery?

A) Fiber diameter
B) Glycolytic activity
C) Maximum contraction velocity
D) Mitochondrial content
E) Myosin ATPase activity

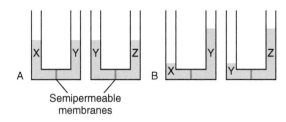

Semipermeable
membranes

46. In the experiment illustrated in part **A** of the above figure, equal volumes of solutions X, Y, and Z are placed into the compartments of the two U-shaped vessels shown. The two compartments of each vessel are separated by semipermeable membranes (i.e., impermeable to ions and large polar molecules). Part **B** illustrates the fluid distribution across the membranes at equilibration. Assuming complete dissociation, identify each of the solutions shown.

	Solution X	Solution Y	Solution Z
A)	1 M $CaCl_2$	1 M NaCl	1 M glucose
B)	1 M glucose	1 M NaCl	1 M $CaCl_2$
C)	1 M NaCl	2 M glucose	3 M $CaCl_2$
D)	2 M NaCl	1 M NaCl	Pure water
E)	Pure water	1 M $CaCl_2$	2 M glucose

Questions 47 and 48

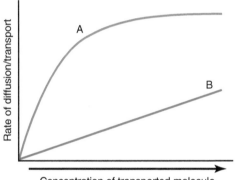

47. Trace A best describes the kinetics of which event?

    A) Movement of CO_2 across the plasma membrane
    B) Movement of O_2 across a lipid bilayer
    C) Na^+ flux through an open nicotinic acetylcholine receptor channel
    D) Transport of K^+ into a muscle cell
    E) Voltage-dependent movement of Ca^{++} into the terminal of a motor neuron

48. Trace B best describes the kinetics of which of the following events?

    A) Na^+-dependent transport of glucose into an epithelial cell
    B) Transport of Ca^{++} into the sarcoplasmic reticulum of a smooth muscle cell
    C) Transport of K^+ into a muscle cell
    D) Transport of Na^+ out of a nerve cell
    E) Transport of O_2 across an artificial lipid bilayer

Questions 49 and 50

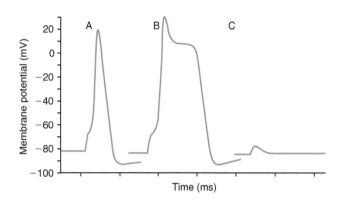

49. Trace A in the above figure represents a typical action potential recorded under control conditions from a normal nerve cell in response to a depolarizing stimulus. Which of the following perturbations would explain the conversion of the response shown in trace A to the action potential shown in trace B?

    A) Blockade of voltage-sensitive Na^+ channels
    B) Blockade of voltage-sensitive K^+ channels
    C) Blockade of Na-K "leak" channels
    D) Replacement of the voltage-sensitive K^+ channels with "slow" Ca^{++} channels
    E) Replacement of the voltage-sensitive Na^+ channels with "slow" Ca^{++} channels

50. Which of the following perturbations would account for the failure of the same stimulus to elicit an action potential in trace C?

    A) Blockade of voltage-sensitive Na^+ channels
    B) Blockade of voltage-sensitive K^+ channels
    C) Blockade of Na-K "leak" channels
    D) Replacement of the voltage-sensitive K^+ channels with "slow" Ca^{++} channels
    E) Replacement of the voltage-sensitive Na^+ channels with "slow" Ca^{++} channels

51. A 17-year-old soccer player sustained a fracture to the left tibia. After her lower leg has been in a cast for 8 weeks, she is surprised to find that the left gastrocnemius muscle is significantly smaller in circumference than it was before the fracture. What is the most likely explanation?

    A) Decrease in the number of individual muscle fibers in the left gastrocnemius
    B) Decrease in blood flow to the muscle caused by constriction from the cast
    C) Temporary reduction in actin and myosin protein synthesis
    D) Increase in glycolytic activity in the affected muscle
    E) Progressive denervation

52. Smooth muscle that exhibits rhythmical contraction in the absence of external stimuli also necessarily exhibits which of the following?

    A) "Slow" voltage-sensitive Ca^{++} channels
    B) Intrinsic pacemaker wave activity
    C) Higher resting cytosolic Ca^{++} concentration
    D) Hyperpolarized membrane potential
    E) Action potentials with "plateaus"

Questions 53–57

    A) Simple diffusion
    B) Facilitated diffusion
    C) Primary active transport
    D) Co-transport
    E) Counter-transport

Match each of the processes described in Questions 53–57 with the correct type of transport listed above. Answers may be used more than once.

53. Ouabain-sensitive transport of Na^+ ions from the cytosol to the extracellular fluid

54. Glucose uptake into skeletal muscle

55. Na^+-dependent transport of Ca^{++} from the cytosol to the extracellular fluid

56. Transport of glucose from the intestinal lumen into an intestinal epithelial cell

57. Movement of Na^+ ions into a nerve cell during the upstroke of an action potential

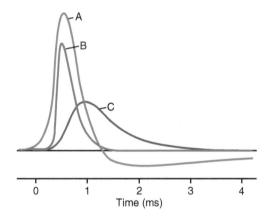

58. Traces A, B, and C in the above figure summarize the changes in membrane potential (V_m) and the underlying membrane permeabilities (P) that occur in a nerve cell over the course of an action potential. Choose the combination below that identifies each of the traces.

	Trace A	Trace B	Trace C
A)	P_K	V_m	P_{Na}
B)	$P_K:P_{Na}$	V_m	P_K
C)	P_{Na}	V_m	P_K
D)	V_m	P_K	P_{Na}
E)	V_m	P_{Na}	P_K

59. If the intracellular concentration of a membrane-permeant substance doubles from 10 to 20 millimolar and the extracellular concentration remains at 5 millimolar, the rate of diffusion of that substance across the plasma membrane will increase by a factor of how much?

    A) 2
    B) 3
    C) 4
    D) 5
    E) 6

60. An apparently healthy 15-year-old boy dies during a minor surgical procedure while under general anesthesia. The boy's grandfather had also died during a surgical procedure. A clinical assessment team determines that the child had malignant hyperthermia (MH). MH is an inherited disease in which triggering agents, such as certain anesthetics, stimulate calcium release from storage sites in muscle, leading to elevated concentrations of myoplasmic calcium. The MH crisis is most likely to be associated with which of the following?

    A) Decreased anaerobic metabolism
    B) Decreased CO_2 production by muscles
    C) Decreased lactic acid production by muscles
    D) Defective calsequestrin
    E) Defective dihydropyridine receptors
    F) Defective ryanodine receptors

61. A 24-year-old woman is admitted as an emergency to University Hospital after an automobile accident in which severe lacerations to the left wrist severed a major muscle tendon. The severed ends of the tendon were overlapped by 6 cm to facilitate suturing and reattachment. Which of the following would be expected after 6 weeks compared with the preinjured muscle? Assume that series growth of sarcomeres cannot be completed within 6 weeks.

	Passive Tension	Maximal Active Tension
A)	Decrease	Decrease
B)	Decrease	Increase
C)	Increase	Increase
D)	Increase	Decrease
E)	No change	No change

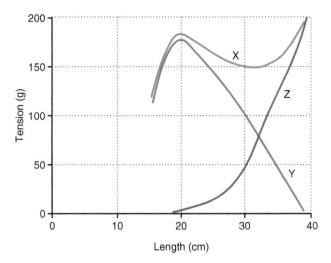

62. The length-tension diagram above was obtained from a skeletal muscle with equal numbers of red and white fibers. Supramaximal tetanic stimuli were used to initiate an isometric contraction at each muscle length studied. The resting length was 20 cm. What is the maximum amount of active tension that the muscle is capable of generating at a preload of 100 grams?

    A) 145 to 155 grams
    B) 25 to 35 grams
    C) 55 to 65 grams
    D) 95 to 105 grams
    E) Cannot be determined

63. The sensitivity of the smooth muscle contractile apparatus to calcium is known to increase in the steady state under normal conditions. This increase in calcium sensitivity can be attributed to a decrease in the levels of which of the following substances?

    A) Actin
    B) Adenosine triphosphate (ATP)
    C) Calcium-calmodulin complex
    D) Calmodulin
    E) Myosin light chain phosphatase (MLCP)

64. Which of the following best describes the correct temporal order of events for skeletal muscle?

	First	Second	Third
A)	Muscle action potential	Muscle contraction	Nerve action potential
B)	Muscle action potential	Nerve action potential	Muscle contraction
C)	Muscle contraction	Muscle action potential	Nerve action potential
D)	Muscle contraction	Nerve action potential	Muscle action potential
E)	Nerve action potential	Muscle action potential	Muscle contraction
F)	Nerve action potential	Muscle contraction	Muscle action potential

65. Which of the following best describes a physiological difference between the contraction of smooth muscle compared with the contraction of cardiac muscle and skeletal muscle?

    A) Ca^{++} independent
    B) Does not require an action potential
    C) Requires more energy
    D) Shorter in duration

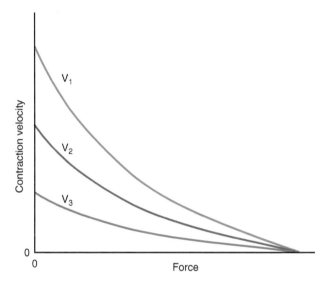

66. The above figure shows the force-velocity relationship for isotonic contractions of skeletal muscle. The differences in the three curves result from differences in which of the following?

    A) Frequency of muscle contraction
    B) Hypertrophy
    C) Muscle mass
    D) Myosin ATPase activity
    E) Recruitment of motor units

67. A 12-year-old boy presents with a 4-month history of diminished vision and diplopia. He also experiences tiredness toward the end of the day. He has no other symptoms. On examination, the patient has ptosis of the left eye that improves after a period of sleep. Clinical examination is otherwise normal. No evidence of weakness of any other muscles is found. Additional testing indicates the presence of anti-acetylcholine antibodies in the plasma, a normal thyroid function test, and a normal computed tomography scan of the brain and orbit. What is the initial diagnosis?

    A) Astrocytoma
    B) Graves' disease
    C) Hashimoto's thyroiditis
    D) Juvenile myasthenia gravis
    E) Multiple sclerosis

ANSWERS

1. **B)** In contrast to primary and secondary active transport, neither facilitated diffusion nor simple diffusion requires additional energy and, therefore, can work in the absence of ATP. Only facilitated diffusion displays saturation kinetics and involves a carrier protein. By definition, neither simple nor facilitated diffusion can move molecules from low to high concentration. The concept of specific inhibitors is not applicable to simple diffusion that occurs through a lipid bilayer without the aid of protein.
   TMP13 p. 47

2. **C)** A 1-millimolar solution has an osmolarity of 1 milliosmole when the solute molecule does not dissociate. However, NaCl and KCl both dissociate into two molecules, and $CaCl_2$ dissociates into three molecules. Therefore, 10-millimolar NaCl has an osmolarity of 20 milliosmoles, 5-millimolar KCl has an osmolarity of 10 milliosmoles, and 10-millimolar $CaCl_2$ has an osmolarity of 30 milliosmoles. These figures add up to 60 milliosmoles.
   TMP13 p. 54

3. **E)** The equilibrium potential for chloride (E_{Cl}^-) can be calculated using the Nernst equation as follows: E_{Cl}^- (in millivolts) = +61 × log (C_i/C_o), where C_i is the intracellular concentration and C_o is the extracellular concentration. Hence, $E_{Cl}^- = +61 \times \log (5/125) = -85$ millivolts.
   TMP13 pp. 52-53

4. **E)** The equilibrium potential for potassium (E_K^+) can be calculated using the Nernst equation as follows: E_K^+ (in millivolts) = −61 X log (C_i/C_o). In this problem, $E_K^+ = -61 \times \log (140/5) = -88$ millivolts.
   TMP13 pp. 52-53

5. **A)** The net driving force on any ion is the difference in millivolts between the membrane potential (V_m) and the equilibrium potential for that ion (E_{ion}). In this cell, $E_K^+ = -88$ millivolts, $E_{Cl}^- = -85$ millivolts, $E_{Na}^+ = +66$ millivolts, and $E_{Ca}^{++} = +145$ millivolts. Therefore, Ca^{++} is the ion with the equilibrium potential farthest from V_m. This means that Ca^{++} would have the greatest tendency to cross the membrane and enter the cell through an open channel in this hypothetical cell.
   TMP13 pp. 52-53

6. **B)** If a membrane is permeable to only a single ion, V_m is equal to the equilibrium potential for that ion. In this hypothetical cell, $E_K = -88$ millivolts. If the extracellular K^+ concentration is reduced by half, $E_K = 61 \times \log (2.5/140) = -107$ millivolts, which is a hyperpolarization of 19 millivolts.
   TMP13 p. 53

7. **B)** A solution of 140-millimolar NaCl has an osmolarity of 280 milliosmoles, which is iso-osmotic relative to "normal" intracellular osmolarity. If red blood cells were placed in 140-millimolar NaCl alone, no change in cell volume would occur because intracellular and extracellular osmolarities would be equal. The presence of 20-millimolar urea, however, increases the solution's osmolarity and makes it hypertonic relative to the intracellular solution. Water will initially move out of the cell, but because the plasma membrane is permeable to urea, urea will diffuse into the cell and equilibrate across the plasma membrane. As a result, water will re-enter the cell, and the cell will return to its original volume.
   TMP13 p. 54

8. **D)** Tonicity and osmolarity are different. Osmolarity is merely another measure of solute concentration. Tonicity depends on the cell membrane and the solute and is determined by the behavior of the cells. The fact that red blood cells placed into the test solution gained volume (swelled) indicates that the test solution is hypotonic. The solution would be considered isotonic had the cells neither swelled nor shrank and would be considered hypertonic had cell volume decreased. In contrast, the osmolarity of the test solution cannot be determined by the behavior of the cells. Permeant molecules such as urea can easily permeate the cell membrane, causing its concentration to become equal on both sides of the membrane, which means that placing cells into a solution containing urea (but no other solute) has an effect similar to placing cells into pure water. In other words, the cells will swell and burst regardless of whether the concentration of urea (or other permeant molecule) is less than that of a red blood cell (hypo-osmotic), the same as a red blood cell (iso-osmotic), or greater than a red blood cell (hyperosmotic).
   TMP13 p. 54

9. **D)** Skeletal muscle contraction is tightly regulated by the concentration of Ca^{++} in the sarcoplasm. As long as sarcoplasmic Ca^{++} is sufficiently high, none of the remaining events—removal of acetylcholine from the neuromuscular junction, removal of Ca^{++} from the presynaptic terminal, closure of the acetylcholine receptor channel, and return of the dihydropyridine receptor to its resting conformation—would have any effect on the contractile state of the muscle.
   TMP13 p. 94

10. C) In a normal cell of the body, intracellular concentrations of sodium, calcium, and chloride are less than the extracellular concentrations, whereas potassium has a higher intracellular concentration compared with its extracellular concentration. The figure shows that transporter Y moves sodium down its concentration gradient into the cell and moves calcium against its concentration gradient out of the cell. The energy required to move calcium ions against their concentration gradient is supplied by the sodium concentration gradient (which was established using ATP) and is a typical example of secondary active transport. Transporter X in the figure moves both potassium and sodium against their concentration gradients, which is primary active transport and requires use of ATP at the pump. Transporter Z suggests that chloride can move in either direction across the cell membrane but only by simple diffusion through the water-filled membrane channel.

TMP13 pp. 57-58

11. B) An important characteristic of visceral smooth muscle is its ability to contract in response to stretch. Stretch results in depolarization and potentially the generation of action potentials. These action potentials, coupled with normal slow-wave potentials, stimulate rhythmical contractions. Like skeletal muscle, smooth muscle contraction is dependent on both actin and ATP. However, the cross-bridge cycle in smooth muscle is considerably slower than in skeletal muscle, which allows for a higher maximal force of contraction.

TMP13 p. 99

12. D) The resting potential of any cell is dependent on the concentration gradients of the permeant ions and their relative permeabilities (Goldman equation). In the myelinated nerve fiber, as in most cells, the resting membrane is predominantly permeable to K^+. The negative membrane potential observed in most cells (including nerve cells) is due primarily to the relatively high intracellular concentration and high permeability of K^+.

TMP13 pp. 62-63

13. D) In smooth muscle, the binding of four Ca^{++} ions to the protein calmodulin permits the interaction of the Ca^{++}-calmodulin complex with myosin light chain kinase. This interaction activates myosin light chain kinase, resulting in the phosphorylation of the myosin light chains and, ultimately, muscle contraction. In skeletal muscle, the activating Ca^{++} signal is received by the protein troponin C. Like calmodulin, each molecule of troponin C can bind with up to four Ca^{++} ions. Binding results in a conformational change in the troponin C protein that dislodges the tropomyosin molecule and exposes the active sites on the actin filament.

TMP13 p. 99

14. B) The nonpermeant molecule glucose cannot move through the biological membrane in either direction. Because side Y in the figure has a greater initial concentration of glucose molecules compared with side X, water will move down its concentration gradient by osmosis from side X to side Y, which will cause a decrease in the volume of side X and an increase in the volume of side Y. The total volume of sides X and Y will not change, which excludes answers D and E.

TMP13 pp. 52, 54

15. A) Muscle fibers involved in fine motor control are generally innervated by small motor neurons with relatively small motor units, including those that innervate single fibers. These neurons fire in response to a smaller depolarizing stimulus compared with motor neurons with larger motor units. As a result, during weak contractions, increases in muscle contraction can occur in small steps, allowing for fine motor control. This concept is called the *size principle*.

TMP13 p. 85

16. B) A neurotransmitter is considered to be a ligand, so when a neurotransmitter binds to its receptor on an ion channel, causing the channel to open, the channel is said to be ligand gated; voltage-gated channels open and close in response to changes in electrical potential across the cell membrane. The mechanism of transport through all water-filled channels is simple diffusion. Secondary active transport, primary active transport, and facilitated diffusion require special transport proteins rather than water-filled channels in the membrane.

TMP13 pp. 49-50

17. A) Recall that the Nernst potential of an ion can be calculated as follows: E_{ion} (in millivolts) = $\pm$ 61 $\times$ log (intracellular concentration/extracellular concentration). In the case of potassium, the intracellular concentration is relatively high, the extracellular concentration is relatively low, and the Nernst potential (also called the equilibrium potential) for potassium normally averages about −90 millivolts in a typical neuron. An increase in extracellular potassium concentration (with no change in intracellular concentration) would cause the potassium Nernst potential to become less negative, according to the Nernst equation. The resting membrane potential therefore would also become less negative because this is dictated by the potassium Nernst potential in normal cells of the body. The sodium extracellular concentration is elevated in this problem, which would cause the sodium Nernst potential to increase above its typical normal value of +61 millivolts; however, the Nernst potential of sodium has relatively little impact on resting membrane compared with potassium because the membrane permeability to sodium is about 100 times lower compared with potassium.

TMP13 pp. 53, 63-64

18. **B)** The physical lengths of the actin and myosin filaments do not change during contraction. Therefore, the A band, which is composed of myosin filaments, does not change either. The distance between Z disks decreases, but the Z disks themselves do not change. Only the I band decreases in length as the muscle contracts.

TMP13 p. 78

19. **E)** The equilibrium potential of an ion (also called the Nernst potential) is the membrane potential at which there is no net movement of that ion across the cell membrane. The various ions (Q, R, and S) will move across the cell membrane in the direction required to reach their individual equilibrium potentials given the resting membrane potential of −90 millivolts. Negatively charged Q ions must move out of the cell (outward) to achieve an equilibrium potential of −75 millivolts (i.e., negatively charged ions must be removed from the cell to cause the membrane potential to change from a resting value of −90 millivolts to a value of −75 millivolts). Because the positively charged R ion has an equilibrium potential of +75 millivolts, the R ion must move into the cell to cause the membrane potential to change from −90 millivolts to +75 millivolts. Ion S is a positively charged ion with an equilibrium potential of −85 mV; this ion must move into the cell (inward) to cause the membrane potential to change from −90 millivolts to −85 millivolts.

TMP13 pp. 52-53

20. **B)** Muscle contraction is dependent on an elevation of intracellular Ca^{++} concentration. As the twitch frequency increases, the initiation of a subsequent twitch can occur before the previous twitch has subsided. As a result, the amplitude of the individual twitches is summed. At very high twitch frequencies, the muscle exhibits tetanic contraction. Under these conditions, intracellular Ca^{++} accumulates and supports sustained maximal contraction.

TMP13 p. 85

21. **B)** Prolonged or repeated maximal contraction results in a concomitant increase in the synthesis of contractile proteins and an increase in muscle mass. This increase in mass, or hypertrophy, is observed at the level of individual muscle fibers.

TMP13 p. 87

22. **E)** Facilitated diffusion and both primary and secondary active transport all involve protein transporters or carriers that must undergo some rate-limited conformational change. The rate of simple diffusion is linear with solute concentration.

TMP13 p. 48

23. **B)** The velocity of an action potential increases in proportion to the diameter of the axon for both myelinated and non-myelinated axons. Myelination increases the velocity of an action potential by several orders of magnitude more compared with the effect of an increase in axon diameter, which means that a large myelinated axon has the highest velocity of conduction. Therefore, even though unmyelinated axon E has the greatest diameter, myelinated axon B can conduct an action potential at a much greater velocity.

TMP13 pp. 71-72

24. **D)** At point B in this action potential, V_m has reached threshold potential and has triggered the opening of voltage-gated Na^+ channels. The resulting Na^+ influx is responsible for the rapid, self-perpetuating depolarization phase of the action potential.

TMP13 p. 67

25. **C)** The rapid depolarization phase is terminated at point D by the inactivation of the voltage-gated Na^+ channels and the opening of the voltage-gated K^+ channels. The latter results in the efflux of K^+ from the cytosol into the extracellular fluid and repolarization of the cell membrane.

TMP13 p. 67

26. **B)** The velocity of an action potential is a function of the physical characteristics of the axon (e.g., myelination, axon diameter). A given axon will always conduct any action potential at the same velocity under normal conditions. Therefore, stimulation of the axon with a 25-millivolt pulse or 100 millivolts will produce an action potential with the same velocity, which is why action potentials are said to be "all or none." However, the level of stimulation must be sufficient to achieve a critical threshold level of potential before an action potential can be initiated in an axon.

TMP13 p. 69

27. **D)** The slower cycling rate of the cross-bridges in smooth muscle means that a higher percentage of possible cross-bridges is active at any point in time. The more active cross-bridges there are, the greater the force that is generated. Although the relatively slow cycling rate means that it takes longer for the myosin head to attach to the actin filament, it also means that the myosin head remains attached longer, prolonging muscle contraction. Because of the slow cross-bridge cycling rate, smooth muscle actually requires less energy to maintain a contraction compared with skeletal muscle.

TMP13 p. 99

28. **E)** The stimulation of either adenylate or guanylate cyclase induces smooth muscle relaxation. The cyclic nucleotides produced by these enzymes stimulate cyclic adenosine monophosphate– and cyclic guanosine monophosphate–dependent kinases, respectively. These kinases phosphorylate, among other things, enzymes that remove Ca^{++} from the cytosol, and in doing so they

inhibit contraction. In contrast, either a decrease in K^+ permeability or an increase in Na^+ permeability results in membrane depolarization and contraction. Likewise, inhibition of the sarcoplasmic reticulum Ca^{++}-ATPase, one of the enzymes activated by cyclic nucleotide-dependent kinases, would also favor muscle contraction. Smooth muscle does not express troponin.

TMP13 p. 104

29. **D)** Muscle B is characteristic of a slow-twitch muscle (type 1) composed of predominantly slow-twitch muscle fibers. These fibers are smaller in size and are innervated by smaller nerve fibers. They typically have a more extensive blood supply, a greater number of mitochondria, and large amounts of myoglobin, all of which support high levels of oxidative phosphorylation.

TMP13 p. 84

30. **C)** Muscle contraction is triggered by an increase in sarcoplasmic Ca^{++} concentration. The delay between the termination of the depolarizing pulse and the onset of muscle contraction, also called the "lag," reflects the time necessary for the depolarizing pulse to be translated into an increase in sarcoplasmic Ca^{++} concentration. This process involves a conformational change in the voltage-sensing, or dihydropyridine receptor, located on the T tubule membrane, along with the subsequent conformational change in the ryanodine receptor on the sarcoplasmic reticulum and the release of Ca^{++} from the sarcoplasmic reticulum.

TMP13 pp. 93-94

31. **B)** Myasthenia gravis is an autoimmune disease in which antibodies damage postsynaptic nicotinic acetylcholine receptors. This damage prevents the firing of an action potential in the postsynaptic membrane. Tensilon is a readily reversible acetylcholinesterase inhibitor that increases acetylcholine levels in the neuromuscular junction, thereby increasing the strength of muscle contraction.

TMP13 p. 93

32. **A)** Myasthenia gravis is an autoimmune disease characterized by the presence of anti-acetylcholine receptor antibodies in the plasma. Overexertion can cause junction fatigue, and both a decrease in the density of voltage-sensitive Ca^{++} channels in the presynaptic membrane and botulinum toxicity can cause muscle weakness. However, these effects are presynaptic and therefore would not be reversed by acetylcholinesterase inhibition. Although the macro-motor units formed during reinnervation after poliomyelitis compromise the patient's fine motor control, they do not affect muscle strength.

TMP13 p. 93

33. **E)** Neostigmine is an acetylcholinesterase inhibitor. Administration of this drug would increase the amount of ACh present in the synapse and its ability to sufficiently depolarize the postsynaptic membrane and trigger an action potential. Botulinum toxin antiserum is effective only against botulinum toxicity. Curare blocks the nicotinic ACh receptor and causes muscle weakness. Atropine is a muscarinic ACh receptor antagonist, and halothane is an anesthetic gas. Neither atropine nor halothane has any effect on the neuromuscular junction.

TMP13 p. 93

34. **E)** The velocity of muscle shortening is greater in type II glycolytic muscles compared with type I oxidative muscles; however, the student must assume that all muscles shown have similar proportions of type I and II fibers because this was not stated in the problem. Another factor that affects the velocity of muscle shortening is muscle length—a longer muscle contracts at a faster velocity compared with a shorter muscle. Muscle 1 on the figure has the highest velocity of contraction, so it must correspond to muscle E in the answer choices because muscle E is the longest. The diameter of the muscle is immaterial in this problem because the maximum velocity of shortening occurs at a force of 0.

TMP13 pp. 81-82

35. **B)** In this figure, "active" or contraction-dependent tension is the difference between total tension (trace A) and the passive tension contributed by noncontractile elements (trace C). The length-tension relationship in intact muscle resembles the biphasic relationship observed in individual sarcomeres and reflects the same physical interactions between actin and myosin filaments.

TMP13 p. 81

36. **E)** "Active" tension is maximal at normal physiological muscle lengths. At this point, there is optimal overlap between actin and myosin filaments to support maximal cross-bridge formation and tension development.

TMP13 p. 81

37. **C)** Trace C represents the passive tension contributed by noncontractile elements, including fascia, tendons, and ligaments. This passive tension accounts for an increasingly large portion of the total tension recorded in intact muscle as it is stretched beyond its normal length.

TMP13 p. 81

38. **B)** Smooth muscle contraction is regulated by both Ca^{++} and myosin light chain phosphorylation. When the cytosolic Ca^{++} concentration decreases after the initiation of contraction, myosin kinase becomes inactivated. However, cross-bridge formation continues, even in the absence of Ca^{++}, until the myosin light chains are dephosphorylated through the action of myosin light chain phosphatase.

TMP13 p. 100

39. C) The normal miniature end-plate potentials indicate sufficient synthesis and packaging of ACh and the presence and normal function of ACh receptor channels. The most likely explanation for this patient's symptoms is a presynaptic deficiency—in this case, an impairment of the voltage-sensitive Ca^{++} channels responsible for the increase in cytosolic Ca^{++} that triggers the release of ACh into the synapse. The increase in postsynaptic depolarization observed after exercise is indicative of an accumulation of Ca^{++} in the presynaptic terminal after multiple action potentials have reached the nerve terminal.
    TMP13 p. 91

40. B) Inhibition of the presynaptic voltage-sensitive Ca^{++} channels is most consistent with the presence of antibodies against this channel. Antibodies against the ACh receptor, a mutation in the ryanodine receptor, and residual ACh in the junction are all indicative of postsynaptic defects. Although it is a presynaptic defect, a deficit of ACh vesicles is unlikely in this scenario, given the normal miniature end-plate potentials recorded in the postsynaptic membrane.
    TMP13 p. 89

41. B) Botulinum toxin inhibits muscle contraction presynaptically by decreasing the amount of ACh released into the neuromuscular junction. In contrast, curare acts postsynaptically, blocking the nicotinic ACh receptors and preventing the excitation of the muscle cell membrane. Tetrodotoxin blocks voltage-sensitive Na^+ channels, affecting both the initiation and the propagation of action potentials in the motor neuron. Both ACh and neostigmine stimulate muscle contraction.
    TMP13 p. 92

42. D) During an action potential in a nerve cell, V_m approaches E_{Na} during the rapid depolarization phase when the permeability of the membrane to Na^+ (P_{Na}) increases relative to its permeability to K^+ (P_K). In a "typical" cell, E_{Na} is close to 60 millivolts. V_m is closest to E_{Na} at point D in this figure. At this point, the ratio of P_{Na} to P_K is the greatest.
    TMP13 p. 67

43. F) The driving force for Na^+ is greatest at the point at which V_m is the farthest from E_{Na}. If E_{Na} is very positive (approximately 60 millivolts), V_m is farthest from E_{Na} at point F, or when the cell is the most hyperpolarized.
    TMP13 p. 67

44. F) Generally, V_m is closest to the equilibrium potential of the most permeant ion. In nerve cells, $P_K \gg P_{Na}$ at rest. As a result, V_m is relatively close to E_K. During the after-potential or the hyperpolarization phase of the action potential, the ratio of P_K to P_{Na} is even greater than it is at rest because of the residual opening of voltage-gated K^+ channels and the inactivation of the voltage-gated Na^+ channels. $P_K:P_{Na}$ is greatest at point F, at which point V_m comes closest to E_K.
    TMP13 p. 67

45. D) Muscle fibers have significant plasticity, which means that their characteristics can change depending on the frequency at which they are stimulated. When a nerve that innervates a predominantly fast type II muscle is anastomosed to a predominantly slow type I muscle, the type I muscle is converted to a type II muscle. Compared with type I muscle fibers, type II fibers have a larger diameter, higher glycolytic activity, greater maximum velocity of contraction, lower mitochondrial content, and higher myosin ATPase activity. Therefore, only mitochondrial content decreases when a type I fiber is converted to a type II fiber.
    TMP13 p. 84

46. B) The redistribution of fluid volume shown in part **B** reflects the net diffusion of water, or osmosis, because of differences in the osmolarity of the solutions on either side of the semipermeable membrane. Osmosis occurs from solutions of high water concentration to low water concentration or from low osmolarity to high osmolarity. In part **B**, osmosis has occurred from X to Y and from Y to Z. Therefore, the osmolarity of solution Z is higher than that of solution Y, and the osmolarity of solution Y is higher than that of solution X.
    TMP13 p. 54

47. D) Trace A reflects the kinetics of a process that is limited by an intrinsic V_{max}. Of the choices provided, only the transport of K^+, which occurs through the activity of the Na^+, K^+-ATPase, is the result of an active transport event. The movement of CO_2 and O_2 through a biological membrane and the movement of Ca^{++} and Na^+ through ion channels are all examples of simple diffusion.
    TMP13 p. 51

48. E) Trace B is indicative of a process not limited by an intrinsic V_{max}. This excludes active transport and facilitated diffusion. Therefore, of the choices provided, only the rate of transport of O_2 across an artificial lipid bilayer via simple diffusion would be accurately reflected by trace B.
    TMP13 p. 51

49. E) These so-called slow Ca^{++} channels have a slower inactivation rate, thereby lengthening the time during which they are open. This phenomenon, in turn, delays the repolarization phase of the action potential, creating a "plateau" before the channels inactivate.
    TMP13 p. 67 (see also Chapter 9)

50. A) In the absence of hyperpolarization, the inability of an otherwise excitatory stimulus to initiate an action potential is most likely the result of the blockade of the voltage-gated channels responsible for the generation of the all-or-none depolarization. In nerve cells, these channels are the voltage-gated Na^+ channels.
    TMP13 p. 66

51. C) Skeletal muscle continuously remodels in response to its level of use. When a muscle is inactive for an extended period, the rate of synthesis of the contractile proteins in individual muscle fibers decreases, resulting in an overall reduction in muscle mass. This reversible reduction in muscle mass is called *atrophy*.
TMP13 p. 87

52. B) An intrinsic rhythmical "pacemaker" is necessary for a muscle to contract spontaneously and rhythmically. Intestinal smooth muscle, for example, exhibits a rhythmical slow-wave potential that transiently depolarizes and repolarizes the muscle membrane. This slow wave does not stimulate contraction itself, but if the amplitude is sufficient, it can trigger one or more action potentials that result in Ca^{++} influx and contraction. Although they are typical of smooth muscle, neither "slow" voltage-sensitive Ca^{++} channels nor action potentials with "plateaus" play a necessary role in rhythmical contraction. A high resting cytosolic Ca^{++} concentration would support a sustained contraction, and hyperpolarization would favor relaxation.
TMP13 p. 104

53. C) Ouabain inhibits Na^+, K^+-ATPase. This ATP-dependent enzyme transports three Na^+ ions out of the cell for every two K^+ ions it transports into the cell. It is a classic example of primary active transport.
TMP13 p. 56

54. B) Glucose is transported into skeletal muscle cells via insulin-dependent facilitated diffusion.
TMP13 p. 52 (see also Chapter 79)

55. E) The activity of Na^+, K^+-ATPase maintains the relatively high K^+ concentration inside the cell and the relatively high Na^+ concentration in the extracellular fluid. This large concentration gradient for Na^+ across the plasma membrane, together with the net negative charge on the inside of the cell, continuously drives Na^+ ions from the extracellular fluid into the cytosol. This energy is used to transport other molecules, such as Ca^{++}, against their concentration gradients. Because ATP is required to maintain the Na^+ gradient that drives this counter-transport, this type of transport is called *secondary active transport*.
TMP13 p. 55

56. D) Much like Na^+-Ca^{++} counter-transport, the strong tendency for Na^+ to move across the plasma membrane into the cytosol can be harnessed by transport proteins and used to co-transport molecules against their concentration gradients into the cytosol. An example of this type of secondary co-transport is the transport of glucose into intestinal epithelial cells.
TMP13 p. 55

57. A) During the rapid depolarization phase of a nerve action potential, voltage-sensitive Na^+ channels open and allow the influx of Na^+ ions into the cytosol. Transport through membrane channels is an example of simple diffusion.
TMP13 pp. 47-48 (see also Chapter 5)

58. E) Trace A exhibits the characteristic shape of an action potential, including the rapid depolarization followed by a rapid repolarization that temporarily overshoots the resting potential. Trace B best illustrates the change in P_{Na} that occurs during an action potential. The rapid increase in P_{Na} closely parallels the rapid depolarization phase of the action potential. Trace C best illustrates the slow onset of the increase in P_K that reflects the opening of the voltage-gated K^+ channels.
TMP13 pp. 67-68

59. B) Net diffusion of a substance across a permeable membrane is proportional to the concentration difference of the substance on either side of the membrane. Initially, the concentration difference is 5 millimolar (10 millimolar – 5 millimolar). When the intracellular concentration doubles to 20 millimolar, the concentration difference becomes 15 millimolar (20 millimolar – 5 millimolar). The concentration difference has tripled; therefore, the rate of diffusion would also increase by a factor of 3.
TMP13 p. 52

60. F) In malignant hyperthermia, defective ryanodine receptors respond to certain halogenated anesthetics by opening their associated calcium channels within the muscle fiber and thus causing an increase in myoplasmic calcium. This increase in calcium concentration causes continuous contraction of the muscles. The result is increased body temperature, increased anaerobic metabolism, increased CO_2 production, and increased lactic acid production. Calsequestrin is a protein molecule that binds calcium within the sarcoplasmic reticulum of the muscle fiber; it is not affected by halogenated anesthetics. In addition, dihydropyridine receptors are activated by the skeletal muscle fiber action potential, but they are not affected by halogenated anesthetics.
TMP13 p. 94

61. D) Stretching the muscle to facilitate reattachment of the tendons leads to an increase in passive tension or preload. This increase in passive tension increases the muscle length beyond its ideal length, which in turn leads to a decrease in the maximal active tension that can be generated by the muscle. The reason maximal active tension decreases is that interdigitation of actin and myosin filaments decreases when the muscle is stretched; the interdigitation of a muscle is normally optimal at its resting length.
TMP13 p. 81

62. C) The figure shows the relationship between preload or passive tension (curve Z), total tension (curve X), and active tension (curve Y). Active tension cannot be measured directly: it is the difference between total tension and passive tension. To answer this question, the student must first find where 100 grams intersects the preload curve (passive tension curve) and then move down to the active tension curve. One can see that a preload of 100 grams is associated with a total tension of a little more than 150 grams and an active tension of a little more than 50 grams. Note that active tension equals total tension minus passive tension, as previously discussed. Drawing these three curves in a manner that is mathematically correct is not an easy task. The student should thus recognize that active tension may not equal total tension minus passive tension at all points on the figure shown here, as well as on United States Medical Licensing Examination figures.

TMP13 p. 81

63. E) Smooth muscle is unique in its ability to generate various degrees of tension at a constant concentration of intracellular calcium. This change in calcium sensitivity of smooth muscle can be attributed to differences in the activity of MLCP. Smooth muscle contracts when the myosin light chain is phosphorylated by the actions of myosin light chain kinase (MLCK). MLCP is a phosphatase that can dephosphorylate the myosin light chain, rendering it inactive and therefore attenuating the muscle contraction. Choice A: Both actin and myosin are important components of the smooth muscle contractile apparatus, much like that of skeletal muscle and cardiac muscle, but these components do not play a role in calcium sensitivity. Choice B: ATP is required for smooth muscle contraction. Decreased ATP levels would be expected to decrease the ability of smooth muscle to contract even in the face of high calcium levels. Choice C: The calcium-calmodulin complex binds with MLCK, which leads to phosphorylation of the myosin light chain. A decrease in the calcium-calmodulin complex should attenuate the contraction of smooth muscle. Choice D: Again, the binding of calcium ions to calmodulin is an initial step in the activation of the smooth muscle contractile apparatus.

TMP13 p. 100

64. E) An action potential from a motor neuron causes ACh to be released from its terminal at the neuromuscular junction. The ACh binds to and opens cation channels on the muscle membrane, causing it to depolarize. The muscle membrane reaches a threshold value, causing voltage gated sodium channels to open, and a muscle action potential follows. The muscle action potential leads to contraction of the muscle.

TMP13 pp. 93-94

65. B) Smooth muscle can be stimulated to contract without the generation of an action potential, whereas both cardiac muscle and skeletal muscle require an action potential. Smooth muscle can contract in response to any stimulus that increases the cytosolic Ca^{++} concentration, which includes Ca^{++} channel openers, subthreshold depolarization, and a variety of tissue factors and circulating hormones that stimulate the release of intracellular Ca^{++} stores. Smooth muscle contraction uses less energy and lasts longer compared with that of skeletal muscle and cardiac muscle. Smooth muscle contraction is heavily Ca^{++} dependent.

TMP13 pp. 100-101

66. D) The figure shows that the maximum velocity of shortening (V_{max}) occurs when there is no afterload on the muscle (force = 0). Increasing afterload decreases the velocity of shortening until a point is reached where shortening does not occur (isometric contraction) and contraction velocity is thus 0 (where curves intersect the X-axis). The maximum velocity of shortening is dictated by the ATPase activity of the muscle, increasing to high levels when the ATPase activity is elevated. Choice A: Increasing the frequency of muscle contraction will increase the load that a muscle can lift within the limits of the muscle, but it will not affect the velocity of contraction. Choices B, C, and E: Muscle hypertrophy, increasing muscle mass, and recruiting additional motor units will increase the maximum load that a muscle can lift, but they will not affect the maximum velocity of contraction.

TMP13 p. 81

67. D) Myasthenia gravis is an acquired autoimmune disease causing skeletal muscle fatigue and weakness. The disease is associated with (caused by) IgG antibodies to ACh receptors at postsynaptic membranes of neuromuscular junctions. The major symptom is muscle weakness, which gets worse with activity. Patients often feel well in the morning but become weaker as the day goes on. The muscle weakness usually causes symptoms of double vision (diplopia) and drooping eyelids (ptosis). The presence of anti-ACh antibodies in the plasma is specific for myasthenia gravis and thus rules out the other answer choices. In addition, the normal computed tomography scan of the brain and orbit specifically rules out the possibility of an astrocytoma (choice A)—that is, a brain tumor—that could compress cranial nerves. Double vision commonly occurs in Graves' disease (choice B), but the thyroid test was normal (which also rules out Hashimoto's thyroiditis, choice C). Multiple sclerosis (choice E) is commonly associated with a spastic weakness of the legs, but again, the presence of anti-ACh antibodies is specific for myasthenia gravis.

TMP13 p. 92

The Heart

Questions 1–4

A 60-year-old woman has a resting heart rate of 70 beats per minute, arterial pressure of 130/85 mm Hg, and normal body temperature. Use the pressure-volume diagram of her left ventricle below to answer Questions 1–4.

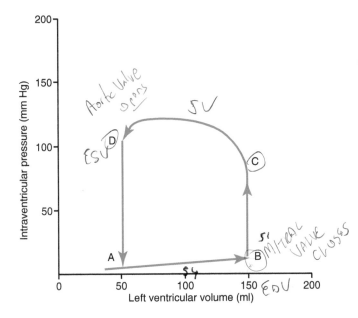

[handwritten annotations: Aortic Valve opens, SV, ESV, D, C, A, B, S1 MITRAL VALVE CLOSES, S4, EDV]

1. What is her cardiac output in milliliters per minute?

A) 2000
B) 3000
C) 4000
D) 6000
E) 7000

[handwritten: CO = SV × HR]

2. When does the first heart sound occur in the ventricular pressure–volume relationship?

A) At point B
B) Between point A and point B
C) Between point B and point C
D) Between point C and point D
E) Between point D and point A

3. When does the fourth heart sound occur in the ventricular pressure–volume relationship?

A) At point D
B) Between point A and point B
C) Between point B and point C
D) Between point C and point D
E) Between point D and point A

[handwritten: 55-70%]

4. What is her ventricular ejection fraction?

A) 33%
B) 50%
C) 60%
D) 67%
E) 80%

[handwritten: EF = SV/EDV = 1U 2/1S 3 = 100/150]

5. Which statement about cardiac muscle is most accurate?

A) The T-tubules of cardiac muscle can store much less calcium than the T-tubules in skeletal muscle
B) The strength and contraction of cardiac muscle depends on the amount of calcium surrounding cardiac myocytes
C) In cardiac muscle, the initiation of the action potential causes an immediate opening of slow calcium channels *[handwritten: fast sodium]*
D) Cardiac muscle repolarization is caused by opening of sodium channels *[handwritten: delayed K+ channel]*
E) Mucopolysaccharides inside the T-tubules bind chloride ions

6. A 30-year-old man has an ejection fraction of 0.25 and an end-systolic volume of 150 milliliters. What is his end-diastolic volume?

A) 50 milliliters
B) 100 milliliters
C) 125 milliliters
D) 200 milliliters
E) 250 milliliters

[handwritten: .25 = (X-150)/X; .25x = x - 50; .25x ≠ 150 = x; 150 = .75x]

7. In a resting adult, the typical ventricular ejection fraction has what value?

A) 20%
B) 30%
C) 40%
D) 60%
E) 80%

8. In which phase of the ventricular muscle action potential is the potassium permeability the highest?

   A) 0
   B) 1
   C) 2
   (D) 3
   E) 4

9. A 60-year-old man's ECG shows that he has an R-R interval of 1.5 seconds at rest. Which statement best explains his condition?

   A) He has fever
   B) He has a normal heart rate
   C) He has decreased parasympathetic stimulation of the S-A node
   D) He is a trained athlete at rest
   E) He has normal polarization of the S-A node

10. Which of the following is most likely to cause the heart to go into spastic contraction?

   A) Increased body temperature
   B) Increased sympathetic activity
   C) Decreased extracellular fluid potassium ions
   D) Excess extracellular fluid potassium ions – DILATED
   E) Excess extracellular fluid calcium ions

11. What happens at the end of ventricular isovolumic relaxation?

   A) The A-V valves close
   B) The aortic valve opens – START!
   C) The aortic valve closes
   (D) The mitral valve opens   end
   E) The pulmonary valve closes

12. Which event is associated with the first heart sound?

   A) Closing of the aortic valve
   B) Inrushing of blood into the ventricles during diastole
   C) Beginning of diastole
   D) Opening of the A-V valves
   (E) Closing of the A-V valves

13. Which condition will result in a dilated, flaccid heart?

   A) Excess calcium ions in the blood
   (B) Excess potassium ions in the blood
   C) Excess sodium ions in the blood
   D) Increased sympathetic stimulation
   E) Increased norepinephrine concentration in the blood

14. A 25-year-old well-conditioned athlete weighs 80 kilograms (176 pounds). During maximal sympathetic stimulation, what is the plateau level of his cardiac output function curve?

   A) 3 liters per minute
   B) 5 liters per minute
   C) 10 liters per minute
   D) 13 liters per minute
   E) 25 liters per minute

15. Which phase of the cardiac cycle follows immediately after the beginning of the QRS wave?

   A) Isovolumic relaxation
   B) Ventricular ejection
   C) Atrial systole
   D) Diastasis
   (E) Isovolumic contraction

16. Which of the following structures will have the slowest rate of conduction of the cardiac action potential?

   A) Atrial muscle – also fast
   B) Anterior internodal pathway – also fast
   C) A-V bundle fibers
   D) Purkinje fibers – FASTEST?
   E) Ventricular muscle – also fast

17. What is the normal total delay of the cardiac impulse in the A-V node + bundle?

   A) 0.22 second
   B) 0.18 second
   C) 0.16 second
   (D) 0.13 second
   E) 0.09 second

18. Sympathetic stimulation of the heart does which of the following?

   A) Releases acetylcholine at the sympathetic endings
   B) Decreases sinus nodal discharge rate
   C) Decreases excitability of the heart
   (D) Releases norepinephrine at the sympathetic endings
   E) Decreases cardiac contractility

19. If the S-A node discharges at 0.00 seconds, when will the action potential normally arrive at the epicardial surface at the base of the left ventricle?

   A) 0.22 second
   B) 0.18 second
   C) 0.16 second
   D) 0.12 second
   E) 0.09 second

20. Which condition at the A-V node will cause a decrease in heart rate?

   A) Increased sodium permeability
   B) Decreased acetylcholine levels
   C) Increased norepinephrine levels
   (D) Increased potassium permeability
   E) Increased calcium permeability

21. Which statement best explains how sympathetic stimulation affects the heart?

   A) The permeability of the S-A node to sodium decreases
   B) The permeability of the A-V node to sodium decreases
   C) The permeability of the S-A node to potassium increases
   (D) There is an increased rate of upward drift of the resting membrane potential of the S-A node
   E) The permeability of the cardiac muscle to calcium decreases

22. What is the membrane potential (threshold level) at which the S-A node discharges?

    A) −40 millivolt
    B) −55 millivolt
    C) −65 millivolt
    D) −85 millivolt
    E) −105 millivolt

23. Which condition at the S-A node will cause heart rate to decrease?

    A) Increased norepinephrine level
    B) Increased sodium permeability
    C) Increased calcium permeability
    D) Increased potassium permeability
    E) Decreased acetylcholine level

24. In which phase of the ventricular muscle action potential is the sodium permeability the highest?

    A) 0   − Na+
    B) 1
    C) 2   − Ca++
    D) 3   − K+
    E) 4

25. If the S-A node discharges at 0.00 seconds, when will the action potential normally arrive at the A-V bundle (bundle of His)?

    A) 0.22 second
    B) 0.18 second
    C) 0.16 second
    D) 0.12 second
    E) 0.09 second

    arrives to AV .03
    delayed .09
    .12

26. If the Purkinje fibers, situated distal to the A-V junction, become the pacemaker of the heart, what is the expected heart rate?

    A) 30/min
    B) 50/min
    C) 60/min
    D) 70/min
    E) 80/min

    SA − 60−100
    AV − 40−60
    Purkinje − 20−40

27. If the S-A node discharges at 0.00 seconds, when will the action potential normally arrive at the A-V node?

    A) 0.03 second
    B) 0.09 second
    C) 0.12 second
    D) 0.16 second
    E) 0.80 second

28. What is the delay between the S-A node discharge and arrival of the action potential at the ventricular septum?

    A) 0.80 second
    B) 0.16 second
    C) 0.12 second
    D) 0.09 second
    E) 0.03 second

29. A patient had an ECG at the local emergency department. The attending physician stated that the patient had an A-V nodal rhythm. What is the likely heart rate?

    A) 30/min
    B) 50/min
    C) 65/min
    D) 75/min
    E) 85/min

30. Which condition at the A-V node will cause a decrease in heart rate?

    A) Increased sodium permeability
    B) Decreased acetylcholine level
    C) Increased norepinephrine level
    D) Increased potassium permeability
    E) Increased calcium permeability

31. When recording lead aVL on an ECG, which is the positive electrode?

    A) Left arm
    B) Left leg
    C) Right leg
    D) Left arm + left leg
    E) Right arm + left leg

    aVL = (+) L Arm

32. When recording lead II on an ECG, the right arm is the negative electrode and the positive electrode is the

    A) Left arm
    B) Left leg
    C) Right leg
    D) Left arm + left leg
    E) Right arm + left leg

    Lead II − (+) Lot Leg

33. Sympathetic stimulation of the heart normally causes which condition?

    A) Acetylcholine release at the sympathetic endings
    B) Decreased heart rate
    C) Decreased rate of conduction of the cardiac impulse
    D) Decreased force of contraction of the atria
    E) Increased force of contraction of the ventricles

Questions 34 and 35

A 70-year-old woman had an ECG at her annual checkup. Use her lead II recording below to answer Questions 34 and 35.

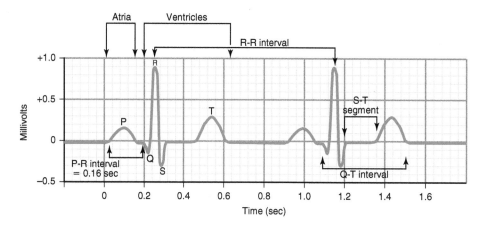

34. What is her heart rate in beats per minute?

    A) 70
    B) 78
    C) 84
    D) 94
    E) 104

35. According to Einthoven's law, if the QRS voltage in lead III is 0.4 millivolt, what is the QRS voltage in lead I?

    A) 0.05 millivolt
    B) 0.50 millivolt
    C) 1.05 millivolts
    D) 1.25 millivolts
    E) 2.05 millivolts

36. What is the normal QT interval?

    A) 0.03 second
    B) 0.13 second
    C) 0.16 second
    D) 0.20 second
    E) 0.35 second

37. When recording lead II on an ECG, the negative electrode is the

    A) Right arm
    B) Left leg
    C) Right leg
    D) Left arm + left leg
    E) Right arm + left leg

38. When recording lead I on an ECG, the right arm is the negative electrode and the positive electrode is the

    A) Left arm
    B) Left leg
    C) Right leg
    D) Left arm + left leg
    E) Right arm + left leg

39. A 65-year-old man had an ECG at a local emergency department after a biking accident. His weight was 80 kilograms (176 pounds), and his aortic blood pressure was 160/90 mm Hg. The QRS voltage was 0.5 millivolt in lead I and 1.5 millivolts in lead III. What is the QRS voltage in lead II?

    A) 0.5 millivolt
    B) 1.0 millivolt
    C) 1.5 millivolts
    D) 2.0 millivolts
    E) 2.5 millivolts

40. A ventricular depolarization wave, when traveling −60 degrees in the frontal plane, will cause a large negative deflection in which lead?

    A) aVR
    B) aVL
    C) Lead II
    D) Lead III
    E) aVF

Questions 41–43

A 60-year-old woman had an ECG recorded at a local emergency department after an automobile accident. Her weight was 70 kilograms (154 pounds), and her aortic blood pressure was 140/80 mm Hg. Use this information and the figure below to answer Questions 41–43.

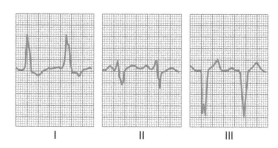

    I   II   III

41. What is the mean electrical axis calculated from standard leads I, II, and III shown in the woman's ECG?

    A) −90 degrees
    B) −50 degrees
    C) −12 degrees
    D) +100 degrees
    E) +170 degrees

42. What is the heart rate using lead I for the calculation?

    A) 70
    B) 88
    C) 100
    D) 112
    E) 148

43. What is her likely diagnosis?

    A) Tricuspid valve stenosis
    B) Left bundle branch block
    C) Pulmonary valve stenosis
    D) Pulmonary valve insufficiency
    E) Aortic insufficiency

44. Which condition will usually result in left axis deviation in an ECG?

    A) Systemic hypertension
    B) Pulmonary valve stenosis
    C) Pulmonary valve regurgitation
    D) Rightward angulation of the heart
    E) Pulmonary hypertension

45. A ventricular depolarization wave, when traveling 60 degrees in the frontal plane, will cause a large positive deflection in which of the following leads?

    A) aVR
    B) aVL
    C) Lead I
    D) Lead II
    E) aVF

Questions 46 and 47

A 50-year-old woman was admitted to a local emergency department after a motorcycle accident. The following ECG was obtained.

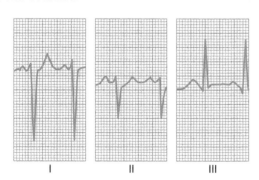

| I | II | III |

46. What is her heart rate? Use lead I for the calculation.

    A) 56
    B) 66
    C) 76
    D) 103
    E) 152

47. What type of murmur is present in this patient?

    A) Aortic valve insufficiency
    B) Left bundle branch block
    C) Pulmonary valve stenosis
    D) Right bundle branch block
    E) Systemic hypertension

48. Mr. Smith had an ECG at a local hospital, but his records were lost. The ECG technician remembered that the QRS deflection was large and positive in lead II and 0 in aVL. What is his mean electrical axis in the frontal plane?

    A) 90 degrees
    B) 60 degrees
    C) 0 degree
    D) −60 degrees
    E) −90 degrees

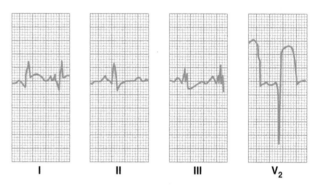

| I | II | III | V₂ |

49. A 70-year-old woman came to a hospital emergency department because she was experiencing chest pain. Based on the ECG shown above, what is the likely diagnosis?

    A) Acute anterior infarction in the left ventricle of the heart
    B) Acute anterior infarction in the right ventricle of the heart
    C) Acute posterior infarction in the left ventricle of the heart
    D) Acute posterior infarction in the right ventricle of the heart
    E) Right ventricular hypertrophy

50. A 55-year-old man underwent an ECG at an annual physical, and his net deflection (R wave minus Q or S wave) in standard limb lead I was −1.2 millivolts. Standard limb lead II has a net deflection of +1.2 millivolts. What is the mean electrical axis of his QRS?

    A) −30 degrees
    B) +30 degrees
    C) +60 degrees
    D) +120 degrees
    E) −120 degrees

51. During the T-P interval in an ECG of a patient with a damaged cardiac muscle, which of the following is true?

    A) The entire ventricle is depolarized
    B) The entire ventricle is depolarized except for the damaged cardiac muscle
    C) About half the ventricle is depolarized
    D) The entire ventricle is repolarized
    E) The entire ventricle is repolarized except for the damaged cardiac muscle

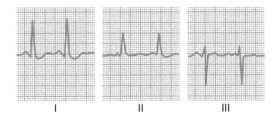

                I   II   III

52. A 50-year-old man is a new employee at ABC Software. The above ECG was recorded during a routine physical examination. What is his likely diagnosis?

    A) Chronic systemic hypertension
    B) Chronic pulmonary hypertension
    C) Second-degree heart block
    D) Paroxysmal tachycardia
    E) Tricuspid valve stenosis

53. A 30-year-old man had an ECG at his physician's office, but his records were lost. The ECG technician remembered that the QRS deflection was large and positive in lead aVF and 0 in lead I. What is the mean electrical axis in the frontal plane?

    A) 90 degrees
    B) 60 degrees
    C) 0 degree
    D) −60 degrees
    E) −90 degrees

54. A 60-year-old woman tires easily. Her ECG shows a QRS complex that is positive in the aVF lead and negative in standard limb lead I. What is a likely cause of this condition?

    A) Chronic systemic hypertension
    B) Pulmonary hypertension
    C) Aortic valve stenosis
    D) Aortic valve regurgitation

55. A 65-year-old patient with a heart murmur has a mean QRS axis of 120 degrees, and the QRS complex lasts 0.18 second. What is the likely diagnosis?

    A) Aortic valve stenosis
    B) Aortic valve regurgitation
    C) Pulmonary valve stenosis
    D) Right bundle branch block
    E) Left bundle branch block

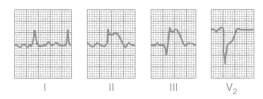

         I   II   III   V₂

56. A 60-year-old woman came to the hospital emergency department and reported chest pain. Based on the ECG tracing shown above, what is the most likely diagnosis?

    A) Acute anterior infarction in the base of the heart
    B) Acute anterior infarction in the apex of the heart
    C) Acute posterior infarction in the base of the heart
    D) Acute posterior infarction in the apex of the heart
    E) Right ventricular hypertrophy

57. A 50-year-old man has been having fainting "spells" for about 2 weeks. During the episodes, his ECG shows a ventricular rate of 25 beats/min and 100 P waves per minute. After about 30 seconds of fainting, a normal sinus rhythm recurs. What is his likely diagnosis?

    A) Atrial flutter
    B) First-degree A-V block
    C) Second-degree A-V block
    D) Third-degree A-V block
    E) Stokes-Adams syndrome

58. An 80-year-old man had an ECG taken at his local doctor's office, and the diagnosis was atrial fibrillation. Which condition is likely in someone with atrial fibrillation?

    A) Ventricular fibrillation, which normally accompanies atrial fibrillation
    B) Strong P waves on the ECG
    C) An irregular and fast rate of ventricular contraction
    D) A normal atrial "a" wave
    E) A smaller atrial volume than normal

59. Circus movements in the ventricle can lead to ventricular fibrillation. Which condition in the ventricular muscle will increase the tendency for circus movements?

    A) Decreased refractory period
    B) Low extracellular potassium concentration
    C) Increased refractory period
    D) Shorter conduction pathway (decreased ventricular volume)
    E) Increase in parasympathetic impulses to the heart

60. A 50-year-old man has a blood pressure of 140/85 mm Hg and weighs 90.7 kilograms (200 pounds). He reports that he is not feeling well, his ECG has no P waves, he has a heart rate of 46 beats/min, and the QRS complexes occur regularly. What is his likely condition?

    A) First-degree heart block
    B) Second-degree heart block
    C) Third-degree heart block
    D) Sinoatrial heart block
    E) Sinus bradycardia

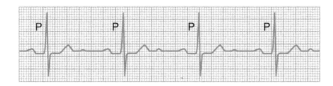

61. The following ECG tracing was obtained for a 60-year-old man who weighs 99.8 kilograms (220 pounds). Standard lead II is shown above. What is his diagnosis?

    A) A-V nodal rhythm
    B) First-degree A-V heart block
    C) Second-degree A-V heart block
    D) Third-degree A-V heart block
    E) Atrial flutter

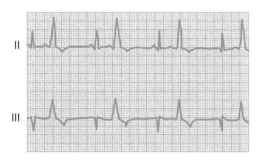

62. A 35-year-old woman had unusual sensations in her chest after she smoked a cigarette. Her ECG tracing is shown above. What is the likely diagnosis?

    A) Premature contraction originating in the atrium
    B) Premature contraction originating high in the A-V node
    C) Premature contraction originating low in the A-V node
    D) Premature contraction originating in the apex of the ventricle
    E) Premature contraction originating in the base of the ventricle

Questions 63 and 64
A 55-year-old man had the below ECG tracing recorded at his doctor's office at a routine physical examination. Use this tracing to answer Questions 63 and 64.

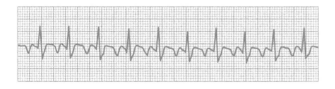

63. What is his diagnosis?

    A) Normal ECG
    B) Atrial flutter
    C) A high A-V junctional pacemaker
    D) A middle A-V junctional pacemaker
    E) A low A-V junctional pacemaker

64. What is his ventricular heart rate in beats/min?

    A) 37.5
    B) 60
    C) 75
    D) 100
    E) 150

65. What decreases the risk of ventricular fibrillation?

    A) A dilated heart
    B) An increased ventricular refractory period
    C) Decreased electrical conduction velocity
    D) Exposure of the heart to 60-cycle alternating current
    E) Epinephrine administration

66. Which of the following will usually result in an inverted P wave that occurs after the QRS complex?

    A) Premature contraction originating in the atrium
    B) Premature contraction originating high in the A-V junction
    C) Premature contraction originating in the middle of the A-V junction
    D) Premature contraction originating low in the A-V junction
    E) Atrial fibrillation

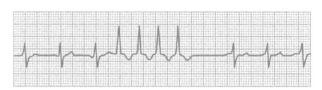

67. A 65-year-old woman who had a myocardial infarction 10 days ago returned to her family physician's office and reported that her pulse rate felt rapid. Based on the above ECG tracing, what is the likely diagnosis?

    A) Stokes-Adams syndrome
    B) Atrial fibrillation
    C) A-V nodal tachycardia
    D) Atrial paroxysmal tachycardia
    E) Ventricular paroxysmal tachycardia

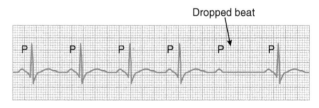

68. A 65-year-old man had the above ECG tracing recorded at his annual physical examination. What is the likely diagnosis?

    A) Atrial paroxysmal tachycardia
    B) First-degree A-V block
    C) Second-degree A-V block
    D) Third-degree A-V block
    E) Atrial flutter

69. A 60-year-old woman has been diagnosed with atrial fibrillation. Which statement best describes this condition?

A) The ventricular rate of contraction is 140 beats/min
B) The P waves of the ECG are pronounced
C) Ventricular contractions occur at regular intervals
D) The QRS waves are more pronounced than normal
E) The atria are smaller than normal

70. What occurs after electrical shock of the heart with a 60-cycle alternating current?

A) A normal arterial pressure
B) A decreased ventricular refractory period
C) Increased electrical conduction velocity
D) A shortened conduction pathway around the heart
E) Normal cardiac output

71. A 55-year-old man has been diagnosed with Stokes-Adams syndrome. Two minutes after the syndrome starts to cause active blockade of the cardiac impulse, which of the following is the pacemaker of the heart?

A) Sinus node
B) A-V node
C) Purkinje fibers
D) Cardiac septum
E) Left atrium

Questions 72 and 73

A man had a myocardial infarction at age 55 years. He is now 63 years old. Use the standard limb lead I tracing on his ECG shown below to answer Questions 72 and 73.

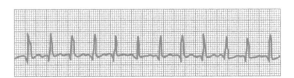

72. What is his heart rate?

A) 40 beats/min
B) 50 beats/min
C) 75 beats/min
D) 100 beats/min
E) 150 beats/min

73. What is his current diagnosis?

A) Sinus tachycardia
B) First-degree heart block
C) Second-degree heart block
D) ST segment depression
E) Third-degree heart block

74. Which statement best describes a patient with premature atrial contraction?

A) The pulse taken from the radial artery immediately after the premature contraction will be weak
B) Stroke volume immediately after the premature contraction will be increased
C) The P wave is never seen
D) The probability of these premature contractions occurring is decreased in people with a large caffeine intake
E) It causes the QRS interval to be lengthened

75. If the origin of the stimulus that causes atrial paroxysmal tachycardia is near the A-V node, which statement about the P wave in standard limb lead I is most accurate?

A) The P wave will originate in the sinus node
B) The P wave will be upright
C) The P wave will be inverted
D) The P wave will be missing

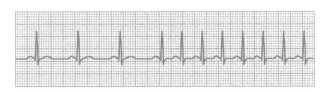

76. A 45-year-old man had the above ECG recorded at his annual physical. What is the likely diagnosis?

A) Atrial paroxysmal tachycardia
B) First-degree A-V block
C) Second-degree A-V block
D) Ventricular paroxysmal tachycardia
E) Atrial flutter

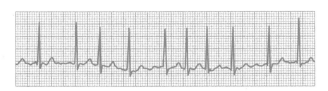

77. A 60-year-old woman sees her physician for her annual physical examination. The physician ordered an ECG, which is shown above. What is the likely diagnosis?

A) First-degree A-V block
B) Second-degree A-V block
C) Third-degree A-V block
D) Atrial paroxysmal tachycardia
E) Atrial fibrillation

Questions 78 and 79

An 80-year-old man went to his family physician for his annual checkup. Use the ECG tracing shown below to answer Questions 78 and 79.

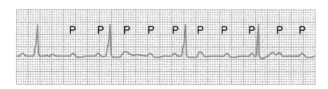

78. What is his heart rate?

   A) 105
   B) 95
   C) 85
   D) 75
   E) 37

79. What is the likely diagnosis?

   A) Left bundle branch block
   B) First-degree A-V block
   C) Second-degree A-V block
   D) Electrical alternans
   E) Complete A-V block

1. **E)** This patient has a heart rate of 70 beats per minute. The cardiac output can be determined by using the following formula: cardiac output = heart rate × stroke volume. The stroke volume can be determined from the figure, which is the volume change during the C-D segment, or 100 milliliters. By using this formula, you can determine that the cardiac output is 7000 milliliters per minute.
    TMP13 p. 118

2. **A)** During the diastolic filling phase, the mitral and tricuspid valves open and blood flows into the ventricles. At point B the isovolumic contraction phase begins, which closes the A-V valves. The closing of these valves causes the first heart sound.
    TMP13 p. 114

3. **B)** Between points A and B is the period of ventricular filling. The vibration of the ventricular walls makes this sound after atrial contraction forces more blood into the ventricles.
    TMP13 p. 114

4. **D)** The ejection fraction is the stroke volume/end-diastolic volume. Stroke volume is 100 milliliters, and the end-systolic volume at point D is 150 milliliters. Thus, the ejection fraction is 0.667, or in terms of percentage, 66.7%.
    TMP13 p. 118

5. **B)** The cardiac muscle stores much more calcium in its tubular system than does skeletal muscle and is much more dependent on extracellular calcium than is the skeletal muscle. An abundance of calcium is bound by the mucopolysaccharides inside the T-tubule. This calcium is necessary for contraction of cardiac muscle, and its strength of contraction depends on the calcium concentration surrounding the cardiac myocytes. At the initiation of the action potential, the fast sodium channels open first, which is followed later by opening of the slow calcium channels.
    TMP13 p. 111

6. **D)** The end-diastolic volume is always greater than the end-systolic volume. Multiplication of the ejection fraction by the end-diastolic volume provides the stroke volume, which is 50 milliliters in this problem. Therefore, the end-diastolic volume is 50 milliliters greater than the end-systolic volume and has a value of 200 milliliters.
    TMP13 p. 118

7. **D)** The typical ejection fraction is 60%, and lower values are indicative of a weakened heart.
    TMP13 p. 115

8. **D)** During phase 3 of the ventricular muscle action potential, the potassium permeability of ventricular muscle greatly increases, which causes a more negative membrane potential.
    TMP13 p. 113

9. **D)** Heart rate is determined by the formula 60/R-R interval. The heart rate for this patient is 40 beats per minute. This heart rate is slow, which would occur in a trained athlete. A fever would increase heart rate. Excess parasympathetic stimulation and hyperpolarization of the S-A node both decrease heart rate.
    TMP13 p. 121

10. **E)** The heart goes into spastic contraction after a large increase in the calcium ion concentration surrounding the cardiac myofibrils, which occurs if the extracellular fluid calcium ion concentration increases too much. An excess potassium concentration in the extracellular fluids causes the heart to become dilated because of the decrease in resting membrane potential of the cardiac muscle fibers.
    TMP13 p. 121

11. **D)** At the end of isovolumic relaxation, the mitral and tricuspid valves open, which is followed by the period of diastolic filling.
    TMP13 pp. 117-118

12. **E)** As seen in Chapter 9, the first heart sound by definition occurs just after the ventricular pressure exceeds the atrial pressure, which causes the A-V valves to mechanically close. The second heart sound occurs when the aortic and pulmonary valves close.
    TMP13 p. 114

13. **B)** Having excess potassium ions in the blood and extracellular fluid causes the heart to become dilated and flaccid and also slows the heart. This effect is important because of a decrease in the resting membrane potential in the cardiac muscle fibers. As the membrane potential decreases, the intensity of the action potential decreases, which makes the contraction of the heart progressively weaker. Excess calcium ions in the blood and sympathetic stimulation and increased norepinephrine concentration of the blood all cause the heart to contract vigorously.
    TMP13 p. 121

14. **E)** The normal plateau level of the cardiac output function curve is 13 L/min. This level decreases in any kind of cardiac failure and increases markedly during sympathetic stimulation.
     TMP13 p. 121

15. **E)** Immediately after the QRS wave, the ventricles begin to contract, and the first phase that occurs is isovolumic contraction. Isovolumic contraction occurs before the ejection phase and increases the ventricular pressure enough to mechanically open the aortic and pulmonary valves.
     TMP13 p. 118

16. **C)** The atrial and ventricular muscles have a relatively rapid rate of conduction of the cardiac action potential, and the anterior internodal pathway also has fairly rapid conduction of the impulse. However, the A-V bundle myofibrils have a slow rate of conduction because their sizes are considerably smaller than the sizes of the normal atrial and ventricular muscle. In addition, their slow conduction is partly caused by diminished numbers of gap junctions between successive muscle cells in the conducting pathway, causing a great resistance to conduction of the excitatory ions from one cell to the next.
     TMP13 p. 124

17. **D)** The impulse from the S-A node travels rapidly through the internodal pathways and arrives at the A-V node at 0.03 second, at the A-V bundle at 0.12 second, and at the ventricular septum at 0.16 second. The total delay is thus 0.13 second.
     TMP13 p. 127

18. **D)** Increased sympathetic stimulation of the heart increases heart rate, atrial contractility, and ventricular contractility and also increases norepinephrine release at the ventricular sympathetic nerve endings. It does not release acetylcholine. It does cause an increased sodium permeability of the A-V node, which increases the rate of upward drift of the membrane potential to the threshold level for self-excitation, thus increasing the heart rate.
     TMP13 pp. 121, 128

19. **A)** After the S-A node discharges, the action potential travels through the atria, through the A-V bundle system, and finally to the ventricular septum and throughout the ventricle. The last place that the impulse arrives is at the epicardial surface at the base of the left ventricle, which requires a transit time of 0.22 second.
     TMP13 p. 127

20. **D)** The increase in potassium permeability causes a hyperpolarization of the A-V node, which will decrease the heart rate. Increases in sodium permeability will actually partially depolarize the A-V node, and an increase in norepinephrine levels increases the heart rate.
     TMP13 p. 110

21. **D)** During sympathetic stimulation, the permeabilities of the S-A node and the A-V node increase. In addition, the permeability of cardiac muscle to calcium increases, resulting in an increased contractile strength. Furthermore, an upward drift of the resting membrane potential of the S-A node occurs. Increased permeability of the S-A node to potassium does not occur during sympathetic stimulation.
     TMP13 p. 128

22. **A)** The normal resting membrane potential of the S-A node is –55 millivolts. As the sodium leaks into the membrane, an upward drift of the membrane potential occurs until it reaches –40 millivolts. This is the threshold level that initiates the action potential at the S-A node.
     TMP13 p. 124

23. **D)** Increases in sodium and calcium permeability at the S-A node result in an increase in heart rate. An increased potassium permeability causes a hyperpolarization of the S-A node, which causes the heart rate to decrease.
     TMP13 p. 128

24. **A)** Sodium permeability is highest during phase 0. Calcium permeability is highest during phase 2, and potassium is most permeable in phase 3.
     TMP13 p. 124

25. **D)** The action potential arrives at the A-V bundle at 0.12 second. It arrives at the A-V node at 0.03 second and is delayed 0.09 second in the A-V node, which results in an arrival time at the bundle of His of 0.12 second.
     TMP13 p. 127

26. **A)** If the Purkinje fibers are the pacemaker of the heart, the heart rate ranges between 15 and 40 beats/min. In contrast, the rate of firing of the A-V nodal fibers are 40 to 60 times a minute, and the sinus node fires at 70 to 80 times per minute. If the sinus node is blocked for some reason, the A-V node will take over as the pacemaker, and if the A-V node is blocked, the Purkinje fibers will take over as the pacemaker of the heart.
     TMP13 pp. 127-128

27. **A)** It takes 0.03 second for the action potential to travel from the S-A node to the A-V node.
     TMP13 p. 127

28. **B)** The impulse coming from the S-A node to the A-V node arrives at 0.03 second. Then there is a total delay of 0.13 second in the A-V node and bundle system, allowing the impulse to arrive at the ventricular septum at 0.16 second.
     TMP13 p. 127

29. **B)** The normal rhythm of the A-V node is 40 to 60 beats per minute. Purkinje fibers have a rhythm of 15 to 40 beats per minute.
TMP13 p. 127

30. **D)** An increase in potassium permeability causes a decrease in the membrane potential of the A-V node. Thus, it will be extremely hyperpolarized, making it much more difficult for the membrane potential to reach its threshold level for conduction, resulting in a decrease in heart rate. Increases in sodium and calcium permeability and norepinephrine levels increase the membrane potential, causing a tendency to increase the heart rate.
TMP13 p. 128

31. **A)** By convention, the left arm is the positive electrode for lead aVL of an ECG.
TMP13 p. 136

32. **B)** By convention, the left leg is the positive electrode for lead II of an ECG.
TMP13 pp. 134-135

33. **E)** Sympathetic stimulation of the heart normally causes an increased heart rate, increased rate of conduction of the cardiac impulse, and increased force of contraction in the atria and ventricles. However, it does not cause acetylcholine release at the sympathetic endings because they contain norepinephrine. Parasympathetic stimulation causes acetylcholine release. The sympathetic nervous system firing increases in the permeability of the cardiac muscle fibers, the S-A node, and the A-V node to sodium and calcium.
TMP13 p. 128

34. **A)** The heart rate can be calculated by 60 divided by the R-R interval, which is 0.86 second. This results in a heart rate of 70 beats/min.
TMP13 p. 133

35. **B)** Einthoven's law states that the voltage in lead I plus the voltage in lead III is equal to the voltage in lead II. In this case the voltage in lead II is 0.9 millivolt and the voltage in lead III is 0.4 millivolt. The lead I voltage is thus 0.5 (0.9 – 0.4 millivolt = 0.5 millivolt).
TMP13 p. 135

36. **E)** The contraction of the ventricles lasts almost from the beginning of the Q wave and continues to the end of the T wave. This interval is called the Q-T interval and ordinarily lasts about 0.35 second.
TMP13 p. 133

37. **A)** By convention, the right arm is the negative electrode for lead II of an ECG.
TMP13 p. 135

38. **A)** By convention, the left arm is the negative electrode for lead I of an ECG.
TMP13 p. 134

39. **D)** Einthoven's law states that the voltage in lead I plus the voltage in lead III is equal to the voltage in lead II, which in this case is 2.0 millivolts.
TMP13 p. 135

40. **D)** Different ECG lead axes are shown in the figure. Lead III has a positive portion at 120 degrees and a negative portion at –60 degrees. Therefore, lead III has correct axes for this question.
TMP13 p. 140

41. **B)** The mean electrical axis can be determined by plotting the resultant voltage of the QRS for leads I, II, and III. The result is shown below and has a value of –50 degrees.
TMP13 pp. 144-145

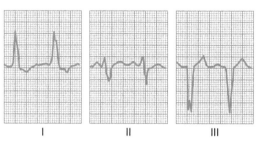

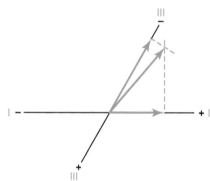

42. **B)** The heart rate can be calculated by 60 divided by the R-R interval, which is 0.68 second. This calculation results in a heart rate of 88 beats/min.
TMP13 p. 133

43. **B)** In the figure, the QRS width is greater than 0.12 second, which indicates a bundle branch block. Right bundle branch block is not a listed answer. The correct answer is therefore left bundle branch block.
TMP13 p. 146

44. **A)** Systemic hypertension results in a left axis deviation because of the enlargement of the left ventricle. Pulmonary valve stenosis and pulmonary valve regurgitation result in an enlarged right ventricle and right axis deviation. A rightward angulation of the heart will cause a rightward shift in the mean electrical axis. Pulmonary hypertension causes enlargement of the right heart and thus causes right axis deviation.
TMP13 p. 145

45. D) Lead II has a positive vector at the 60-degree angle. The negative end of lead II is at −120 degrees.
TMP13 p. 140

46. D) Note in the figure below that the QRS complex has a large negative deflection in lead I and a positive deflection in lead III, which indicates that there is a rightward axis deviation. Heart rate is calculated by 60/R-R interval and is 103 beats per minute.
TMP13 pp. 133, 146

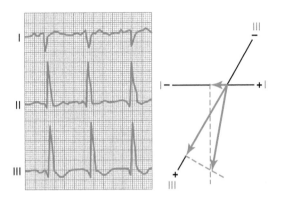

47. C) The right axis deviation in this patient has to occur because of a change in muscle mass in the right ventricle, which occurs in pulmonary valve stenosis. Aortic valve insufficiency and systemic hypertension will cause a left axis shift. The QRS width is not greater than 0.12 second, so the patient does not have bundle branch block.
TMP13 p. 146

48. B) The patient has a mean electrical axis of 60 degrees because of the large deflection in lead II and zero in lead aVL. The axis of aVL is −30 degrees, which is perpendicular to lead II, and this indicates that the axis must be 60 degrees.
TMP13 p. 148

49. A) This patient has an acute anterior infarction in the left ventricle of the heart. This diagnosis can be determined by plotting the currents of injury from the different leads (see figure below). The limb leads are used to determine whether the infarction is coming from the left or right side of the ventricle and from the base or inferior part of the ventricle. The chest leads are used to determine whether it is an anterior or posterior infarct. When we analyze the currents of injury, a negative potential, caused by the current of injury, occurs in lead I and a positive potential, caused by the

current of injury, occurs in lead III. This is determined by subtracting the J point from the TP segment. The negative end of the resultant vector originates in the ischemic area, which is therefore the left side of the heart. In lead V_2, the chest lead, the electrode is in a field of very negative potential, which occurs in patients with an anterior lesion.
TMP13 pp. 150-151

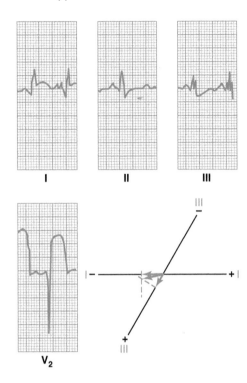

50. D) The QRS wave plotted on lead I was −1.2 millivolts, and lead II was +1.2 millivolts, so the absolute value of the deflections was the same. Therefore, the mean electrical axis must be exactly halfway in between these two leads, which is halfway between the lead II axis of 60 degrees and the lead I negative axis of 180 degrees, which provides a value of 120 degrees.
TMP13 p. 144

51. E) During the T-P interval in a patient with a damaged ventricle, the only area depolarized is the damaged muscle. Therefore, the remainder of the ventricle is repolarized. At the J point the entire ventricle is depolarized in a patient with a damaged cardiac muscle or in a patient with a normal cardiac muscle. The area of the heart that is damaged will not repolarize but remains depolarized at all times.
TMP13 p. 150

52. A) Note in the figure below that the QRS complex has a positive deflection in lead I and a negative in lead III, which indicates that there is a leftward axis deviation, which occurs during chronic systemic hypertension. Pulmonary hypertension increases the ventricular mass on the right side of the heart, which gives a right axis deviation.

TMP13 p. 145

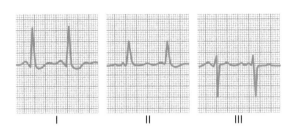

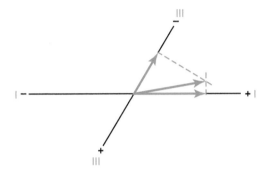

53. A) Because the deflection in this ECG is 0 in lead I, the axis has to be 90 degrees away from this lead. Therefore, the mean electrical axis must be +90 degrees or −90 degrees. Because the aVF lead has a positive deflection, the mean electrical axis must be at +90 degrees.

TMP13 p. 140

54. B) The ECG from this patient has a positive deflection in aVF and a negative deflection in standard limb lead I. Therefore, the mean electrical axis is between 90 degrees and 180 degrees, which is a rightward shift in the ECG mean electrical axis. Systemic hypertension, aortic valve stenosis, and aortic valve regurgitation cause hypertrophy of the left ventricle and thus a leftward shift in the mean electrical axis. Pulmonary hypertension causes a rightward shift in the axis and is therefore characterized by this ECG.

TMP13 p. 146

55. D) A QRS axis of 120 degrees indicates a rightward shift. Because the QRS complex is 0.18 second, this indicates a conduction block. Therefore, the diagnosis that fits with these characteristics is a right bundle branch block.

TMP13 p. 146

56. D) In the figure below, the current of injury is plotted at the bottom of the graph. This is not a plot of the QRS voltages but the current of injury voltages. They are plotted for leads II and III, which are both negative, and the resultant vector is nearly vertical. The negative end of the vector points to where the current of injury originated, which is in the apex of the ventricle. The elevation of the TP segment above the J point indicates a posterior lesion. Therefore, the ECG is consistent with acute posterior infarction in the apex of the ventricle.

TMP13 p. 151

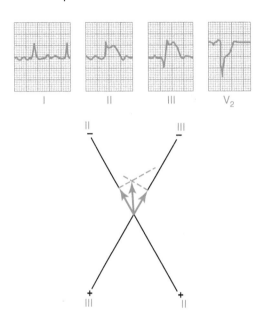

57. E) This patient has a difference in the atrial rate of 100 and in the ventricular rate of 25. The 25 rate in the ventricles is indicative of a rhythm starting in the Purkinje fibers. A-V block is occurring, but it comes and goes, which is only fulfilled by Stokes-Adams syndrome.

TMP13 p. 157

58. C) A person with atrial fibrillation has a rapid, irregular heart rate. The P waves are missing or are very weak. The atria exhibit circus movements, and atrial volume is often increased, causing the atrial fibrillation.

TMP13 pp. 164-165

59. A) Circus movements occur in ventricular muscle, particularly in persons with a dilated heart or decreases in conduction velocity. High extracellular potassium and sympathetic stimulation, not parasympathetic stimulation, increase the tendency for circus movements. A longer refractory period tends to prevent circus movements of the heart, because when the impulses travel around the heart and contact the area of ventricular muscle that has a longer refractory period, the action potential stops at this point.

TMP13 pp. 161-162

60. **D)** When a patient has no P waves and a low heart rate, it is likely that the impulse leaving the sinus node is totally blocked before entering the atrial muscle, which is called sinoatrial block. The ventricles pick up the new rhythm, usually initiated in the A-V node at this point, which results in a heart rate of 40 to 60 per minute. In contrast, during sinus bradycardia, P waves are still associated with each QRS complex. In first-, second-, and third-degree heart block, P waves are present in each of these instances, although some are not associated with QRS complex.

   TMP13 p. 156

61. **B)** By definition, first-degree A-V heart block occurs when the P-R interval exceeds a value of 0.20 second but without any dropped QRS waves. This ECG shows first degree block. In this figure the P-R interval is about 0.30 second, which is considerably prolonged. However, there are no dropped QRS waves. During second-degree A-V block, QRS waves are dropped.

   TMP13 p. 157

62. **E)** In the figure below, note that the premature ventricular contractions (PVCs) have a wide and tall QRS wave in the ECG. The mean electrical axis of the premature contraction can be determined by plotting these large QRS complexes on the standard limb leads. The PVC originates at the negative end of the resultant mean electrical axis, which is at the base of the ventricle. Notice that the QRS of the PVC is wider and much taller than the normal QRS waves in this ECG.

   TMP13 p. 159

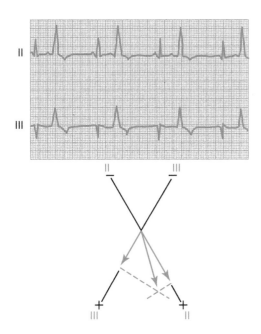

63. **B)** This patient has atrial flutter, which is characterized by several P waves for each QRS complex. This ECG has two P waves for every QRS. Notice the rapid heart rate, which is characteristic of atrial flutter.

   TMP13 p. 165

64. **E)** The average ventricular rate is 150 beats/min in this ECG, which is typical of atrial flutter. Once again notice that the heart rate is irregular because of the inability of the impulses to quickly pass through the A-V node because of its refractory period.

   TMP13 p. 133

65. **B)** A dilated heart increases the risk of occurrence of ventricular fibrillation because of an increase in the likelihood of circus movements. Also, if the conduction velocity decreases, it will take a longer period for the impulse to travel around the heart, which decreases the risk of ventricular fibrillation. Exposure of the heart to 60-cycle alternating current or epinephrine administration increases the irritability of the heart. If the refractory period is long, the likelihood of re-entrant type of pathways decreases, because when the impulse travels around the heart, the ventricles remain in a refractory period.

   TMP13 pp. 161-162

66. **D)** An inverted P wave occurs in patients with a premature contraction originating in the A-V junction. If the P wave occurs after the QRS complex, the junctional contraction started low in the A-V junction. Junctional contractions originating high in the A-V junction will have a P wave that occurs before the QRS, and likewise one originating in the middle of junction occurs during the QRS.

   TMP13 p. 157

67. **E)** The term "paroxysmal" means that the heart rate becomes rapid in paroxysms, with the paroxysm beginning suddenly and lasting for a few seconds, a few minutes, a few hours, or much longer. Then the paroxysm usually ends as suddenly as it began and the pacemaker shifts back to the S-A node. The mechanism by which this phenomenon is believed to occur is by a re-entrant circus movement feedback pathway that sets up an area of local repeated self–re-excitation. The ECG shown is ventricular paroxysmal tachycardia. That the origin is in the ventricles can be determined because of the changes in the QRS complex, which have high voltages and look much different than the preceding normal QRS complexes. This is very characteristic of a ventricular irritable locus.

   TMP13 pp. 160-161

68. **C)** Notice in this ECG that a P wave precedes each of the first four QRS complexes. After that we see a P wave but a dropped QRS wave, which is characteristic of second-degree A-V block.

   TMP13 p. 157

69. **A)** A person with atrial fibrillation has a rapid, irregular heart rate. The P waves are missing or are very weak. The atria exhibit circus movements and often are very enlarged, causing the atrial fibrillation.

   TMP13 pp. 164-165

70. **B)** Ventricular fibrillation often occurs in a heart exposed to a 60-cycle alternating current. An increased conduction velocity through the heart muscle or a shortened conduction pathway around the heart decreases the probability of re-entrant pathways. A shortened ventricular refractory period increases the possibility of fibrillation. Thus, when the electrical stimulus travels around the heart and reaches the ventricular muscle that was again initially stimulated, the risk of ventricular fibrillation increases because the muscle will be out of the refractory period.
  TMP13 p. 162

71. **B)** During a Stokes-Adams syndrome attack, total A-V block suddenly begins, and the duration of the block may be a few seconds or even several weeks. The new pacemaker of the heart is distal to the point of blockade but is usually deep in the A-V node or the A-V bundle.
  TMP13 p. 157

72. **E)** The heart rate can be determined by 60 divided by the R-R interval, which gives a value of 150 beats/min. This patient has tachycardia, which is defined as a heart rate greater than 100 beats/min.
  TMP13 p. 133

73. **A)** The relationship between the P waves and the QRS complexes appears to be normal, and there are no missing beats. Therefore, this patient has a sinus rhythm, and there is no heart block. There is also no ST segment depression in this patient. Because we have normal P and QRS and T waves, this condition is sinus tachycardia.
  TMP13 p. 156

74. **A)** The heartbeat immediately following a premature atrial contraction weakens because the diastolic period is very short in this condition. Therefore, the ventricular filling time is very short, and thus the stroke volume decreases. The P wave is usually visible in this arrhythmia unless it coincides with the QRS complex. The probability of these premature contractions increases in people with toxic irritation of the heart and local ischemic areas.
  TMP13 p. 158

75. **C)** During atrial paroxysmal tachycardia, the impulse is initiated by an ectopic focus somewhere in the atria. If the point of initiation is near the A-V node, the P wave travels backward toward the S-A node and then forward into the ventricles at the same time. Therefore, the P wave will be inverted.
  TMP13 p. 160

76. **A)** This ECG has characteristics of atrial paroxysmal tachycardia, which means that the tachycardia may come and go at random times. The basic shape of the QRS complex and its magnitude are virtually unchanged from the normal QRS complexes, which eliminates the possibility of ventricular paroxysmal tachycardia. This ECG is not characteristic of atrial flutter because there is only one P wave for each QRS complex.
  TMP13 p. 160

77. **E)** First-, second-, and third-degree heart blocks, as well as atrial paroxysmal tachycardia, all have P waves in the ECG. However, there are usually no evident P waves during atrial fibrillation, and the heart rate is irregular. Therefore, this ECG is characteristic of atrial fibrillation.
  TMP13 pp. 164-165

78. **E)** This patient's heart rate is 37 beats/min, which can be determined by dividing 60 by the R-R interval. This is characteristic of some types of A-V block.
  TMP13 p. 133

79. **E)** This ECG is characteristic of complete A-V block, which is also called third-degree A-V block. The P waves seem to be totally dissociated from the QRS complexes, because sometimes there are three P waves and sometimes two P waves between QRS complexes. First-degree A-V block causes a lengthened P-R interval, and second-degree A-V block has long P-R intervals with dropped beats. However, this does not seem to be occurring in this ECG, because there is no relationship between the ORS waves and the P waves.
  TMP13 p. 157

The Circulation

1. Listed below are the hydrostatic and oncotic pressures within a microcirculatory bed.

   Π_c

   P_c Plasma colloid osmotic pressure = 25 mm Hg
   Capillary hydrostatic pressure = 25 mm Hg
   Venous hydrostatic pressure = 5 mm Hg
   Arterial pressure = 80 mm Hg
   Interstitial fluid hydrostatic pressure = −5 mm Hg P_i
   Interstitial colloid osmotic pressure = 10 mm Hg Π_i
   Capillary filtration coefficient = 10 ml/min/mm Hg

   What is the rate of net fluid movement across the capillary wall?

   $$J_v = K_f (P_c - P_i) - (\Pi_c - \Pi_i)$$

   $$K_f \times [P_c - \Pi_c + \Pi_i - P_i]$$

   $$25 - 25 + 10 - (-5)$$

   A) 25 ml/min
   B) 50 ml/min
   C) 100 ml/min
   D) 150 ml/min
   E) 200 ml/min

2. A healthy 60-year-old woman with a 10-year history of hypertension stands up from a supine position. Which set of cardiovascular changes is most likely to occur in response to standing up from a supine position?

	Sympathetic Nerve Activity	Parasympathetic Nerve Activity	Heart Rate
A)	↑	↑	↑
B)	↑	↑	↓
C)	↑	↓	↓
D)	↑	↓	↑
E)	↓	↓	↓
F)	↓	↓	↑
G)	↓	↑	↑
H)	↓	↑	↓

3. In an experimental study, administration of a drug decreases the diameter of arterioles in the muscle bed of an animal subject. Which set of physiological changes would be expected to occur in response to the decrease in diameter?

	Vascular Conductance	Capillary Filtration	Blood Flow
A)	↑	↑	↑
B)	↑	↓	↑
C)	↑	↓	↓
D)	↑	↑	↓
E)	↓	↓	↓
F)	↓	↑	↓
G)	↓	↑	↑
H)	↓	↓	↑

   ↓ + ↓ capillary hydrostatic pressure

4. A 60-year-old woman has experienced dizziness for the past 6 months when getting out of bed in the morning and when standing up. Her mean arterial pressure is 130/90 mm Hg while lying down and 95/60 while sitting. Which set of physiological changes would be expected in response to moving from a supine to an upright position?

	Parasympathetic Nerve Activity	Plasma Renin Activity	Sympathetic Activity
A)	↑	↑	↑
B)	↑	↓	↑
C)	↑	↓	↓
D)	↑	↑	↓
E)	↓	↓	↓
F)	↓	↑	↓
G)	↓	↑	↑
H)	↓	↓	↑

5. A 35-year-old woman visits her family practitioner for an examination. She has a blood pressure of 160/75 mm Hg and a heart rate of 74 beats/min. Further tests by a cardiologist reveal that the patient has moderate aortic regurgitation. Which set of changes would be expected in this patient?

	Pulse Pressure	Systolic Pressure	Stroke Volume
A)	↑	↑	↑
B)	↑	↓	↑
C)	↑	↓	↓
D)	↑	↑	↓
E)	↓	↓	↓
F)	↓	↑	↓
G)	↓	↑	↑
H)	↓	↓	↑

6. A healthy 27-year-old female medical student runs a 5K race. Which set of physiological changes is most likely to occur in this woman's skeletal muscles during the race?

	Arteriole Diameter	Vascular Conductance	Tissue Oxygen Concentration
A)	↑	↑	↑
B)	↑	↑	↓
C)	↑	↓	↓
D)	↑	↓	↑
E)	↓	↓	↓
F)	↓	↓	↑
G)	↓	↑	↑
H)	↓	↑	↓

7. Cognitive stimuli such as reading, problem solving, and talking all result in significant increases in cerebral blood flow. Which set of changes in cerebral tissue concentrations is the most likely explanation for the increase in cerebral blood flow?

	Carbon Dioxide	pH	Adenosine
A)	↑	↑	↑
B)	↑	↓	↑
C)	↑	↓	↓
D)	↑	↑	↓
E)	↓	↓	↓
F)	↓	↑	↓
G)	↓	↑	↑
H)	↓	↓	↑

8. Histamine is infused into the brachial artery. Which set of microcirculatory changes would be expected in the infused arm?

	Capillary Water Permeability	Capillary Hydrostatic Pressure	Capillary Filtration Rate
A)	↑	↑	↑
B)	↑	↑	↓
C)	↑	↓	↓
D)	↑	↓	↑
E)	↓	↓	↓
F)	↓	↓	↑
G)	↓	↑	↑
H)	↓	↑	↓

9. An increase in shear stress in a blood vessel results in which change?

A) Decreased endothelin production
B) Decreased cyclic guanosine monophosphate production
C) Increased nitric oxide release
D) Increased renin production
E) Decreased prostacyclin production

10. A 65-year-old man with a 10-year history of essential hypertension is being treated with an angiotensin-converting enzyme (ACE) inhibitor. Which set of changes would be expected to occur in response to the ACE inhibitor drug therapy?

	Plasma Renin Concentration	Total Peripheral Resistance	Renal Sodium Excretory Function
A)	↑	↑	↑
B)	↑	↑	↓
C)	↑	↓	↓
D)	↑	↓	↑
E)	↓	↓	↓
F)	↓	↓	↑
G)	↓	↑	↑
H)	↓	↑	↓

11. The diameter of a precapillary arteriole is increased in a muscle vascular bed. A decrease in which of the following would be expected?

A) Capillary filtration rate
B) Vascular conductance
C) Capillary blood flow
D) Capillary hydrostatic pressure
E) Arteriolar resistance

12. A 55-year-old man with a history of normal health visits his physician for a checkup. The physical examination reveals that his blood pressure is 170/98 mm Hg. Further tests indicate that he has renovascular hypertension as a result of stenosis in the left kidney. Which set of findings would be expected in this man with renovascular hypertension?

	Total Peripheral Resistance	Plasma Renin Activity	Plasma Aldosterone Concentration
A)	↑	↑	↑
B)	↑	↓	↑
C)	↑	↓	↓
D)	↑	↑	↓
E)	↓	↓	↓
F)	↓	↑	↓
G)	↓	↑	↑
H)	↓	↓	↑

13. Under control conditions, flow through a blood vessel is 100 ml/min with a pressure gradient of 50 mm Hg. What would be the approximate flow through the vessel after increasing the vessel diameter by 50%, assuming that the pressure gradient is maintained at 50 mm Hg?
    A) 100 ml/min
    B) 150 ml/min
    C) 300 ml/min
    D) 500 ml/min
    E) 700 ml/min

14. A 24-year-old woman delivers a 6-pound, 8-ounce baby girl. The newborn is diagnosed as having patent ductus arteriosus. Which set of changes would be expected in this baby?

	Pulse Pressure	Stroke Volume	Systolic Pressure
A)	↑	↑	↑
B)	↑	↓	↑
C)	↑	↓	↓
D)	↑	↑	↓
E)	↓	↓	↓
F)	↓	↑	↓
G)	↓	↑	↑
H)	↓	↓	↑

15. A 72-year-old man had surgery to remove an abdominal tumor. Pathohistological studies revealed that the tumor mass contained a large number of vessels. The most likely stimulus for the growth of vessels in a solid tumor is an increase in which of the following?
    A) Growth hormone
    B) Plasma glucose concentration
    C) Angiostatin growth factor
    D) Vascular endothelial growth factor
    E) Tissue oxygen concentration

16. Which set of changes would be expected to cause the greatest increase in the net movement of sodium across a muscle capillary wall?

	Wall Permeability to Sodium	Wall Surface Area	Concentration Difference Across Wall
A)	↑	↑	↑
B)	↑	↑	↓
C)	↑	↓	↓
D)	↑	↓	↑
E)	↓	↓	↓
F)	↓	↓	↑
G)	↓	↑	↑
H)	↓	↑	↓

17. While participating in a cardiovascular physiology laboratory, a medical student isolates an animal's carotid artery proximal to the carotid bifurcation and partially constricts the artery with a tie around the vessel. Which set of changes would be expected to occur in response to constriction of the carotid artery?

	Heart Rate	Sympathetic Nerve Activity	Total Peripheral Resistance
A)	↑	↑	↑
B)	↑	↑	↓
C)	↑	↓	↓
D)	↑	↓	↑
E)	↓	↓	↓
F)	↓	↓	↑
G)	↓	↑	↑
H)	↓	↑	↓

18. A 35-year-old woman visits her family practice physician for an examination. She has a mean arterial blood pressure of 105 mm Hg and a heart rate of 74 beats/min. Further tests by a cardiologist reveal that the patient has moderate aortic valve stenosis. Which set of changes would be expected in this patient?

	Pulse Pressure	Stroke Volume	Systolic Pressure
A)	↑	↑	↑
B)	↑	↓	↑
C)	↑	↓	↓
D)	↑	↑	↓
E)	↓	↓	↓
F)	↓	↑	↓
G)	↓	↑	↑
H)	↓	↓	↑

19. A 60-year-old man visits his family practitioner for an annual examination. He has a mean blood pressure of 130 mm Hg and a heart rate of 78 beats/min. His plasma cholesterol level is in the upper 25th percentile, and he is diagnosed as having atherosclerosis. Which set of changes would be expected in this patient?

	Pulse Pressure	Arterial Compliance	Systolic Pressure
A)	↑	↑	↑
B)	↑	↓	↑
C)	↑	↓	↓
D)	↑	↑	↓
E)	↓	↓	↓
F)	↓	↑	↓
G)	↓	↑	↑
H)	↓	↓	↑

20. While participating in a cardiovascular physiology laboratory, a medical student isolates the carotid artery of an animal and partially constricts the artery with a tie around the vessel. Which set of changes would be expected to occur in response to constriction of the carotid artery?

	Sympathetic Nerve Activity	Renal Blood Flow	Total Peripheral Resistance
A)	↑	↑	↑
B)	↑	↓	↑
C)	↑	↓	↓
D)	↑	↑	↓
E)	↓	↓	↓
F)	↓	↑	↓
G)	↓	↑	↑
H)	↓	↓	↑

21. Which mechanism would tend to decrease capillary filtration rate?

A) Increased capillary hydrostatic pressure
B) Decreased plasma colloid osmotic pressure
C) Increased interstitial colloid osmotic pressure
D) Decreased capillary water permeability
E) Decreased arteriolar resistance

22. A 72-year-old man had surgery to remove an abdominal tumor. Findings of pathohistological studies reveal that the tumor mass contains a large number of blood vessels. The most likely stimulus for the growth of vessels in a solid tumor is an increase in which of the following?

A) Growth hormone
B) Plasma glucose concentration
C) Angiostatin growth factor
D) Tissue oxygen concentration
E) Vascular endothelial growth factor (VEGF)

23. The diameter of a precapillary arteriole is decreased in a muscle vascular bed. Which change in the microcirculation would be expected?

A) Decreased capillary filtration rate
B) Increased interstitial volume
C) Increased lymph flow
D) Increased capillary hydrostatic pressure
E) Decreased arteriolar resistance

24. A 50-year-old man has a 3-year history of hypertension. He reports fatigue and occasional muscle cramps. There is no family history of hypertension. The patient has not had any other significant medical problems in the past. Examination reveals a blood pressure of 168/104 mm Hg. Additional laboratory tests indicate that the patient has primary hyperaldosteronism. Which set of findings would be expected in this man with primary hyperaldosteronism hypertension?

	Extracellular Fluid Volume	Plasma Renin Activity	Plasma Potassium Concentration
A)	↑	↑	↑
B)	↑	↓	↑
C)	↑	↓	↓
D)	↑	↑	↓
E)	↓	↓	↓
F)	↓	↑	↓
G)	↓	↑	↑
H)	↓	↓	↑

25. An increase in which of the following would tend to increase lymph flow?

A) Hydraulic conductivity of the capillary wall   ↑ Filtration ↑
B) Plasma colloid osmotic pressure — ↓ Filtration
C) Capillary hydrostatic pressure   — ↑ Filtration
D) Arteriolar resistance
E) A and C

26. In control conditions, flow through a blood vessel is 100 ml/min under a pressure gradient of 50 mm Hg. What would be the approximate flow through the vessel after increasing the vessel diameter to four times normal, assuming that the pressure gradient was maintained at 50 mm Hg?

A) 300 ml/min
B) 1600 ml/min
C) 1000 ml/min
D) 16,000 ml/min
E) 25,600 ml/min

27. A 50-year-old woman has a renal blood flow of 1200 ml/min and hematocrit of 50. Her arterial pressure is 125 mm Hg, and her renal venous pressure is 5 mm Hg. She also has a plasma colloid osmotic pressure of 25 mm Hg and a glomerular capillary hydrostatic pressure of 50 mm Hg. What is the total renal vascular resistance (in mm Hg/ml/min) in this woman?

    A) 0.05
    B) 0.10
    C) 0.50
    D) 1.00
    E) 1.50

28. An increase in which of the following would be expected to decrease blood flow in a vessel?

    A) Pressure gradient across the vessel
    B) Radius of the vessel
    C) Plasma colloid osmotic pressure
    D) Viscosity of the blood
    E) Plasma sodium concentration

29. Assuming that vessels A to D are the same length, which one has the greatest flow?

	Pressure Gradient	Radius	Viscosity
A)	100	1	10
B)	50	2	5
C)	25	4	2
D)	10	6	1

30. A 22-year-old man enters the hospital emergency department after severing a major artery in a motorcycle accident. It is estimated that he has lost approximately 700 milliliters of blood. His blood pressure is 90/55 mm Hg. Which set of changes would be expected in response to hemorrhage in this man?

	Heart Rate	Sympathetic Nerve Activity	Total Peripheral Resistance
A)	↑	↑	↑
B)	↑	↓	↑
C)	↑	↓	↓
D)	↑	↑	↓
E)	↓	↓	↓
F)	↓	↑	↓
G)	↓	↑	↑
H)	↓	↓	↑

31. A healthy 28-year-old woman stands up from a supine position. Moving from a supine to a standing position results in a transient decrease in arterial pressure that is detected by arterial baroreceptors located in the aortic arch and carotid sinuses. Which set of cardiovascular changes is most likely to occur in response to activation of the baroreceptors?

	Mean Circulatory Filling Pressure	Strength of Cardiac Contraction	Sympathetic Nerve Activity
A)	↑	↑	↑
B)	↑	↓	↑
C)	↑	↓	↓
D)	↑	↑	↓
E)	↓	↓	↓
F)	↓	↑	↓
G)	↓	↑	↑
H)	↓	↓	↑

32. An ACE inhibitor is administered to a 65-year-old man with a 20-year history of hypertension. The drug lowered his arterial pressure and increased his plasma levels of renin and bradykinin. Which mechanism would best explain the decrease in arterial pressure?

    A) Inhibition of angiotensin I
    B) Decreased conversion of angiotensinogen to angiotensin I
    C) Increased plasma levels of bradykinin
    D) Increased plasma levels of renin
    E) Decreased formation of angiotensin II

33. A 25-year-old man enters the hospital emergency department after severing a major artery during a farm accident. It is estimated that the patient has lost approximately 800 milliliters of blood. His mean blood pressure is 65 mm Hg, and his heart rate is elevated as a result of activation of the chemoreceptor reflex. Which set of changes in plasma concentration would be expected to cause the greatest activation of the chemoreceptor reflex?

	Oxygen	Carbon Dioxide	Hydrogen
A)	↑	↑	↑
B)	↑	↓	↑
C)	↑	↓	↓
D)	↑	↑	↓
E)	↓	↓	↓
F)	↓	↑	↓
G)	↓	↑	↑
H)	↓	↓	↑

34. Under normal physiological conditions, blood flow to the skeletal muscles is determined mainly by which of the following?

    A) Sympathetic nerves
    B) Angiotensin II
    C) Vasopressin
    D) Metabolic needs
    E) Capillary osmotic pressure

35. A healthy 22-year-old female medical student has an exercise stress test at a local health club. An increase in which of the following is most likely to occur in this woman's skeletal muscles during exercise?

    A) Vascular conductance
    B) Blood flow
    C) Carbon dioxide concentration
    D) Arteriolar diameter
    E) All the above

36. Which of the following segments of the circulatory system has the highest velocity of blood flow?

    A) Aorta
    B) Arteries
    C) Capillaries
    D) Venules
    E) Veins

37. Listed below are the hydrostatic and oncotic pressures within a microcirculatory bed.

    Plasma colloid osmotic pressure = 25 mm Hg
    Capillary hydrostatic pressure = 25 mm Hg
    Venous hydrostatic pressure = 5 mm Hg
    Arterial pressure = 80 mm Hg
    Interstitial hydrostatic pressure = –5 mm Hg
    Interstitial colloid osmotic pressure = 5 mm Hg
    Filtration coefficient = 15 ml/min/mm Hg

What is the filtration rate (ml/min) of the capillary wall?

    A) 100   ιs(
    B) 150
    C) 200
    D) 250
    E) 300

38. Which blood vessel has the highest vascular resistance?

	Blood Flow (ml/min)	Pressure Gradient (mm Hg)
A)	1000	100
B)	1200	60
C)	1400	20
D)	1600	80
E)	1800	40

39. A twofold increase in which of the following would result in the greatest increase in the transport of oxygen across the capillary wall?

    A) Capillary hydrostatic pressure
    B) Intercellular clefts in the capillary wall
    C) Oxygen concentration gradient
    D) Plasma colloid osmotic pressure
    E) Capillary wall hydraulic permeability

40. A balloon catheter is advanced from the superior vena cava into the heart and inflated to increase atrial pressure by 5 mm Hg. An increase in which of the following would be expected to occur in response to the elevated atrial pressure?

    A) Atrial natriuretic peptide
    B) Angiotensin II
    C) Aldosterone
    D) Renal sympathetic nerve activity

41. Which of the following vessels has the greatest total cross-sectional area in the circulatory system?

    A) Aorta
    B) Small arteries
    C) Capillaries
    D) Venules
    E) Vena cava

42. An increase in atrial pressure results in which of the following?

    A) Decrease in plasma atrial natriuretic peptide
    B) Increase in plasma angiotensin II concentration
    C) Increase in plasma aldosterone concentration
    D) Increase in sodium excretion

43. Autoregulation of tissue blood flow in response to an increase in arterial pressure occurs as a result of which of the following?

    A) Decrease in vascular resistance
    B) Initial decrease in vascular wall tension
    C) Excess delivery of nutrients such as oxygen to the tissues
    D) Decrease in tissue metabolism

44. Which component of the circulatory system contains the largest percentage of the total blood volume?

    A) Arteries
    B) Capillaries
    C) Veins
    D) Pulmonary circulation
    E) Heart

45. Which set of changes would be expected to occur 2 weeks after a 50% reduction in renal artery pressure?

	Plasma Renin	Plasma Aldosterone Concentration	Glomerular Filtration Rate
A)	↑	↑	↑
B)	↑	↑	↓
C)	↑	↓	↓
D)	↑	↓	↑
E)	↓	↓	↓
F)	↓	↓	↑
G)	↓	↑	↑
H)	↓	↑	↓

46. An increase in which of the following tends to decrease capillary filtration rate?

    A) Capillary hydrostatic pressure
    B) Plasma colloid osmotic pressure
    C) Interstitial colloid osmotic pressure
    D) Venous hydrostatic pressure
    E) Arteriolar diameter

47. An increase in which of the following would be expected to occur in a person 2 weeks after an increase in sodium intake?

    A) Angiotensin II
    B) Aldosterone
    C) Potassium excretion
    D) Atrial natriuretic peptide

48. A decrease in which of the following tends to increase lymph flow?

    A) Capillary hydrostatic pressure
    B) Interstitial hydrostatic pressure
    C) Plasma colloid osmotic pressure
    D) Lymphatic pump activity
    E) Arteriolar diameter

49. A decrease in the production of which of the following would most likely result in chronic hypertension?

    A) Aldosterone
    B) Thromboxane
    C) Angiotensin II
    D) Nitric oxide

50. Which of the following capillaries has the lowest capillary permeability to plasma molecules?

    A) Glomerular
    B) Liver
    C) Muscle
    D) Intestinal
    E) Brain

51. Which of the following would be expected to occur during a Cushing reaction caused by brain ischemia?

    A) Increase in parasympathetic activity
    B) Decrease in arterial pressure
    C) Decrease in heart rate
    D) Increase in sympathetic activity

52. Which of the following tends to increase the net movement of glucose across a capillary wall?

    A) Increase in plasma sodium concentration
    B) Increase in the concentration difference of glucose across the wall
    C) Decrease in wall permeability to glucose
    D) Decrease in wall surface area without an increase in the number of pores
    E) Decrease in plasma potassium concentration

53. A 65-year-old man has congestive heart failure. He has a cardiac output of 4 L/min, arterial pressure of 115/85 mm Hg, and a heart rate of 90 beats/min. Further tests by a cardiologist reveal that the patient has a right atrial pressure of 10 mm Hg. An increase in which of the following would be expected in this patient?

    A) Plasma colloid osmotic pressure
    B) Interstitial colloid osmotic pressure
    C) Arterial pressure
    D) Cardiac output
    E) Vena cava hydrostatic pressure

54. Which set of changes would be expected to occur in response to a direct increase in renal arterial pressure in kidneys without an intact tubuloglomerular feedback system?

	Glomerular Filtration	Sodium Excretion	Water Excretion Rate
A)	↑	↑	↑
B)	↑	↑	↓
C)	↑	↓	↓
D)	↑	↓	↑
E)	↓	↓	↓
F)	↓	↓	↑
G)	↓	↑	↑
H)	↓	↑	↓

55. Which part of the circulation has the highest compliance?

    A) Capillaries
    B) Large arteries
    C) Veins
    D) Aorta
    E) Small arteries

56. A decrease in which of the following tends to increase pulse pressure?

    A) Systolic pressure
    B) Stroke volume
    C) Arterial compliance
    D) Venous return
    E) Plasma volume

57. Using the following data, calculate the filtration coefficient for the capillary bed.

    Plasma colloid osmotic pressure = 30 mm Hg
    Capillary hydrostatic pressure = 40 mm Hg
    Interstitial hydrostatic pressure = 5 mm Hg
    Interstitial colloid osmotic pressure = 5 mm Hg
    Filtration rate = 150 ml/min
    Venous hydrostatic pressure = 10 mm Hg

    A) 10 ml/min/mm Hg
    B) 15 ml/min/mm Hg
    C) 20 ml/min/mm Hg
    D) 25 ml/min/mm Hg
    E) 30 ml/min/mm Hg

58. Which set of physiological changes would be expected to occur in a person who stands up from a supine position?

	Venous Hydrostatic Pressure in Legs	Heart Rate	Renal Blood Flow
A)	↑	↑	↑
B)	↑	↑	↓
C)	↑	↓	↓
D)	↓	↓	↓
E)	↓	↓	↑
F)	↓	↑	↑

59. Blood flow to a tissue remains relatively constant despite a reduction in arterial pressure (autoregulation). Which of the following would be expected to occur in response to the reduction in arterial pressure?

A) Decreased conductance
B) Decreased tissue carbon dioxide concentration
C) Increased tissue oxygen concentration
D) Decreased vascular resistance
E) Decreased arteriolar diameter

60. Which of the following would have the slowest rate of net movement across the capillary wall?

A) Sodium
B) Albumin
C) Glucose
D) Oxygen

61. An increase in which of the following tends to increase capillary filtration rate?

A) Capillary wall hydraulic conductivity
B) Arteriolar resistance
C) Plasma colloid osmotic pressure
D) Interstitial hydrostatic pressure
E) Plasma sodium concentration

62. The tendency for turbulent flow is greatest in which of the following?

A) Arterioles
B) Capillaries
C) Small arterioles
D) Aorta

63. A 60-year-old man has a mean arterial blood pressure of 130 mm Hg, a heart rate of 78 beats/min, a right atrial pressure of 0 mm Hg, and a cardiac output of 3.5 L/min. He also has a pulse pressure of 35 mm Hg and a hematocrit of 40. What is the approximate total peripheral vascular resistance in this man?

A) 17 mm Hg/L/min
B) 1.3 mm Hg/L/min
C) 13 mm Hg/L/min
D) 27 mm Hg/L/min
E) 37 mm Hg/L/min

64. Which pressure is normally negative in a muscle capillary bed in the lower extremities?

A) Plasma colloid osmotic pressure
B) Capillary hydrostatic pressure
C) Interstitial hydrostatic pressure
D) Interstitial colloid osmotic pressure
E) Venous hydrostatic pressure

65. What would tend to increase a person's pulse pressure?

A) Decreased stroke volume
B) Increased arterial compliance
C) Hemorrhage
D) Patent ductus
E) Decreased venous return

66. Movement of solutes such as Na⁺ across the capillary walls occurs primarily by which process?

A) Filtration
B) Active transport
C) Vesicular transport
D) Diffusion

67. What would decrease venous hydrostatic pressure in the legs?

A) Increase in right atrial pressure
B) Pregnancy
C) Movement of leg muscles
D) Presence of ascitic fluid in the abdomen

68. A nitric oxide donor is infused into the brachial artery of a 22-year-old man. Which set of microcirculatory changes would be expected in the infused arm?

	Capillary Hydrostatic Pressure	Interstitial Hydrostatic Pressure	Lymph Flow
A)	↑	↑	↑
B)	↑	↑	↓
C)	↑	↓	↓
D)	↑	↓	↑
E)	↓	↓	↓
F)	↓	↓	↑
G)	↓	↑	↑
H)	↓	↑	↓

69. What often occurs in decompensated heart failure?

A) Increased renal loss of sodium and water
B) Decreased mean systemic filling pressure
C) Increased norepinephrine in cardiac sympathetic nerves
D) Orthopnea
E) Weight loss

70. Which condition often occurs in progressive hemorrhagic shock?

A) Vasomotor center failure
B) Increased urine output
C) Tissue alkalosis
D) Decreased capillary permeability
E) Increased mean systemic filling pressure

71. A 50-year-old woman received an overdose of furosemide, and her arterial pressure decreased to 70/40. Her heart rate is 120, and her respiratory rate is 30/min. What therapy would you recommend?

    A) Whole blood infusion
    B) Plasma infusion
    C) Infusion of a balanced electrolyte solution
    D) Infusion of a sympathomimetic drug
    E) Administration of a glucocorticoid

72. A 30-year-old woman comes to a local emergency department with severe vomiting. She has pale skin, tachycardia, an arterial pressure of 70/45, and trouble walking. What therapy do you recommend to prevent shock?

    A) Infusion of packed red blood cells
    B) Administration of an antihistamine
    C) Infusion of a balanced electrolyte solution
    D) Infusion of a sympathomimetic drug
    E) Administration of a glucocorticoid

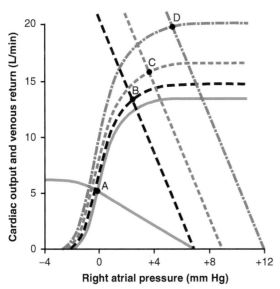

Modified from Guyton AC, Jones CE, Coleman TB: Circulatory Physiology: Cardiac Output and Its Regulation, 2nd ed. Philadelphia: WB Saunders, 1973.

73. In the above figure, for the cardiac output and venous return curves defined by the solid red lines (with the equilibrium at A), which of the following options is true?

    A) Mean systemic filling pressure is 12 mm Hg
    B) Right atrial pressure is 2 mm Hg
    C) Resistance to venous return is 1.4 mm Hg/L/min
    D) Pulmonary arterial flow is approximately 7 L/min
    E) Resistance to venous return is 0.71 mm Hg/L/min

74. A 30-year-old man is resting, and his sympathetic output increases to maximal values. Which set of changes would be expected in response to this increased sympathetic output?

	Resistance to Venous Return	Mean Systemic Filling Pressure	Venous Return
A)	↑	↑	↑
B)	↑	↓	↑
C)	↑	↓	↓
D)	↑	↑	↓
E)	↓	↓	↓
F)	↓	↑	↓
G)	↓	↑	↑
H)	↓	↓	↑

75. If a patient has an oxygen consumption of 240 ml/min, a pulmonary vein oxygen concentration of 180 ml/L of blood, and a pulmonary artery oxygen concentration of 160 ml/L of blood units, what is the cardiac output in L/min?

    A) 8
    B) 10
    C) 12
    D) 16
    E) 20

76. What normally causes the cardiac output curve to shift to the right along the right atrial pressure axis?

    A) Changing intrapleural pressure to –1 mm Hg
    B) Increasing mean systemic filling pressure
    C) Taking a patient off a mechanical ventilator and allowing normal respiration
    D) Decreasing intrapleural pressure to –7 mm Hg
    E) Breathing against a negative pressure

77. What normally causes the cardiac output curve to shift to the left along the right atrial pressure axis?

    A) Surgically opening the chest
    B) Severe cardiac tamponade
    C) Breathing against a negative pressure
    D) Playing a trumpet
    E) Positive pressure breathing

78. What will elevate the plateau of the cardiac output curve?

    A) Surgically opening the thoracic cage
    B) Connecting a patient to a mechanical ventilator
    C) Cardiac tamponade
    D) Increasing parasympathetic stimulation of the heart
    E) Increasing sympathetic stimulation of the heart

79. What is normally associated with an increased cardiac output?

    A) Increased parasympathetic stimulation
    B) Atrioventricular (A-V) fistula
    C) Decreased blood volume
    D) Polycythemia
    E) Severe aortic regurgitation

80. Which condition would be expected to decrease mean systemic filling pressure?

    A) Norepinephrine administration
    B) Increased blood volume
    C) Increased sympathetic stimulation
    D) Increased venous compliance
    E) Skeletal muscle contraction

81. Which statement about resistance to venous return (RVR) is true?

    A) An increase in venous resistance causes an increase in RVR
    B) Increased parasympathetic stimulation causes an increase in RVR
    C) An increase in RVR causes an increase in venous return
    D) Sympathetic inhibition causes an increase in RVR
    E) Changes in arterial resistance have a greater effect on RVR than do equal changes in venous resistance

82. In which condition would you expect a decreased resistance to venous return?

    A) Anemia
    B) Increased venous resistance
    C) Increased arteriolar resistance
    D) Increased sympathetic output
    E) Obstruction of veins

83. What is normally associated with an increased cardiac output?

    A) Increased venous compliance
    B) Cardiac tamponade
    C) Surgically opening the chest
    D) Moderate anemia
    E) Severe aortic stenosis

84. In which condition would you normally expect to find a decreased cardiac output?

    A) Hyperthyroidism
    B) Beriberi
    C) A-V fistula
    D) Anemia
    E) Acute myocardial infarction

85. At the onset of exercise, what normally occurs?

    A) Decreased cerebral blood flow
    B) Increased venous constriction
    C) Decreased coronary blood flow
    D) Decreased mean systemic filling pressure
    E) Increased parasympathetic impulses to the heart

86. What will usually increase the plateau level of the cardiac output curve?

    A) Myocarditis
    B) Severe cardiac tamponade
    C) Decreased parasympathetic stimulation of the heart

D) Myocardial infarction
E) Mitral stenosis

87. If a person has been exercising for 1 hour, which organ will have the smallest decrease in blood flow?

    A) Brain
    B) Intestines
    C) Kidneys
    D) Nonexercising skeletal muscle
    E) Pancreas

88. What increases the risk of adverse cardiac events?

    A) Decreased blood levels of low-density lipoprotein (LDL)
    B) Decreased blood levels of high-density lipoprotein (HDL)
    C) Female gender
    D) Moderate hypotension
    E) Decreased blood triglycerides

89. Which vasoactive agent is usually the most important controller of coronary blood flow?

    A) Adenosine
    B) Bradykinin
    C) Prostaglandins
    D) Carbon dioxide
    E) Potassium ions

90. What will elevate the plateau of the cardiac output curve?

    A) Surgically opening the thoracic cage
    B) Connecting a patient to a mechanical ventilator
    C) Cardiac tamponade
    D) Increasing parasympathetic stimulation of the heart
    E) Increasing sympathetic stimulation of the heart

91. Which statement about coronary blood flow is most accurate?

    A) Normal resting coronary blood flow is 500 ml/min
    B) The majority of flow occurs during systole
    C) During systole, the percentage decrease in sub-endocardial flow is greater than the percentage decrease in epicardial flow
    D) Adenosine release will normally decrease coronary flow

92. Which condition normally causes arteriolar vasodilation during exercise?

    A) Decreased plasma potassium ion concentration
    B) Increased histamine release
    C) Decreased plasma nitric oxide concentration
    D) Increased plasma adenosine concentration
    E) Decreased plasma osmolality

93. At the onset of exercise, the mass sympathetic nervous system strongly discharges. What would you expect to occur?

    A) Increased sympathetic impulses to the heart
    B) Decreased coronary blood flow
    C) Decreased cerebral blood flow
    D) Reverse stress relaxation
    E) Venous dilation

94. Which of the following blood vessels is responsible for transporting the majority of venous blood flow that leaves the ventricular heart muscle?

    A) Anterior cardiac veins
    B) Coronary sinus
    C) Bronchial veins
    D) Azygos vein
    E) Thebesian veins

95. A 70-year-old man with a weight of 100 kilograms (220 pounds) and a blood pressure of 160/90 has been told by his doctor that he has angina caused by myocardial ischemia. Which treatment would be beneficial to this man?

    A) Increased dietary calcium
    B) Isometric exercise
    C) A beta-1 receptor stimulator
    D) Angiotensin II infusion
    E) Nitroglycerin

96. Which event normally occurs during exercise?

    A) Arteriolar dilation in non-exercising muscle
    B) Decreased sympathetic output
    C) Venoconstriction
    D) Decreased release of epinephrine by the adrenals
    E) Decreased release of norepinephrine by the adrenals

97. What is the most frequent cause of decreased coronary blood flow in patients with ischemic heart disease?

    A) Increased adenosine release
    B) Atherosclerosis
    C) Coronary artery spasm
    D) Increased sympathetic tone of the coronary arteries
    E) Occlusion of the coronary sinus

98. A 60-year-old man sustained an ischemia-induced myocardial infarction and died from ventricular fibrillation. In this patient, what factor was most likely to increase the tendency of the heart to fibrillate after the infarction?

    A) Low potassium concentration in the heart extracellular fluid
    B) A decrease in ventricular diameter
    C) Increased sympathetic stimulation of the heart
    D) Low adenosine concentration
    E) Decreased parasympathetic stimulation of the heart

99. A 60-year-old man has been told by his doctor that he has angina caused by myocardial ischemia. Which treatment would be beneficial to this man?

    A) Angiotensin-converting enzyme inhibition
    B) Isometric exercise
    C) Chelation therapy such as ethylenediamine tetraacetic acid (EDTA)
    D) Beta receptor stimulation
    E) Increased dietary calcium

100. What is one of the major causes of death after myocardial infarction?

    A) Increased cardiac output
    B) A decrease in pulmonary interstitial volume
    C) Fibrillation of the heart
    D) Increased cardiac contractility

101. Which statement about the results of sympathetic stimulation is most accurate?

    A) Epicardial flow increases
    B) Venous resistance decreases
    C) Arteriolar resistance decreases
    D) Heart rate decreases
    E) Venous reservoirs constrict

102. What is normally associated with the chronic stages of compensated heart failure? Assume the patient is resting.

    A) Dyspnea
    B) Decreased right atrial pressure
    C) Decreased heart rate
    D) Sweating
    E) Increased mean systemic filling pressure

103. What normally occurs in a person with unilateral left heart failure?

    A) Decreased pulmonary artery pressure
    B) Decreased left atrial pressure
    C) Decreased right atrial pressure
    D) Edema of feet
    E) Increased mean pulmonary filling pressure

104. What normally causes renal sodium retention during compensated heart failure?

    A) Increased formation of angiotensin II
    B) Increased release of atrial natriuretic factor
    C) Sympathetic vasodilation of the afferent arterioles
    D) Increased glomerular filtration rate
    E) Increased formation of antidiuretic hormone (ADH)

105. Which intervention would normally be beneficial to a patient with acute pulmonary edema?

    A) Infuse a vasoconstrictor drug
    B) Infuse a balanced electrolyte solution
    C) Administer furosemide
    D) Administer a bronchoconstrictor
    E) Infuse whole blood

106. A 60-year-old man had a heart attack 2 days ago, and his blood pressure has continued to decrease. He is now in cardiogenic shock. Which therapy would be most beneficial?

A) Placing tourniquets on all four limbs
B) Administering a sympathetic inhibitor
C) Administering furosemide
D) Administering a blood volume expander
E) Increasing dietary sodium intake

107. If a 21-year-old male patient has a cardiac reserve of 300% and a maximum cardiac output of 16 L/min, what is his resting cardiac output?

A) 3 L/min
B) 4 L/min
C) 5.33 L/min
D) 6 L/min
E) 8 L/min

108. Which of the following occurs during heart failure and causes an increase in renal sodium excretion?

A) Increased aldosterone release
B) Increased atrial natriuretic factor release
C) Decreased glomerular filtration rate
D) Increased angiotensin II release
E) Decreased mean arterial pressure

109. Which intervention would be appropriate therapy for a patient in cardiogenic shock?

A) Placing tourniquets on the four limbs
B) Withdrawing a moderate amount of blood from the patient
C) Administering furosemide
D) Infusing a vasoconstrictor drug

110. Which condition normally accompanies acute unilateral right heart failure?

A) Increased right atrial pressure
B) Increased left atrial pressure
C) Increased urinary output
D) Increased cardiac output
E) Increased arterial pressure

111. What is normally associated with the chronic stages of compensated heart failure? Assume the patient is resting.

A) Decreased mean systemic filling pressure
B) Increased right atrial pressure
C) Increased heart rate
D) Sweating
E) Dyspnea

112. Patients with pulmonary edema often have dyspnea because of accumulation of fluid in the lungs. Which of the following would normally be the most beneficial for a patient with acute pulmonary edema?

A) Infusing furosemide
B) Infusing dobutamine

C) Infusing saline solution
D) Infusing norepinephrine
E) Infusing whole blood

113. Which of the following is associated with compensated heart failure?

A) Increased cardiac output
B) Increased blood volume
C) Decreased mean systemic filling pressure
D) Normal right atrial pressure

114. Which condition is normally associated with an increase in mean systemic filling pressure?

A) Decreased blood volume
B) Congestive heart failure
C) Sympathetic inhibition
D) Venous dilation

115. Which condition normally occurs during the early stages of compensated heart failure?

A) Increased right atrial pressure
B) Normal heart rate
C) Decreased angiotensin II release
D) Decreased aldosterone release
E) Increased urinary output of sodium and water

116. What often occurs during decompensated heart failure?

A) Hypertension
B) Increased mean pulmonary filling pressure
C) Decreased pulmonary capillary pressure
D) Increased cardiac output
E) Increased norepinephrine in the endings of the cardiac sympathetic nerves

117. Which of the following often occurs in decompensated heart failure?

A) Increased renal loss of sodium and water
B) Decreased mean systemic filling pressure
C) Increased norepinephrine in cardiac sympathetic receptors
D) Orthopnea
E) Weight loss

118. An 80-year-old male patient at a local hospital was diagnosed with a heart murmur. A chest radiograph showed an enlarged heart but no edema fluid in the lungs. The mean QRS axis of his ECG was 170 degrees. His pulmonary wedge pressure was normal. What is the diagnosis?

A) Mitral stenosis
B) Aortic stenosis
C) Pulmonary valve stenosis
D) Tricuspid stenosis
E) Mitral regurgitation

119. The fourth heart sound is associated with which mechanism?
    A) In-rushing of blood into the ventricles from atrial contraction
    B) Closing of the A-V valves
    C) Closing of the pulmonary valve
    D) Opening of the A-V valves
    E) In-rushing of blood into the ventricles in the early to middle part of diastole

120. A 40-year-old woman has been diagnosed with a heart murmur. A "blowing" murmur of relatively high pitch is heard maximally over the left ventricle. The chest radiograph shows an enlarged heart. Arterial pressure in the aorta is 140/40 mm Hg. What is the diagnosis?
    A) Aortic valve stenosis
    B) Aortic valve regurgitation
    C) Pulmonary valve stenosis
    D) Mitral valve stenosis
    E) Tricuspid valve regurgitation

121. In which disorder will left ventricular hypertrophy normally occur?
    A) Pulmonary valve regurgitation
    B) Tricuspid regurgitation
    C) Mitral stenosis
    D) Tricuspid stenosis
    E) Aortic stenosis

122. Which heart murmur is heard during systole?
    A) Aortic valve regurgitation
    B) Pulmonary valve regurgitation
    C) Tricuspid valve stenosis
    D) Mitral valve stenosis
    E) Patent ductus arteriosus

123. An increase in left atrial pressure is most likely to occur in which heart murmur?
    A) Tricuspid stenosis
    B) Pulmonary valve regurgitation
    C) Aortic stenosis
    D) Tricuspid regurgitation
    E) Pulmonary valve stenosis

124. A 50-year-old female patient at a local hospital has been diagnosed with a heart murmur. A murmur of relatively low pitch is heard maximally over the second intercostal space to the right of the sternum. The chest radiograph shows an enlarged heart. The mean QRS axis of the ECG is –45 degrees. What is the diagnosis?
    A) Mitral valve stenosis
    B) Aortic valve stenosis
    C) Pulmonary valve stenosis
    D) Tricuspid valve stenosis
    E) Tricuspid valve regurgitation

125. A 40-year-old female patient has been diagnosed with a heart murmur of relatively high pitch heard maximally in the second intercostal space to the left of the sternum. The mean QRS axis of his ECG is 150 degrees. The arterial blood oxygen content is normal. What is the likely diagnosis?
    A) Aortic stenosis
    B) Aortic regurgitation
    C) Pulmonary valve regurgitation
    D) Mitral stenosis
    E) Tricuspid stenosis

126. In which condition will right ventricular hypertrophy normally occur?
    A) Tetralogy of Fallot
    B) Mild aortic stenosis
    C) Mild aortic insufficiency
    D) Mitral stenosis
    E) Tricuspid stenosis

127. Which heart murmur is only heard during diastole?
    A) Patent ductus arteriosus
    B) Aortic stenosis
    C) Tricuspid valve regurgitation
    D) Interventricular septal defect
    E) Mitral stenosis

128. A person with which condition is most likely to have low arterial oxygen content?
    A) Tetralogy of Fallot
    B) Pulmonary artery stenosis
    C) Tricuspid insufficiency
    D) Patent ductus arteriosus
    E) Tricuspid stenosis

129. Which of the following is associated with the first heart sound?
    A) Inrushing of blood into the ventricles as a result of atrial contraction
    B) Closing of the A-V valves
    C) Closing of the pulmonary valve
    D) Opening of the A-V valves
    E) Inrushing of blood into the ventricles in the early to middle part of diastole

130. A 50-year-old woman had an echocardiogram. The results indicated a thickened right ventricle. Other data indicated that the patient had severely decreased arterial oxygen content and equal systolic pressures in both cardiac ventricles. What condition is present?
    A) Interventricular septal defect
    B) Tetralogy of Fallot
    C) Pulmonary valve stenosis
    D) Pulmonary valve regurgitation
    E) Patent ductus arteriosus

131. Which heart murmur is only heard during diastole?

    A) Patent ductus arteriosus
    B) Mitral regurgitation
    C) Tricuspid valve stenosis
    D) Interventricular septal defect
    E) Aortic stenosis

132. Which mechanism is associated with the third heart sound?

    A) Inrushing of blood into the ventricles as a result of atrial contraction
    B) Closing of the A-V valves
    C) Closing of the pulmonary valve
    D) Opening of the A-V valves
    E) Inrushing of blood into the ventricles in the early to middle part of diastole

133. Which condition often occurs in a person with progressive hemorrhagic shock?

    A) Increased capillary permeability
    B) Stress relaxation of veins
    C) Tissue alkalosis
    D) Increased urine output
    E) Increased mean systemic filling pressure

134. In which condition will administration of a sympathomimetic drug be the therapy of choice to prevent shock?

    A) Spinal cord injury
    B) Shock due to excessive vomiting
    C) Hemorrhagic shock
    D) Shock caused by excess diuretics

135. The blood pressure of a 60-year-old man decreased to 55/35 mm Hg during induction of anesthesia. His ECG still shows a normal sinus rhythm. What initial therapy do you recommend?

    A) Infusion of packed red blood cells
    B) Infusion of plasma
    C) Infusion of a balanced electrolyte solution
    D) Infusion of a sympathomimetic drug
    E) Administration of a glucocorticoid

136. A 65-year-old man enters a local emergency department a few minutes after receiving an influenza inoculation. He has pallor, tachycardia, arterial pressure of 80/50, and trouble walking. What therapy do you recommend to prevent shock?

    A) Infusion of blood
    B) Administration of an antihistamine
    C) Infusion of a balanced electrolyte solution such as saline
    D) Infusion of a sympathomimetic drug
    E) Administration of tissue plasminogen activator

137. Which condition often occurs in compensated hemorrhagic shock? Assume systolic pressure is 48 mm Hg.

    A) Decreased heart rate
    B) Stress relaxation of veins
    C) Decreased ADH release
    D) Decreased absorption of interstitial fluid through the capillaries
    E) Central nervous system (CNS) ischemic response

138. If a patient undergoing spinal anesthesia experiences a large decrease in arterial pressure and goes into shock, what would be the therapy of choice?

    A) Plasma infusion
    B) Blood infusion
    C) Saline solution infusion
    D) Glucocorticoid infusion
    E) Infusion of a sympathomimetic drug

139. A 25-year-old man who has been in a motorcycle wreck enters the emergency department. His clothes are very bloody, and his arterial pressure is decreased to 70/40. His heart rate is 120, and his respiratory rate is 30/min. Which therapy would the physician recommend?

    A) Infusion of blood
    B) Infusion of plasma
    C) Infusion of a balanced electrolyte solution
    D) Infusion of a sympathomimetic drug
    E) Administration of a glucocorticoid

140. In which type of shock does cardiac output often increase?

    A) Hemorrhagic shock
    B) Anaphylactic shock
    C) Septic shock   _ ↑ metabolic rate.
    D) Neurogenic shock

141. A 20-year-old man who has been hemorrhaging as a result of a gunshot wound enters a local emergency department. He has pale skin, tachycardia, an arterial pressure of 60/40, and trouble walking. Unfortunately, the blood bank is out of whole blood. Which therapy would the physician recommend to prevent shock?

    A) Administration of a glucocorticoid
    B) Administration of an antihistamine
    C) Infusion of a balanced electrolyte solution
    D) Infusion of a sympathomimetic drug
    E) Infusion of plasma

142. A 10-year-old girl in the hospital had an intestinal obstruction, and her arterial pressure decreased to 70/40. Her heart rate is 120, and her respiratory rate is 30/min. Which therapy would the physician recommend?

    A) Infusion of blood
    B) Infusion of plasma
    C) Infusion of a balanced electrolyte solution
    D) Infusion of a sympathomimetic drug
    E) Administration of a glucocorticoid

143. What often occurs during progressive shock?

    A) Patchy areas of necrosis in the liver
    B) Decreased tendency for blood to clot
    C) Increased glucose metabolism
    D) Decreased release of hydrolases by lysosomes
    E) Decreased capillary permeability

144. Release of which substance causes vasodilation and increased capillary permeability during anaphylactic shock?

    A) Histamine
    B) Bradykinin
    C) Nitric oxide
    D) Atrial natriuretic factor
    E) Adenosine

1. **D)** The rate of net fluid movement across a capillary wall is calculated as capillary filtration coefficient × net filtration pressure. Net filtration pressure = capillary hydrostatic pressure − plasma colloid osmotic pressure + interstitial colloid osmotic pressure − interstitial hydrostatic pressure. Thus, the rate of net fluid movement across the capillary wall is 150 ml/min.

    Filtration rate = Capillary filtration coefficient (K_f)
                       × Net filtration pressure
    Filtration rate = K_f × [Pc − Πc + Πi − P_i]
    Filtration rate = 10 ml/min/mm Hg
                       × [25 − 25 + 10 − (−5)]
    Filtration rate = 10 × 15 = 150 ml/min

    TMP13 p. 194

2. **D)** Moving from a supine to a standing position causes an acute fall in arterial pressure that is sensed by arterial baroreceptors located in the carotid bifurcation and aortic arch. Activation of the arterial baroreceptors leads to an increase in sympathetic outflow to the heart and peripheral vasculature and a decrease in parasympathetic outflow to the heart. The increase in sympathetic activity to peripheral vessels results in an increase in total peripheral resistance. The increase in sympathetic activity and decrease in parasympathetic outflow to the heart result in an increase in heart rate.
    TMP13 pp. 220-221

3. **E)** Administration of a drug that decreases the diameter of arterioles in a muscle bed increases the vascular resistance. The increased vascular resistance decreases vascular conductance and blood flow. The reduction in arteriolar diameter also leads to a decrease in capillary hydrostatic pressure and capillary filtration rate.
    TMP13 pp. 175 and 194

4. **G)** Moving from a supine to a standing position causes an acute fall in arterial pressure that is sensed by arterial baroreceptors located in the carotid sinuses and aortic arch. Activation of the baroreceptors results in a decrease in parasympathetic activity (or vagal tone) and an increase in sympathetic activity, which leads to an increase in plasma renin activity (or renin release).
    TMP13 pp. 219-222

5. **A)** The difference between systolic pressure and diastolic pressure is the pulse pressure. The two major factors that affect pulse pressure are the stroke volume output of the heart and the compliance of the arterial tree. In patients with moderate aortic regurgitation (due to incomplete closure of aortic valve), the blood that is pumped into the aorta immediately flows back into the left ventricle. The backflow of blood into the left ventricle increases stroke volume and systolic pressure. The rapid backflow of blood also results in a decrease in diastolic pressure. Thus, patients with moderate aortic regurgitation have high systolic pressure, low diastolic pressure, and high pulse pressure.
    TMP13 pp. 180-181

6. **B)** The increase in local metabolism during exercise increases oxygen utilization and decreases tissue oxygen concentration. The decrease in tissue oxygen concentration increases arteriolar diameter and increases vascular conductance and blood flow to skeletal muscles.
    TMP13 pp. 204-206

7. **B)** Cognitive stimuli increase cerebral blood flow by decreasing cerebral vascular resistance. The diameter of cerebral vessels is decreased by various metabolic factors in response to cognitive stimuli. Metabolic factors that enhance cerebral blood flow include increases in carbon dioxide, hydrogen ion (decreased pH), and adenosine.
    TMP13 pp. 203-206

8. **A)** Histamine is a vasodilator that is typically released by mast cells and basophils. Infusion of histamine into a brachial artery would decrease arteriolar resistance and increase water permeability of the capillary wall. The decrease in arteriolar resistance would also increase capillary hydrostatic pressure. The increase in capillary hydrostatic pressure and water permeability leads to an increase in capillary filtration rate.
    TMP13 pp. 175 and 194

9. **C)** An increase in shear stress in blood vessels is one of the major stimuli for the release of nitric oxide by endothelial cells. Nitric oxide increases blood flow by increasing cyclic guanosine monophosphate.
    TMP13 p. 208

10. **D)** Angiotensin I is formed by an enzyme (renin) acting on a substrate called angiotensinogen. Angiotensin I is converted to angiotensin II by a converting enzyme. Angiotensin II also has a negative feedback effect on juxtaglomerular cells to inhibit renin secretion. Angiotensin II is a powerful vasoconstrictor and sodium-retaining hormone that increases arterial pressure. Administration of an ACE inhibitor would increase plasma renin concentration, decrease angiotensin II formation, enhance renal sodium excretory function, and decrease total peripheral resistance and arterial pressure.
    TMP13 pp. 234-235

    ↑renin, ↑Na+ excretion
    ↓TPR, ↓Arterial 61
                   Pressure

11. **E)** An increase in the diameter of a precapillary arteriole would decrease arteriolar resistance. The decrease in arteriolar resistance would lead to an increase in vascular conductance and capillary blood flow, hydrostatic pressure, and filtration rate.
TMP13 pp. 175 and 194

12. **A)** Stenosis of one kidney results in the release of renin and the formation of angiotensin II from the affected kidney. Angiotensin II stimulates aldosterone production and increases total peripheral resistance by constricting most of the blood vessels in the body.
TMP13 p. 236

13. **D)** Blood flow in a vessel is directly proportional to the fourth power of the vessel radius. Increasing vessel diameter by 50% (1.5 × control) would increase blood flow 1.5 to the fourth power × normal blood flow (100 ml/min). Thus, blood flow would increase to 100 ml/min × 5.06, or approximately 500 ml/min.
TMP13 p. 175

14. **A)** In patent ductus arteriosus, a large quantity of the blood pumped into the aorta by the left ventricle immediately flows backward into the pulmonary artery and then into the lung and left atrium. The shunting of blood from the aorta results in a low diastolic pressure, while the increased inflow of blood into the left atrium and ventricle increases stroke volume and systolic pressure. The combined increase in systolic pressure and decrease in diastolic pressure results in an increase in pulse pressure.
TMP13 p. 181

15. **D)** A decrease in tissue oxygen tension is thought to be an important stimulus for vascular endothelial growth factor and the growth of blood vessels in solid tumors.
TMP13 pp. 209-210

16. **A)** The net movement of sodium across a capillary wall is directly proportional to the wall permeability to sodium, wall surface area, and concentration gradient across the capillary wall. Thus, increases in permeability to sodium, surface area, and sodium concentration gradient wall would all increase the net movement of sodium across the capillary wall.
TMP13 pp. 190-192

17. **A)** Constriction of the carotid artery decreases blood pressure at the level of the carotid sinus. A decrease in carotid sinus pressure leads to a decrease in carotid sinus nerve impulses to the vasomotor center, which in turn leads to enhanced sympathetic nervous activity and decreased parasympathetic nerve activity. The increase in sympathetic nerve activity results in peripheral vasoconstriction and an increase in total peripheral resistance and heart rate.
TMP13 pp. 220-221

18. **E)** Pulse pressure is the difference between systolic pressure and diastolic pressure. The two major factors that affect pulse pressure are the stroke volume output of the heart and the compliance of the arterial tree. An increase in stroke volume increases systolic and pulse pressure, whereas an increase in compliance of the arterial tree decreases pulse pressure. Moderate aortic valve stenosis results in a decrease in stroke volume, which leads to a decrease in systolic pressure and pulse pressure.
TMP13 pp. 180-181

19. **B)** A person with atherosclerosis would be expected to have decreased arterial compliance. The decrease in arterial compliance would lead to an increase in systolic pressure and pulse pressure.
TMP13 pp. 180-181

20. **B)** Constriction of the carotid artery reduces blood pressure at the carotid bifurcation where the arterial baroreceptors are located. The decrease in arterial pressure activates baroreceptors, which in turn leads to an increase in sympathetic activity and a decrease in parasympathetic activity (or vagal tone). The enhanced sympathetic activity results in constriction of peripheral blood vessels, including the kidneys. The enhanced sympathetic activity leads to an increase in total peripheral resistance and a decrease in renal blood flow. The combination of enhanced sympathetic activity and decreased vagal tone also leads to an increase in heart rate.
TMP13 pp. 219-222

21. **D)** Filtration rate is the product of the filtration coefficient (K_f) and the net pressure across the capillary wall. The net pressure for fluid movement across a capillary wall is promoted by increases in capillary hydrostatic pressure and positive interstitial colloid osmotic pressure, whereas negative plasma colloid osmotic pressure and a positive interstitial hydrostatic pressure oppose filtration. Thus, increased capillary hydrostatic pressure, decreased plasma colloid osmotic pressure, and increased interstitial colloid osmotic pressure would all promote filtration. Decreased arteriolar resistance would also promote filtration by increasing capillary hydrostatic pressure. The filtration coefficient is the product of capillary surface area and the capillary water permeability. A decrease in capillary water permeability would decrease the filtration coefficient and reduce the filtration rate.
TMP13 pp. 193-194

22. **E)** Solid tumors are metabolically active tissues that need increased quantities of oxygen and other nutrients. When metabolism in a tissue is increased for a prolonged period, the vascularity of the tissue also increases. One of the important factors that increases growth of new blood vessels is VEGF. Presumably, a deficiency of tissue oxygen or other nutrients, or both, leads to the formation of VEGF.
TMP13 p. 210

23. **A)** A decrease in the diameter of a precapillary arteriole increases arteriolar resistance while decreasing vascular conductance and capillary blood flow, hydrostatic pressure, filtration rate, interstitial volume, and interstitial hydrostatic pressure.
TMP13 pp. 175 and 194

24. **C)** Excess secretion of aldosterone results in enhanced tubular reabsorption of sodium and secretion of potassium. The increased reabsorption of sodium and water leads to an increase in extracellular fluid volume, which in turn suppresses renin release by the kidney. The increase in potassium secretion leads to a decrease in plasma potassium concentration, or hypokalemia.
TMP13 pp. 235-236

25. **E)** The two main factors that increase lymph flow are an increase in capillary filtration rate and an increase in lymphatic pump activity. An increase in plasma colloid osmotic pressure decreases capillary filtration rate, interstitial volume and hydrostatic pressure, and lymph flow. In contrast, an increase in hydraulic conductivity of the capillary wall and capillary hydrostatic pressure increase capillary filtration rate, interstitial volume and pressure, and lymph flow. An increase in arteriole resistance would decrease capillary hydrostatic pressure, capillary filtration rate, interstitial volume and pressure, and lymph flow.
TMP13 pp. 193-198

26. **E)** According to Poiseuille's law, flow through a vessel increases in proportion to the fourth power of the radius. A fourfold increase in vessel diameter (or radius) would increase 4 to the fourth power, or 256 times normal. Thus, flow through the vessel after increasing the vessel 4 times normal would increase from 100 to 25,600 ml/min.
TMP13 pp. 175-176

27. **B)** Vascular resistance is equal to arterial pressure minus venous pressure divided by blood flow. In this example, arterial pressure is 125 mm Hg, venous pressure is 5 mm Hg, and blood flow is 1200 ml/min. Thus, vascular resistance is equal to 120/1200, or 0.10 mm Hg/ml/min.
TMP13 p. 172

28. **D)** The rate of blood flow is directly proportional to the fourth power of the vessel radius and to the pressure gradient across the vessel. In contrast, the rate of blood flow is inversely proportional to the viscosity of the blood. Thus, an increase in blood viscosity would decrease blood flow in a vessel.
TMP13 pp. 175-176

29. **D)** The flow in a vessel is directly proportional to the pressure gradient across the vessel and to the fourth power of the radius of the vessel. In contrast, blood flow is inversely proportional to the viscosity of the blood. Because blood flow is proportional to the

fourth power of the vessel radius, the vessel with the largest radius (vessel D) would have the greatest flow.
TMP13 p. 176

30. **A)** The arterial baroreceptors are activated in response to a fall in arterial pressure. During hemorrhage, the fall in arterial pressure at the level of the baroreceptors results in enhanced sympathetic outflow from the vasomotor center and a decrease in parasympathetic nerve activity. The increase in sympathetic nerve activity leads to constriction of peripheral blood vessels, increased total peripheral resistance, and a return of blood pressure toward normal. The decrease in parasympathetic nerve activity and sympathetic outflow would result in an increase in heart rate.
TMP13 pp. 219-222

31. **A)** Activation of the baroreceptors leads to an increase in sympathetic activity, which in turn increases heart rate, strength of cardiac contraction, and constriction of arterioles and veins. The increase in venous constriction results in an increase in mean circulatory filling pressure, venous return, and cardiac output.
TMP13 pp. 219-222

32. **E)** The conversion of angiotensin I to angiotensin II is catalyzed by a converting enzyme that is present in the endothelium of the lung vessels and in the kidneys. The converting enzyme also serves as a kininase that degrades bradykinin. Thus, a converting enzyme inhibitor not only decreases the formation of angiotensin II but also inhibits kininases and the breakdown of bradykinin. Angiotensin II is a vasoconstrictor and a powerful sodium-retaining hormone. The major cause for the decrease in arterial pressure in response to an ACE inhibitor is the decrease in formation of angiotensin II.
TMP13 pp. 234-235

33. **G)** When blood pressure falls below 80 mm Hg, carotid and aortic chemoreceptors are activated to elicit a neural reflex to minimize the fall in blood pressure. The chemoreceptors are chemosensitive cells that are sensitive to oxygen lack, carbon dioxide excess, or hydrogen ion excess (or fall in pH). The signals transmitted from the chemoreceptors into the vasomotor center excite the vasomotor center to increase arterial pressure.
TMP13 p. 222

34. **D)** Although sympathetic nerves, angiotensin II, and vasopressin are powerful vasoconstrictors, blood flow to skeletal muscles under normal physiological conditions is mainly determined by local metabolic needs.
TMP13 pp. 206-208

35. **E)** During exercise, tissue levels of carbon dioxide and lactic acid increase. These metabolites dilate blood vessels, decrease arteriolar resistance, and enhance vascular conductance and blood flow.
TMP13 pp. 206-207

36. A) The velocity of blood flow within each segment of the circulatory system is inversely proportional to the total cross-sectional area of the segment. Because the aorta has the smallest total cross-sectional area of all circulatory segments, it has the highest velocity of blood flow.
TMP13 pp. 173-174

37. B) Filtration rate is the product of the filtration coefficient (K_f) and the net pressure across the capillary wall. The net pressure for fluid movement across a capillary wall = capillary hydrostatic pressure – plasma colloid osmotic pressure – interstitial colloid osmotic pressure – interstitial hydrostatic pressure. The net pressure in this question calculates to be 10 mm Hg, and the K_f is 15. Thus, the filtration rate is 15 × 10, or 150 ml/min.
TMP13 pp. 193-194

38. A) Resistance of a vessel = pressure gradient ÷ blood flow of the vessel. In this example, vessel A has the highest vascular resistance (100 mm Hg/1000 ml/min, or 0.1 mm Hg/ml/min).
TMP13 p. 175

39. C) The transport of oxygen across a capillary wall is proportional to the capillary surface area, capillary wall permeability to oxygen, and oxygen gradient across the capillary wall. Thus, a twofold increase in the oxygen concentration gradient would result in the greatest increase in the transport of oxygen across the capillary wall. A twofold increase in intercellular clefts in the capillary wall would not have a significant impact on oxygen transport because oxygen can permeate the endothelial cell wall.
TMP13 pp. 191-192

40. A) Atrial natriuretic peptide is released from myocytes in the atria in response to increases in atrial pressure.
TMP13 p. 222

41. C) The capillaries have the largest total cross-sectional area of all vessels of the circulatory system. The venules also have a relatively large total cross-sectional area, but not as great as the capillaries, which explains the large storage of blood in the venous system compared with that in the arterial system.
TMP13 pp. 172-173

42. D) An increase in atrial pressure would also increase plasma levels of atrial natriuretic peptide, which in turn would decrease plasma levels of angiotensin II and aldosterone and increase sodium excretion.
TMP13 pp. 222-223

43. C) An increase in perfusion pressure to a tissue results in excessive delivery of nutrients such as oxygen to a tissue. The increase in tissue oxygen concentration constricts arterioles and returns blood flow and nutrient delivery toward normal levels.
TMP13 pp. 206-207

44. C) The percentage of total blood volume in the veins is approximately 64%.
TMP13 p. 169

45. B) Constriction of the renal artery increases release of renin, formation of angiotensin II and aldosterone, and arterial pressure. A 50% reduction in renal artery pressure would be below the range of renal autoregulation and would result in a decrease in the glomerular filtration rate.
TMP13 p. 238

46. B) An increase in plasma colloid osmotic pressure would reduce net filtration pressure and capillary filtration rate. Increases in capillary hydrostatic pressure and interstitial colloid osmotic pressure would also favor capillary filtration. An increase in venous hydrostatic pressure and arteriolar diameter would tend to increase capillary hydrostatic pressure and capillary filtration rate.
TMP13 pp. 193-197

47. D) An increase in sodium intake would result in an increase in sodium excretion to maintain sodium balance. Conversely, potassium excretion would only transiently increase after an increase in sodium intake. Angiotensin II and aldosterone would decrease in response to a chronic elevation in sodium intake, whereas plasma atrial natriuretic peptide levels would increase.
TMP13 pp. 236-237

48. C) The rate of lymph flow increases in proportion to the interstitial hydrostatic pressure and the lymphatic pump activity. A decrease in plasma colloid osmotic pressure would increase filtration rate, interstitial volume, interstitial hydrostatic pressure, and lymph flow. A decrease in arteriolar diameter would decrease capillary hydrostatic pressure, capillary filtration, and lymph flow.
TMP13 pp. 193-200

49. D) Nitric oxide is a potent vasodilator and natriuretic substance. Thus, a reduction in nitric oxide production would result in an increase in arterial pressure. In contrast, angiotensin II, thromboxane, and aldosterone are vasoconstrictor and/or antinatriuretic factors. A decrease in the production of these factors would tend to decrease arterial pressure.
TMP13 p. 239

50. E) The brain has tight junctions between capillary endothelial cells that allow only extremely small molecules such as water, oxygen, and carbon dioxide to pass in or out of the brain tissues.
TMP13 p. 190

51. D) The Cushing reaction is a special type of CNS ischemic response that results from increased pressure of the cerebrospinal fluid around the brain in the cranial vault. When the cerebrospinal fluid pressure

rises, it decreases the blood supply to the brain and elicits a CNS ischemic response. The CNS ischemic response includes enhanced sympathetic activity, decreased parasympathetic activity, and increased heart rate, arterial pressure, and total peripheral resistance.
TMP13 p. 223

52. **B)** The factors that determine the net movement of glucose across a capillary wall include the wall permeability to glucose, the glucose concentration gradient across the wall, and the capillary wall surface area. Thus, an increase in the concentration difference of glucose across the wall would enhance the net movement of glucose.
TMP13 pp. 191-192

53. **E)** An increase in atrial pressure of 10 mm Hg would tend to decrease venous return to the heart and increase vena cava hydrostatic pressure. Plasma colloid osmotic pressure, interstitial colloid osmotic pressure, arterial pressure, and cardiac output would generally be low to normal in this patient.
TMP13 pp. 184-185

54. **A)** An increase in renal arterial pressure results in increases in sodium and water excretion. Normally, glomerular filtration rate would be normal or slightly increased in response to an increase in renal artery pressure. However, in the absence of an intact tubuloglomerular feedback system, an important renal autoregulatory mechanism, an increase in renal artery pressure would result in significant increases in glomerular filtration rate.
TMP13 pp. 227-228

55. **C)** The vascular compliance is proportional to the vascular distensibility and the vascular volume of any given segment of the circulation. The compliance of a systemic vein is 24 times that of its corresponding artery because it is about 8 times as distensible and has a volume about 3 times as great.
TMP13 p. 179

56. **C)** The difference between systolic pressure and diastolic pressure is called the pulse pressure. The two main factors that affect pulse pressure are stroke volume and arterial compliance. Pulse pressure is directly proportional to the stroke volume and inversely proportional to the arterial compliance. Thus, a decrease in arterial compliance would tend to increase pulse pressure.
TMP13 pp. 180-181

57. **B)** Filtration coefficient (K_f) = filtration rate ÷ net filtration pressure. Net filtration pressure = capillary hydrostatic pressure – plasma colloid osmotic pressure + interstitial colloid osmotic pressure – interstitial hydrostatic pressure. The net filtration pressure in this example is 10 mm Hg. Thus, K_f = 150 ml/min ÷ 10 mm Hg, or 15 ml/min/mm Hg.
TMP13 pp. 193-198

58. **B)** Moving from a supine to a standing position results in pooling of blood in the lower extremities and a fall in blood pressure. The pooling of blood in the legs increases venous hydrostatic pressure. The fall in arterial pressure activates the arterial baroreceptors, which in turn increases sympathetic nerve activity and decreases parasympathetic nerve activity. The increase in sympathetic activity constricts renal vessels and reduces renal blood flow. The heart rate also increases.
TMP13 pp. 219-222

59. **D)** Reduction in perfusion pressure to a tissue leads to a decrease in tissue oxygen concentration and an increase in tissue carbon dioxide concentration. Both events lead to an increase in arteriolar diameter, decreased vascular resistance, and increased vascular conductance.
TMP13 pp. 206-207

60. **B)** Because oxygen is lipid soluble and can cross the capillary wall with ease, it has the fastest rate of movement across the capillary wall. The ability of lipid-insoluble substances such as sodium, albumin, and glucose to move across a capillary wall depends on the permeability of the capillary to lipid-insoluble substances. Because the capillary wall is relatively impermeable to albumin, it has the slowest rate of net movement across the capillary wall.
TMP13 pp. 191-192

61. **A)** An increase in capillary wall permeability to water would increase capillary filtration rate, whereas increases in arteriolar resistance, plasma colloid osmotic pressure, and interstitial hydrostatic pressure would all decrease filtration rate. Plasma sodium concentration would have no effect on filtration.
TMP13 pp. 193-198

62. **D)** The tendency for turbulent flow occurs at vascular sites where the velocity of blood flow is high. The aorta has the highest velocity of blood flow.
TMP13 pp. 175-176

63. **E)** Total peripheral vascular resistance = arterial pressure – right atrial pressure ÷ cardiac output. In this example, total peripheral vascular resistance = 130 mm Hg ÷ 3.5 L/min, or approximately 37 mm Hg/L/min.
TMP13 pp. 175-176

64. **C)** Interstitial hydrostatic pressure in a muscle capillary bed is normally negative (–3 mm Hg). Pumping by the lymphatic system is the basic cause of the negative pressure.
TMP13 p. 195   ↑SV = ↑PP

65. **A)** The two main factors that affect pulse pressure are stroke volume and arterial compliance. Increases in stroke volume increase pulse pressure, whereas an increase in arterial compliance decreases pulse pressure. Hemorrhage and decreased venous return would decrease stroke volume and pulse pressure. In

↑Compliance = ↓PP

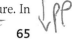

patients with patent ductus, stroke volume and pulse pressure are increased as a result of shunting of blood from the aorta to the pulmonary artery.
TMP13 pp. 180-181

66. **D)** The primary mechanism whereby solutes move across a capillary wall is simple diffusion.
TMP13 p. 191

67. **C)** Movement of the leg muscles causes blood to flow toward the vena cava, which reduces venous hydrostatic pressure. An increase in right atrial pressure would decrease venous return and increase venous hydrostatic pressure. Pregnancy and the presence of ascitic fluid in the abdomen would tend to compress the vena cava and increase venous hydrostatic pressure in the legs.
TMP13 pp. 184-185

68. **A)** Nitric oxide is a vasodilator that is believed to play a role in regulating blood flow. Infusion of a nitric oxide donor into the brachial artery would increase arteriolar diameter and decrease arteriolar resistance. The decrease in arteriolar resistance would also result in an increase in capillary hydrostatic pressure and filtration rate. The increase in filtration rate leads to an increase in interstitial hydrostatic pressure and lymph flow.
TMP13 pp. 170-171, 200-201

69. **D)** In persons with decompensated heart failure, the kidneys retain sodium and water, which causes a weight gain and an increase in blood volume. This effect increases the mean systemic filling pressure, which also stretches the heart. Therefore, a decreased mean systemic filling pressure does not occur in decompensated heart failure. The excess blood volume often will overstretch the sarcomeres of the heart, which will prevent them from achieving their maximal tension. An excess central fluid volume also results in orthopnea, which is the inability to breathe properly except in the upright position.
TMP13 pp. 273-275

70. **A)** During progressive hemorrhagic shock, the vasomotor center often fails, thus reducing sympathetic output. Decreases in arterial pressure will reduce urine output. Decreased blood flow throughout the body causes acidosis because of decreased removal of carbon dioxide. In progressive shock due to hemorrhage, capillary permeability increases and mean systemic filling pressure decreases.
TMP13 p. 296

71. **C)** With an overdose of furosemide there is a large loss of sodium and water from the body, resulting in dehydration and sometimes shock. The optimal therapy is to replenish the electrolytes that were lost as a result of the overdose of the furosemide. Therefore, infusion of a balanced electrolyte solution is the therapy of choice.
TMP13 pp. 301-302

72. **C)** Severe vomiting can lead to a large loss of sodium and water from the body, resulting in dehydration and sometimes shock. The best therapy is to replenish the depleted sodium and water lost by vomiting. Therefore, infusion of a balanced electrolyte solution is the therapy of choice.
TMP13 pp. 301-302

73. **C)** The formula for resistance to venous return is mean systemic filling pressure – right atrial pressure/cardiac output. In this example the mean systemic filling pressure is 7 mm Hg and the right atrial pressure is 0 mm Hg. The cardiac output is 5 L/min. Using these values in the previous formula indicates that the resistance to venous return is 1.4 mm Hg/L/min. Note that this formula only applies to the linear portion of the venous return curve.
TMP13 pp. 253-254

74. **A)** During increases in sympathetic output to maximal values, several changes occur. First, the mean systemic filling pressure increases markedly, but at the same time the resistance to venous return increases. Venous return is determined by the following formula: mean systemic filling pressure – right atrial pressure/resistance to venous return. During maximal sympathetic output, the increase in systemic filling pressure is greater than the increase in resistance to venous return. Therefore, in this formula the numerator has a much greater increase than the denominator, which results in an increase in the venous return.
TMP13 p. 255

75. **C)** This problem concerns the Fick principle for determining cardiac output. The formula for cardiac output is oxygen absorbed per minute by the lungs divided by the arterial-venous oxygen difference. In this problem, oxygen consumption of the body is 240 ml/min, and in a steady-state condition, this would exactly equal the oxygen absorbed by the lungs. Therefore, by inserting these values into the equation, we see that the cardiac output will equal 12 L/min.
TMP13 p. 257

76. **A)** A shift to the right in the cardiac output curve involves an increase in the normal intrapleural pressure of –4 mm Hg. Changing intrapleural pressure to –1 mm Hg will shift the curve to the right. Changing mean systemic filling pressure does not change the cardiac output curve. Taking a patient off of a ventilator, decreasing intrapleural pressure to –7 mm Hg, and breathing against a negative pressure will shift the cardiac output curve to the left.
TMP13 p. 250

77. **C)** Several factors can cause the cardiac output to shift to the right or to the left. Among those are surgically opening the chest, which makes the cardiac output curve shift 4 mm Hg to the right, and severe cardiac

tamponade, which increases the pressure inside the pericardium, thus tending to collapse the heart, particularly the atria. Playing a trumpet or positive pressure breathing tremendously increases the intrapleural pressure, thus collapsing the atria and shifting the cardiac output curve to the right. Breathing against a negative pressure will shift the cardiac output curve to the left.
TMP13 p. 250

78. **E)** The plateau level of the cardiac output curve, which is one measure of cardiac contractility, decreases in several circumstances. Some of these circumstances include severe cardiac tamponade, which increases the pressure in the pericardial space, and increasing parasympathetic stimulation of the heart. Increased sympathetic stimulation of the heart increases the level of the cardiac output curve by increasing heart rate and contractility.
TMP13 p. 247

79. **B)** Cardiac output increases in several conditions because of increased venous return. A-V fistulae also cause a decreased resistance to venous return, thus increasing cardiac output. Cardiac output decreases in patients with hypovolemia, severe aortic regurgitation, and polycythemia. The hematocrit level is high in polycythemia, which increases resistance to venous return.
TMP13 pp. 255-256

80. **D)** Mean systemic filling pressure is a measure of the tightness of fit of the blood in the circulation. Mean systemic filling pressure is increased by factors that increase blood volume and decrease the vascular compliance. Therefore, an decreased venous compliance, not an increased compliance, would cause an increase in mean systemic filling pressure. Norepinephrine administration and sympathetic stimulation cause arteriolar vasoconstriction and decreased vascular compliance, resulting in an increase in mean systemic filling pressure. Increased blood volume and skeletal muscle contraction, which cause a contraction of the vasculature, also increase this filling pressure.
TMP13 pp. 252-253

81. **A)** An increase in venous resistance will increase resistance to venous return to a greater degree than an increase in arterial resistance. Venous return of the heart is equal to the mean systemic filling pressure minus the right atrial pressure divided by the resistance to venous return. Parasympathetic stimulation does not affect resistance to venous return, and sympathetic inhibition will reduce resistance to venous return.
TMP13 pp. 253-254

82. **A)** Anemia will decrease resistance to venous return because of arteriolar dilation. The following mechanisms increase resistance to venous return: increased venous resistance, increased arteriolar resistance, increased sympathetic output, and obstruction of veins.
TMP13 pp. 253-254

83. **D)** Decreased cardiac output can result from a weakened heart or from a decrease in venous return. Increased venous compliance decreases the venous return of blood to the heart. Cardiac tamponade, surgically opening the chest, and severe aortic stenosis will effectively weaken the heart and thus decrease cardiac output. Moderate anemia will cause an arteriolar vasodilation, which increases venous return of blood back to the heart, thus increasing cardiac output.
TMP13 pp. 249, 255

84. **E)** Cardiac output increases in several conditions because of increased venous return. Cardiac output increases in hyperthyroidism because of the increased oxygen use by the peripheral tissues, resulting in arteriolar vasodilation and thus increased venous return. Beriberi causes increased cardiac output because a lack of the vitamin thiamine results in peripheral vasodilation. A-V fistulae also cause a decreased resistance to venous return, thus increasing cardiac output. Anemia, because of the decreased oxygen delivery to the tissues, causes an increase in venous return to the heart and thus an increase in cardiac output. Cardiac output decreases in patients with myocardial infarction.
TMP13 pp. 248-249

85. **B)** During exercise there is very little change in cerebral blood flow, and coronary blood flow increases. Because of the increased sympathetic output, mean systemic filling pressure increases and the veins constrict. During exercise there is also a decrease in parasympathetic impulses to the heart.
TMP13 pp. 255, 260

86. **C)** The plateau level of the cardiac output curve, which is one measure of cardiac contractility, decreases in several circumstances. Some of these include myocarditis, severe cardiac tamponade that increases the pressure in the pericardial space, myocardial infarction, and various valvular diseases such as mitral stenosis. Decreased parasympathetic stimulation of the heart actually moderately increases the level of the cardiac output curve by increasing the heart rate.
TMP13 p. 247

87. **A)** During increases in sympathetic output, the main two organs that maintain their blood flow are the brain and the heart. During exercise for 1 hour, the intestinal flow decreases significantly, as does the renal and pancreatic blood flows. The skeletal muscle blood flow to non-exercising muscles also decreases at this time. Therefore, the cerebral blood flow remains close to its control value.
TMP13 p. 260

88. **B)** Several factors decrease the risk of adverse cardiac events, including decreased levels of LDL, female gender, moderate hypotension, and decreased levels of triglycerides. Decreased levels of HDL will

increase cardiac risks because HDL is a protective cholesterol.
TMP13 pp. 264-265

89. A) Although bradykinin, prostaglandins, carbon dioxide, and potassium ions serve as vasodilators for the coronary artery system, the major controller of coronary blood flow is adenosine. Adenosine is formed as adenosine triphosphate degrades to adenosine monophosphate. Small portions of the adenosine monophosphate are then further degraded to release adenosine into the tissue fluids of the heart muscle, and this adenosine vasodilates the coronary arteries.
TMP13 p. 263

90. E) Sympathetic stimulation directly increases the strength of cardiac contraction and increases the heart rate. In this way the plateau of the Starling curve elevates. Surgically opening the chest and undergoing mechanical ventilation shifts the cardiac output curve to the right. Cardiac tamponade rotates the curve downward, and parasympathetic stimulation depresses the curve.
TMP13 p. 260

91. C) The normal resting coronary blood flow is approximately 225 ml/min. Infusion of adenosine or local release of adenosine normally increases the coronary blood flow. The contraction of the cardiac muscle around the vasculature, particularly in the subendocardial vessels, causes a decrease in blood flow. Therefore, during the systolic phase of the cardiac cycle, the subendocardial flow clearly decreases, while the decrease in epicardial flow is relatively minor.
TMP13 p. 263

92. D) Several factors cause arteriolar vasodilation during exercise, including increases in potassium ion concentration, plasma nitric oxide concentration, plasma adenosine concentration, and plasma osmolality. Although histamine causes arteriolar vasodilation, histamine release does not normally occur during exercise.
TMP13 p. 259

93. A) At the beginning of exercise, increases in sympathetic stimulation of the heart strengthens the heart and increases the heart rate. Coronary and cerebral blood flow are spared from any decrease. Reverse stress relaxation does not occur. Venous constriction occurs, not dilation.
TMP13 p. 260

94. B) The anterior cardiac veins and the thebesian veins both drain venous blood from the heart. However, 75% of the total coronary flow drains from the heart by the coronary sinus.
TMP13 p. 262

95. E) Several drugs have proven to be helpful to patients with myocardial ischemia. Beta receptor blockers (not stimulators) inhibit the sympathetic effects on the heart and are very helpful. ACE inhibition prevents the production of angiotensin II and thus decreases the afterload effect on the heart. Nitroglycerin causes nitric oxide release, resulting in coronary vasodilation. Isometric exercise increases blood pressure markedly and can be harmful, and increased dietary calcium would be of little benefit.
TMP13 p. 269

96. C) During exercise the sympathetic output increases markedly, which causes arteriolar constriction in many places of the body, including non-exercising muscle. The increased sympathetic output also causes venoconstriction throughout the body. During exercise there also is an increased release of norepinephrine and epinephrine by the adrenal glands.
TMP13 pp. 260-261

97. B) Several factors contribute to decreased coronary flow in patients with ischemic heart disease. Some patients will have spasm of the coronary arteries, which acutely decreases coronary flow. However, the major cause of decreased coronary flow is an atherosclerotic narrowing of the lumen of the coronary arteries.
TMP13 p. 264

98. C) Increased sympathetic stimulation excites the cardiac myocytes and makes them much more susceptible to fibrillation. High (not low) potassium increases fibrillation tendency. An increase (not a decrease) in ventricular diameter will allow the cardiac muscle to be out of the refractory period when the cardiac impulse next arrives and can increase the tendency to fibrillate. A low adenosine level will probably only cause some coronary constriction. Decreased parasympathetics will allow the heart rate to increase and has little to do with fibrillation.
TMP13 p. 268

99. A) In a patient with angina due to myocardial ischemia, oxygen use by the heart must be minimized. Oxygen use can be minimized with ACE inhibition, which decreases angiotensin II formation. This will reduce the arterial pressure and decrease myocardial tension and oxygen use. The use of beta sympathetic blockers (not stimulation) will inhibit the effects of excess sympathetic output on the heart, thus reducing wall tension and oxygen use. Isometric exercise should be avoided because of the large increase in arterial pressure that occurs. Chelation therapy with EDTA and increased dietary calcium have little to do with cardiac function.
TMP13 p. 269

100. C) The major causes of death after myocardial infarction include a decrease in cardiac output that prevents tissues of the body from receiving adequate nutrition and oxygen delivery and prevents removal of waste materials. Other causes of death are pulmonary edema, which reduces the oxygenation of the blood, fibrillation of the heart, and rupture of the heart. Cardiac contractility decreases after a myocardial infarction.

TMP13 p. 266

101. **E)** During sympathetic stimulation, venous reservoirs constrict, venous vascular resistance also increases, arterioles constrict (which increases their resistance), and the heart rate increases. The epicardial coronary vessels have a large number of alpha receptors, but the subendocardial vessels have more beta receptors. Therefore, sympathetic stimulation causes at least a slight constriction of the epicardial vessels. This results in a slight decrease in epicardial flow.

TMP13 pp. 260-261, 263

102. **E)** Several factors change during compensated heart failure to stabilize the circulatory system. Because of increased sympathetic output, the heart rate increases during compensated heart failure. The kidneys retain sodium and water, which increases blood volume and thus right atrial pressure. The increased blood volume that results causes an increase in mean systemic filling pressure, which will help to increase the cardiac output. Dyspnea usually will occur only in the early stages of compensated failure.

TMP13 pp. 271-272

103. **E)** In unilateral left heart failure, the kidneys retain sodium and water and thus increase blood volume and the pulmonary veins, in turn, become congested. Therefore, mean pulmonary filling pressure, pulmonary wedge pressure, and left atrial pressure increase. In contrast, in right heart failure, right atrial pressure increases and edema of the lower extremities, including the feet and ankles, occurs.

TMP13 p. 275

104. **A)** In compensated heart failure, an increased release of angiotensin II also occurs, which causes direct renal sodium retention and also stimulates aldosterone secretion that will, in turn, cause further increases in sodium retention by the kidneys. Because of the low arterial pressure that occurs in compensated heart failure, the sympathetic output increases. One of the results is a sympathetic vasoconstriction (not vasodilation) of the afferent arterioles of the kidney. This decreases the glomerular hydrostatic pressure and the glomerular filtration rate, resulting in an increase in sodium and water retention in the body. The excess sodium in the body will increase osmolality, which increases the release of antidiuretic hormone, which causes renal water retention (but not sodium retention).

TMP13 p. 276

105. **C)** During acute pulmonary edema, the increased fluid in the lungs diminishes the oxygen content in the blood. This decreased oxygen weakens the heart even further and also causes arteriolar dilation in the body. This results in increases in venous return of blood to the heart, which cause further leakage of the fluid in the lungs and further decreases in oxygen content in the blood. It is important to interrupt this vicious circle to save a patient's life. This can be interrupted by placing tourniquets on all four limbs, which effectively removes blood volume from the chest. The patient can also breathe oxygen, and a bronchodilator can be administered. Furosemide can be administered to reduce some of the fluid volume in the body and especially in the lungs. One thing you do not want to do is infuse whole blood or an electrolyte solution in this patient because it may exacerbate the pulmonary edema that is already present.

TMP13 p. 277

106. **D)** Cardiogenic shock results from a weakening of the cardiac muscle many times after coronary thrombosis, which can result in a vicious circle because of low cardiac output resulting in a low diastolic pressure. This causes a decrease in coronary flow, which decreases the cardiac strength even more. Therefore, arterial pressure, particularly diastolic pressure, must be increased in patients with cardiogenic shock with either vasoconstrictors or volume expanders. In this patient the best answer is to infuse plasma. Placing tourniquets on all four limbs decreases the central blood volume, which would worsen the condition of the patient in shock.

TMP13 p. 275

107. **B)** This patient has a resting cardiac output of 4 L/min, and his cardiac reserve is 300% of this resting cardiac output or 12 L/min. This gives a total maximum cardiac output of 16 L/min. Therefore, the cardiac reserve is the percentage increase that the cardiac output can be elevated over the resting cardiac output.

TMP13 p. 277

108. **B)** Several factors cause sodium retention during heart failure, including aldosterone release, decreased glomerular filtration rate, and an increased angiotensin II release. A decrease in mean arterial pressure also results in decreases in glomerular hydrostatic pressure and causes a decrease in renal sodium excretion. During heart failure, blood volume increases, resulting in an increased cardiac stretch. In particular, the atrial pressure increases, causing a release of atrial natriuretic factor, resulting in an increase in renal sodium excretion.

TMP13 p. 276

109. **D)** There is a vicious circle of cardiac deterioration in cardiogenic shock. A weakened heart causes a

decreased cardiac output, which decreases arterial pressure. The decreased arterial pressure, particularly the decrease in diastolic pressure, decreases the coronary blood flow and further weakens the heart and thus further decreases cardiac output. The therapy of choice for a patient in cardiogenic shock is to increase the arterial pressure either with a vasoconstrictor drug or with a volume-expanding drug. Placing tourniquets on the four limbs, withdrawing a moderate amount of blood, or administering furosemide decreases the thoracic blood volume and thus worsens the condition of the patient in cardiogenic shock.

   TMP13 p. 275

110. **A)** In unilateral right heart failure, the right atrial pressure decreases and the overall cardiac output decreases, which results in a decrease in arterial pressure and urinary output. However, left atrial pressure does not increase but in fact decreases.

   TMP13 p. 275

111. **B)** During compensated heart failure, many factors combine to increase cardiac output so it returns to normal. The kidneys decrease their urinary output of sodium and water to increase the blood volume. This action, when combined with a depressed cardiac output curve, will increase right atrial pressure. Mean systemic filling pressure increases (not decreases), and the venous return of blood back toward the heart thus increases right atrial pressure. Heart rate is normal, and sweating and dyspnea are absent in the chronic stages of compensated failure.

   TMP13 pp. 274-275

112. **A)** Reduction of fluid in the lungs can prevent rapid deterioration in patients with acute pulmonary edema. Furosemide causes venodilation, which reduces thoracic blood volume and acts as a powerful diuretic. These both reduce excess fluid in the lungs. Blood can actually be removed in moderate quantities from the patient to decrease the volume of blood in the chest. Patients should also breathe oxygen to increase the oxygen levels in the blood. However, they should never be given a volume expander, such as saline, plasma, whole blood, or dextran, because it could worsen the pulmonary edema. Norepinephrine would be of little help in treating pulmonary edema.

   TMP13 pp. 277-278

113. **B)** In compensated heart failure, mean systemic filling pressure increases because of hypervolemia, and cardiac output is often at normal values. The patient has air hunger, called dyspnea, and excess sweating occurs in the early phases of compensated heart failure. However, right atrial pressure becomes elevated to very high values in these patients and is a hallmark of this disease.

   TMP13 pp. 272-273

114. **B)** Mean systemic pressure is increased by factors that increase blood volume or decrease vascular capacity. Sympathetic inhibition and venous dilation both decrease the mean systemic filling pressure. In congestive heart failure, the kidneys retain great quantities of sodium and water, resulting in an increase in blood volume, which causes large increases in mean systemic filling pressure.

   TMP13 p. 272

115. **A)** During compensated heart failure, release of angiotensin II and aldosterone is increased, causing the kidneys retain sodium and water, which increases the blood volume in the body and the venous return of blood to the heart. This situation results in an increase in right atrial pressure. Increased sympathetic output during compensated heart failure will increase heart rate. Air hunger, called dyspnea, occurs during any type of exertion. The patient also has orthopnea, which is the air hunger that occurs from being in a recumbent position.

   TMP13 pp. 272-274

116. **B)** During decompensated heart failure, cardiac output decreases because of weakness of the heart and edema of the cardiac muscle. Pressures in the pulmonary capillary system increase, including the pulmonary capillary pressure and the mean pulmonary filling pressure. Depletion of norepinephrine in the endings of the cardiac sympathetic nerves is another factor that causes weakness of the heart.

   TMP13 pp. 273-274

117. **D)** In decompensated heart failure, the kidneys retain sodium and water, which causes a weight gain and an increase in blood volume. This situation increases the mean systemic filling pressure, which also stretches the heart. Therefore, a decreased mean systemic filling pressure does not occur in decompensated heart failure. The excess blood volume often overstretches the sarcomeres of the heart, which prevents them from achieving their maximal tension. An excess central fluid volume also results in orthopnea, which is the inability to breathe properly except in the upright position.

   TMP13 pp. 273-274

118. **C)** The mean electrical axis of the QRS of this patient is shifted rightward to 170 degrees, which indicates that the right side of the heart is involved. Both aortic stenosis and mitral regurgitation will cause a leftward shift of the QRS axis. Mitral stenosis will not affect the left ventricle, but in severe enough circumstances it could cause an increase in pulmonary artery pressure, which would cause an increase in pulmonary capillary pressure at the same time. Tricuspid stenosis will not affect the right ventricle. Therefore, pulmonary valve stenosis is the only condition that fits this set of symptoms.

   TMP13 pp. 285-286

119. **A)** The fourth heart sound occurs at the end of diastole and is caused by inrushing of blood into the ventricles due to atrial contraction. The first heart sound is caused by closing of the A-V valves. The closing of the aortic and pulmonary valves at the end of systole causes the second heart sound. This initiates a vibration throughout the ventricles, aorta, and pulmonary artery. The third heart sound is caused by inrushing of blood into the ventricles in the early to middle part of diastole.
   TMP13 p. 284

120. **B)** Blowing murmurs of relatively high pitch are usually murmurs associated with valvular insufficiency. The key pieces of data to identify this murmur are the systolic and diastolic pressures. Aortic valve regurgitation typically has a high pulse pressure, which is the systolic - the diastolic pressure, and in this case is 100 mm Hg. Also notice that the diastolic pressure decreases to very low values of 40 mm Hg as the blood leaks back into the left ventricle.
   TMP13 pp. 285-286

121. **E)** Left ventricular hypertrophy occurs when the left ventricle either has to produce high pressure or when it pumps extra volume with each stroke. During aortic regurgitation, extra blood leaks back into the ventricle during the diastolic period. This extra volume must be expelled during the next heartbeat. During mitral regurgitation, some blood gets pumped out into the aorta, while at the same time blood leaks back into the left atrium. Therefore, the left ventricle is pumping extra volume with each heartbeat. During aortic stenosis, the left ventricle must contract very strongly, producing high wall tension to increase the aortic pressure to the values high enough to expel blood into the aorta. During mitral stenosis the ventricle is normal because the atrium produces the extra pressure to get blood through the stenotic mitral valve.
   TMP13 pp. 285-286

122. **E)** Several diastolic murmurs can be heard easily with a stethoscope. During diastole, aortic and pulmonary valve regurgitation occur through the insufficient valves causing the heart murmur at this time. Tricuspid and mitral stenosis are diastolic murmurs because blood flows through the restricted valves during the diastolic period. Patent ductus arteriosus is heard in both systole and diastole.
   TMP13 pp. 285-286

123. **C)** Aortic stenosis has a very high ventricular systolic pressure. Diastolic filling of the ventricle requires a much higher left atrial pressure. However, tricuspid stenosis and regurgitation, pulmonary valve regurgitation, and pulmonary stenosis are associated with an increase in right atrial pressure and should not affect pressure in the left atrium.
   TMP13 pp. 285-286

124. **B)** This patient has a QRS axis of −45 degrees, indicating a leftward axis shift. In other words, the left side of the heart is enlarged. In aortic valve stenosis the left side of the heart is enlarged because of the extra tension the left ventricular walls must exert to expel blood out the aorta. Therefore, these symptoms fit with a patient with aortic stenosis. In pulmonary valve stenosis, the right side of the heart hypertrophies, and in mitral valve stenosis there is no left ventricular hypertrophy. In tricuspid valve regurgitation, the right side of the heart enlarges, and in tricuspid valve stenosis, no ventricular hypertrophy occurs.
   TMP13 pp. 285-286

125. **C)** This patient has a heart murmur heard maximally in the "pulmonary area of cardiac auscultation." The high pitch indicates regurgitation. The rightward axis shift indicates that the right side of the heart has hypertrophied. The two choices that have a rightward axis shift are pulmonary valve regurgitation and tetralogy of Fallot. In tetralogy of Fallot, the arterial blood oxygen content is low, which is not the case with this patient. Therefore, pulmonary valve regurgitation is the correct answer.
   TMP13 pp. 285-286

126. **A)** Right ventricular hypertrophy occurs when the right heart has to pump a higher volume of blood or pump it against a higher pressure. Tetralogy of Fallot is associated with right ventricular hypertrophy because of the increased pulmonary valvular resistance, and this also occurs during pulmonary artery stenosis. Tricuspid insufficiency causes an increased stroke volume by the right heart, which causes hypertrophy. However, tricuspid stenosis does not affect the right ventricle.
   TMP13 pp. 289-290

127. **E)** Mitral stenosis is heard during diastole only. Aortic stenosis, tricuspid valve regurgitation, interventricular septal effect, and patent ductus arteriosis are clearly heard during systole. However, patent ductus arteriosus is also heard during diastole.
   TMP13 p. 285

128. **A)** In tetralogy of Fallot, there is an interventricular septal defect as well as stenosis of either the pulmonary artery or the pulmonary valve. Therefore, it is very difficult for blood to pass into the pulmonary artery and into the lungs to be oxygenated. Instead the blood partially shunts to the left side of the heart, thus bypassing the lungs. This situation results in low arterial oxygen content.
   TMP13 pp. 289-290

129. **B)** The first heart sound by definition is always associated with the closing of the A-V valves. The heart sounds are usually not associated with opening of any of the valves but with the closing of the valves and

the associated vibration of the blood and the walls of the heart. One exception is an opening snap in some mitral valves.

> TMP13 pp. 283-284

130. **B)** In tetralogy of Fallot, an interventricular septal defect and increased resistance in the pulmonary valve or pulmonary artery cause partial blood shunting toward the left side of the heart without going through the lungs. This situation results in a severely decreased arterial oxygen content. The interventricular septal defect causes equal systolic pressures in both cardiac ventricles, which causes right ventricular hypertrophy and a wall thickness very similar to that of the left ventricle.

> TMP13 pp. 289-290

131. **C)** Mitral regurgitation and aortic stenosis are murmurs heard during the systolic period. A ventricular septal defect murmur is normally heard only during the systolic phase. Tricuspid valve stenosis and patent ductus arteriosus murmurs are heard during diastole. However, a patent ductus arteriosus murmur is also heard during systole.

> TMP13 pp. 285-286

132. **E)** The third heart sound is associated with inrushing of blood into the ventricles in the early to middle part of diastole. The next heart sound, the fourth heart sound, is caused by inrushing of blood in the ventricles caused by atrial contraction. The first heart sound is caused by the closing of the A-V valves, and the second heart sound is caused by the closing of the pulmonary and aortic valves.

> TMP13 pp. 283-284

133. **A)** A number of things occur in progressive shock, including increased capillary permeability, which allows fluid to leak out of the vasculature, thus decreasing the blood volume. Other deteriorating factors include vasomotor center failure, peripheral circulatory failure, decreased cellular mitochondrial activity, and acidosis throughout the body. Usually, urine output strikingly decreases; therefore, the increased urinary output answer is incorrect. Tissue pH decreases and reverse stress relaxation of the veins occurs.

> TMP13 pp. 296-297

134. **A)** Sympathomimetic drugs are given to counteract hypotension during a number of conditions. These conditions include spinal cord injury in which the sympathetic output is interrupted. Sympathomimetic drugs are also given during very deep anesthesia, which decreases the sympathetic output, and during anaphylactic shock that results from histamine release and the accompanying vasodilatation. Sympathomimetic drugs, such as norepinephrine, increase blood pressure by causing a vasoconstriction. Shock caused by excess vomiting, hemorrhage, or excessive

administration of diuretics results in fluid volume depletion, resulting in decreased blood volume and decreased mean systemic filling pressure. Administering a balanced electrolyte solution best counteracts this condition.

> TMP13 p. 301

135. **D)** Too deep a level of anesthesia can decrease sympathetic tone and reduce arterial pressure enough to induce shock. To replace the sympathetic tone that was lost, the optimal therapy is infusion of a sympathomimetic drug. Infusion of red blood cells, plasma, or electrolytes would be of little benefit.

> TMP13 pp. 300-301

136. **D)** The patient received an influenza inoculation and quickly went into shock, which leads one to believe that he may be in anaphylactic shock. Anaphylactic shock is a state of extreme vasodilation because of histamine release. Antihistamines would be somewhat helpful, but they are very slow acting, and the patient could die in the meantime. Therefore, a very rapid-acting agent must be used, such as a sympathomimetic drug.

> TMP13 pp. 300-301

137. **E)** In compensated hemorrhagic shock, a number of factors prevent the progression of the shock, including increased heart rate. Also occurring is reverse stress relaxation in which the vasculature, particularly the veins, constrict around the available blood volume. Increased ADH release also occurs, which causes water retention from the kidney but also vasoconstriction of the arterioles. A CNS ischemic response also occurs if the blood pressure drops to very low values, causing an increase in sympathetic output. Increased absorption of interstitial fluid through the capillaries also occurs, which increases the volume in the vasculature.

> TMP13 p. 295

138. **E)** Spinal anesthesia, especially when the anesthesia extends all the way up the spinal cord, can block the sympathetic nervous outflow from the spinal cord. This can be a very potent cause of neurogenic shock. The therapy of choice is to replace the sympathetic tone that was lost in the body. The best way to increase the sympathetic tone is by infusing a sympathomimetic drug.

> TMP13 p. 301

139. **A)** This patient has obviously lost a lot of blood because of the motorcycle wreck. The most advantageous therapy is to replace what was lost in the accident. This would be whole blood, which is much superior to a plasma infusion, because the patient is also receiving red blood cells that have a much superior oxygen-carrying capacity than the plasma component of blood. Sympathetic nerves are firing very

rapidly in this condition, and an infusion of a sympathomimetic agent would be of little advantage.

TMP13 pp. 300-301

140. **C)** In hemorrhagic shock, anaphylactic shock, and neurogenic shock, the venous return of blood to the heart markedly decreases. However, in septic shock the cardiac output increases in many patients because of vasodilation in affected tissues and a high metabolic rate causing vasodilation in other parts of the body.

TMP13 p. 300

141. **E)** This patient has been hemorrhaging, and the optimal therapy is to replace the blood he has lost. Unfortunately, no blood is available, and therefore we must choose next best therapy, which is increasing the volume of his blood. Thus, plasma infusion is the next best therapy because its high colloid osmotic pressure will help the infused fluid stay in the circulation much longer than would a balanced electrolyte solution.

TMP13 pp. 300-301

142. **B)** Intestinal obstruction often causes severe reduction in plasma volume. Obstruction causes a distention of the intestine and partially blocks the venous blood flow in the intestines. This partial blockage results in an increased intestinal capillary pressure, which causes fluid to leak from the capillary into the walls of the intestines and also into the intestinal lumen. The leaking fluid has a high protein content very similar to that of the plasma, which reduces the total plasma protein and the plasma volume. Therefore, the therapy of choice would be to replace the fluid lost by infusing plasma.

TMP13 pp. 300-301

143. **A)** In progressive shock, because of the poor blood flow, the pH in the tissues throughout the body decreases. Many vessels become blocked because of local blood agglutination, which is called "sludged blood." Patchy areas of necrosis also occur in the liver. Mitochondrial activity decreases and capillary permeability increases. There is also an increased release of hydrolases by the lysosomes and a decrease in cellular metabolism of glucose.

TMP13 p. 297

144. **A)** Anaphylaxis is an allergic condition that results from an antigen-antibody reaction that takes place after exposure of an individual to an antigenic substance. The basophils and mast cells in the pericapillary tissues release histamine or histamine-like substances. The histamine causes venous dilation, dilation of arterioles, and greatly increased capillary permeability with rapid loss of fluid and protein into the tissue spaces. This response reduces venous return and often results in anaphylactic shock.

TMP13 pp. 300-301

The Body Fluids and Kidneys

1. Which of the following solutions, when infused intravenously, would result in an increase in extracellular fluid volume, a decrease in intracellular fluid volume, and an increase in total body water after osmotic equilibrium?

    A) 1 Liter of 0.9% sodium chloride (NaCl) solution
    B) 1 Liter of 0.45% NaCl solution
    C) 1 Liter of 3% NaCl solution
    D) 1 Liter of 5% dextrose solution
    E) 1 Liter of pure water

2. Partial obstruction of a major vein draining a tissue would tend to _____ lymph flow rate, _____ interstitial fluid hydrostatic pressure, and _____ interstitial fluid protein concentration in the tissue drained by that vein.

    A) Increase, increase, increase
    B) Increase, increase, decrease
    C) Increase, decrease, decrease
    D) Decrease, decrease, decrease
    E) Decrease, increase, increase
    F) Decrease, increase, decrease

3. A 36-year-old woman reports headaches and frequent urination. Laboratory values reveal the following information.

    Urine specific gravity = 1.003
    Urine protein = negative
    Plasma sodium (Na⁺) = 165 mmol/L
    Plasma potassium (K⁺) = 4.4 mmol/L
    Plasma creatinine = 1.4 mg/dl
    Blood pressure = 88/40 mm Hg
    Heart rate = 115 beats/min

    What is the most likely cause of her elevated plasma Na⁺ concentration?

    A) Primary aldosteronism
    B) Diabetes mellitus
    C) Diabetes insipidus
    D) Simple dehydration due to insufficient water intake and heavy exercise
    E) Bartter's syndrome
    F) Liddle's syndrome

4. After receiving a kidney transplant, a patient has severe hypertension (170/110 mm Hg). A renal arteriogram indicates severe renal artery stenosis in his single remaining kidney, with a reduction in glomerular filtration rate (GFR) to 25% of normal. Which of the following changes, compared with normal, would be expected in this patient, assuming steady-state conditions?

    A) A large increase in plasma sodium concentration
    B) A reduction in urinary sodium excretion to 25% of normal
    C) A reduction in urinary creatinine excretion to 25% of normal
    D) An increase in serum creatinine to about four times normal
    E) Normal renal blood flow in the stenotic kidney due to autoregulation

Questions 5–7

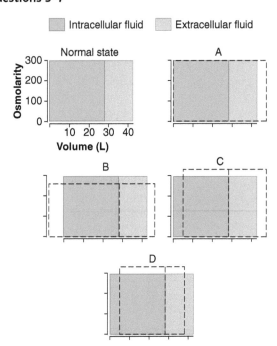

The figure above represents various states of abnormal hydration. In each diagram, the normal state (orange and lavender) is superimposed on the abnormal state (dashed lines) to illustrate the shifts in the volume (width of rectangles) and total osmolarity (height of rectangles) of the extracellular and intracellular fluid compartments. Use this figure to answer Questions 5–7.

5. Which diagram represents the changes (after osmotic equilibrium) in extracellular and intracellular fluid volume and osmolarity after the infusion of 1% dextrose?

A) A
B) B
C) C
D) D

6. Which diagram represents the changes (after osmotic equilibrium) in extracellular and intracellular fluid volume and osmolarity in a patient with the syndrome of inappropriate antidiuretic hormone (ADH; i.e., excessive secretion of ADH)?

A) A
B) B
C) C
D) D

7. Which diagram represents the changes (after osmotic equilibrium) in extracellular and intracellular fluid volumes and osmolarities after the infusion of 3% NaCl?

A) A
B) B
C) C
D) D

8. Which of the following tends to decrease potassium secretion by the cortical collecting tubule?

A) Increased plasma potassium concentration
B) A diuretic that decreases proximal tubule sodium reabsorption
C) A diuretic that inhibits the action of aldosterone (e.g., spironolactone)
D) Acute alkalosis
E) High sodium intake

9. Because the usual rate of phosphate filtration exceeds the transport maximum for phosphate reabsorption, which statement is true?

A) All the phosphate that is filtered is reabsorbed
B) More phosphate is reabsorbed than is filtered
C) Phosphate in the tubules can contribute significantly to titratable acid in the urine
D) The "threshold" for phosphate is usually not exceeded
E) Parathyroid hormone must be secreted for phosphate reabsorption to occur

Questions 10 and 11
Use the following clinical laboratory test results to answer Questions 10 and 11.

Urine flow rate = 1 ml/min
Urine inulin concentration = 100 mg/ml
Plasma inulin concentration = 2 mg/ml
Urine urea concentration = 50 mg/ml
Plasma urea concentration = 2.5 mg/ml

10. What is the GFR?

A) 25 ml/min
B) 50 ml/min
C) 100 ml/min
D) 125 ml/min
E) None of the above

11. What is the net urea reabsorption rate?

A) 0 mg/min
B) 25 mg/min
C) 50 mg/min
D) 75 mg/min
E) 100 mg/min

12. If a patient has a creatinine clearance of 90 ml/min, a urine flow rate of 1 ml/min, a plasma K^+ concentration of 4 mEq/L, and a urine K^+ concentration of 60 mEq/L, what is the approximate rate of K^+ excretion?

A) 0.06 mEq/min
B) 0.30 mEq/min
C) 0.36 mEq/min
D) 3.6 mEq/min
E) 60 mEq/min

13. Given the following measurements, calculate the filtration fraction:

Glomerular capillary hydrostatic pressure (P_G) = 70 mm Hg
Bowman's space hydrostatic pressure (P_B) = 20 mm Hg
Colloid osmotic pressure in the glomerular capillaries (π_G) = 35 mm Hg
Glomerular capillary filtration coefficient (K_f) = 10 ml/min/mm Hg
Renal plasma flow = 428 ml/min

A) 0.16
B) 0.20
C) 0.25
D) 0.30
E) 0.35
F) 0.40

14. In normal kidneys, which of the following is true of the osmolarity of renal tubular fluid that flows through the early distal tubule in the region of the macula densa?

A) Usually isotonic compared with plasma
B) Usually hypotonic compared with plasma
C) Usually hypertonic compared with plasma
D) Hypertonic, compared with plasma, in antidiuresis

15. Which of the following changes would be expected in a patient with diabetes insipidus due to a lack of ADH secretion?

	Plasma Osmolarity Concentration	Plasma Sodium Concentration	Plasma Renin	Urine Volume
A)	↔	↔	↓	↑
B)	↔	↔	↑	↑
C)	↑	↑	↑	↑
D)	↑	↑	↔	↔
E)	↓	↓	↓	↔

16. A 26-year-old woman recently decided to adopt a healthier diet and eat more fruits and vegetables. As a result, her potassium intake increased from 80 to 160 mmol/day. Which of the following conditions would you expect to find 2 weeks after she increased her potassium intake, compared with before the increase?

	Potassium Excretion Rate	Sodium Excretion Rate	Plasma Aldosterone Concentration	Plasma Potassium Concentration
A)	↔	↔	↑	Large increase (>1 mmol/L)
B)	↔	↓	↑	Small increase (<1 mmol/L)
C)	↑2×	↔	↑	Small increase (<1 mmol/L)
D)	↑2×	↑	↓	Large increase (>1 mmol/L)
E)	↑2×	↑	↔	Large increase (>1 mmol/L)

17. When the dietary intake of K^+ increases, body K^+ balance is maintained by an increase in K^+ excretion primarily by which of the following?

A) Decreased glomerular filtration of K^+
B) Decreased reabsorption of K^+ by the proximal tubule
C) Decreased reabsorption of K^+ by the thick ascending limb of the loop of Henle
D) Increased K^+ secretion by the late distal and collecting tubules
E) Shift of K^+ into the intracellular compartment

18. Which of the following would cause the greatest decrease in GFR in a person with otherwise normal kidneys?

A) Decrease in renal arterial pressure from 100 to 80 mm Hg in a normal kidney
B) 50% increase in glomerular capillary filtration coefficient
C) 50% increase in proximal tubular sodium reabsorption
D) 50% decrease in afferent arteriolar resistance
E) 50% decrease in efferent arteriolar resistance
F) 5 mm Hg decrease in Bowman's capsule pressure

19. An 8-year-old boy is brought to your office with extreme swelling of the abdomen. His parents indicate that he had a very sore throat a "month or so" ago and that he has been "swelling up" since that time. He appears to be edematous, and when you check his urine, you find that large amounts of protein are being excreted. Your diagnosis is nephrotic syndrome subsequent to glomerulonephritis. Which of the following changes would you expect to find, compared with normal?

	Thoracic Lymph Flow	Interstitial Fluid Protein Concentration	Interstitial Fluid Hydrostatic Pressure	Plasma Renin Concentration
A)	↑	↓	↑	↑
B)	↑	↓	↑	↔
C)	↑	↓	↔	↑
D)	↓	↑	↔	↔
E)	↓	↓	↓	↓

20. A patient with severe hypertension (blood pressure 185/110 mm Hg) is referred to you. A renal magnetic resonance imaging scan shows a tumor in the kidney, and laboratory findings include a very high plasma renin activity of 12 ng angiotensin I/ml/h (normal = 1). The diagnosis is a renin-secreting tumor. Which of the following changes would you expect to find in this patient, under steady-state conditions, compared with normal?

	Plasma Aldosterone Concentration	Sodium Excretion Rate	Plasma Potassium Concentration	Renal Blood Flow
A)	↔	↓	↓	↑
B)	↔	↔	↓	↑
C)	↑	↔	↓	↓
D)	↑	↓	↔	↓
E)	↑	↓	↓	↔

21. The clinical laboratory returned the following values for arterial blood taken from a patient: plasma pH = 7.28, plasma $HCO_3^- = 32$ mEq/L, and plasma partial pressure of carbon dioxide (P_{CO_2}) = 70 mm Hg. What is this patient's acid-base disorder?

A) Acute respiratory acidosis without renal compensation
B) Respiratory acidosis with partial renal compensation
C) Acute metabolic acidosis without respiratory compensation
D) Metabolic acidosis with partial respiratory compensation

22. The following laboratory values were obtained in a 58-year-old man:

Urine volume = 4320 milliliters of urine collected during the preceding 24 hours
Plasma creatinine = 3 mg/100 ml
Urine creatinine = 50 mg/100 ml
Plasma potassium = 4.0 mmol/L
Urine potassium = 30 mmol/L

What is his approximate GFR, assuming that he collected all of his urine in the 24-hour period?

A) 20 ml/min
B) 30 ml/min
C) 40 ml/min
D) 50 ml/min
E) 60 ml/min
F) 80 ml/min
G) 100 ml/min

Questions 23 and 24

23. A 65-year-old man had a heart attack and experiences cardiopulmonary arrest while being transported to the emergency department. Use the following laboratory values obtained from arterial blood to answer Questions 23 and 24.

Plasma pH = 7.12
Plasma P_{CO_2} = 60 mm Hg
Plasma HCO_3^- concentration = 19 mEq/L

Which of the following options best describes his acid-base disorder?

A) Respiratory acidosis with partial renal compensation
B) Metabolic acidosis with partial respiratory compensation
C) Mixed acidosis: combined metabolic and respiratory acidosis
D) Mixed alkalosis: combined respiratory and metabolic alkalosis

24. In this patient, which of the following laboratory results would be expected, compared with normal?

A) Increased renal excretion of bicarbonate (HCO_3^-)
B) Decreased urinary titratable acid
C) Increased urine pH
D) Increased renal excretion of ammonia (NH_4^+)

25. What would cause the greatest degree of hyperkalemia?

A) Increase in potassium intake from 60 to 180 mmol/day in a person with normal kidneys and a normal aldosterone system
B) Chronic treatment with a diuretic that inhibits the action of aldosterone
C) Decrease in sodium intake from 200 to 100 mmol/day
D) Chronic treatment with a diuretic that inhibits loop of Henle Na^+-$2Cl^-$-K^+ co-transport
E) Chronic treatment with a diuretic that inhibits sodium reabsorption in the collecting ducts

26. Which of the following changes would be expected in a patient with Liddle's syndrome (i.e., excessive activity of amiloride-sensitive sodium channel in the collecting tubule) under steady-state conditions, assuming that the intake of electrolytes remained constant?

	Plasma Renin Concentration	Blood Pressure	Sodium Excretion Concentration	Plasma Aldosterone
A)	↔	↑	↓	↔
B)	↑	↑	↔	↑
C)	↑	↑	↓	↓
D)	↓	↑	↔	↓
E)	↓	↑	↓	↓
F)	↓	↓	↑	↑

27. A patient is referred for treatment of hypertension. After testing, you discover that he has a very high level of plasma aldosterone, and your diagnosis is Conn's syndrome. Assuming no change in electrolyte intake, which of the following changes would you expect to find, compared with normal?

	Plasma pH	Plasma K^+ Concentration	Urine K^+ Excretion	Urine Na^+ Excretion	Plasma Renin Concentration
A)	↑	↓	↔	↔	↓
B)	↓	↓	↔	↔	↓
C)	↑	↓	↑	↓	↓
D)	↑	↑	↔	↓	↑
E)	↑	↑	↑	↑	↑

28. A patient with renal disease had a plasma creatinine of 2 mg/dl during an examination 6 months ago. You note that his blood pressure has increased about 30 mm Hg since his previous visit, and laboratory tests indicate that his plasma creatinine is now 4 mg/dl. Which of the following changes, compared with his previous visit, would you expect to find, assuming steady-state conditions and no changes in electrolyte intake or metabolism?

	Sodium Excretion Rate	Creatinine Excretion Rate	Creatinine Clearance	Filtered Load of Creatinine
A)	↔	↔	↓ by 50%	↓
B)	↔	↔	↓ by 50%	↔
C)	↔	↔	↓ by 75%	↓
D)	↓	↓	↔	↔
E)	↓	↓	↓ by 50%	↓

29. Which change tends to increase GFR?

A) Increased afferent arteriolar resistance
B) Decreased efferent arteriolar resistance
C) Increased glomerular capillary filtration coefficient
D) Increased Bowman's capsule hydrostatic pressure
E) Decreased glomerular capillary hydrostatic pressure

30. Which of the following changes, compared with normal, would you expect to find 3 weeks after a patient ingested a toxin that caused sustained impairment of proximal tubular NaCl reabsorption? Assume that there has been no change in diet or ingestion of electrolytes.

	Glomerular Filtration Rate	Afferent Arteriolar Resistance	Sodium Excretion
A)	↔	↔	↑
B)	↔	↔	↑
C)	↓	↑	↑
D)	↓	↑	↔
E)	↑	↓	↔

31. What is the net renal tubular reabsorption rate of potassium in the patient described in Question 5?

    A) 0.020 mmol/min
    B) 0.040 mmol/min
    C) 0.090 mmol/min
    D) 0.110 mmol/min
    E) 0.200 mmol/min
    F) Potassium is not reabsorbed in this example

32. The maximum clearance rate possible for a substance that is totally cleared from the plasma is equal to which of the following?

    A) GFR
    B) Filtered load of that substance
    C) Urinary excretion rate of that substance
    D) Renal plasma flow
    E) Filtration fraction

33. A patient has the following laboratory values: arterial pH = 7.13, plasma HCO_3^- = 15 mEq/L, plasma chloride concentration = 118 mEq/L, arterial P_{CO_2} = 28 mm Hg, and plasma Na^+ concentration = 141 mEq/L. What is the most likely cause of his acidosis?

    A) Salicylic acid poisoning
    B) Diabetes mellitus
    C) Diarrhea
    D) Emphysema

34. The GFR of a 26-year-old man with glomerulonephritis decreases by 50% and remains at that level. For which substance would you expect to find the greatest increase in plasma concentration?

    A) Creatinine
    B) K^+
    C) Glucose
    D) Na^+
    E) Phosphate
    F) H^+

Questions 35 and 36
Assume the following initial conditions: intracellular fluid volume = 40% of body weight before fluid administration, extracellular fluid volume = 20% of body weight before fluid administration, molecular weight of NaCl = 58.5 g/mol, and no excretion of water or electrolytes.

35. A male patient appears to be dehydrated, and after obtaining a plasma sample, you find that he has hyponatremia, with a plasma sodium concentration of 130 mmol/L and a plasma osmolarity of 260 mOsm/L. You decide to administer 2 L of 3% sodium chloride (NaCl). His body weight was 60 kilograms before the fluid is administered. What is his approximate plasma osmolarity after administration of the NaCl solution and after osmotic equilibrium? Assume the initial conditions previously described.

    A) 273 mOsm/L
    B) 286 mOsm/L
    C) 300 mOsm/L
    D) 310 mOsm/L
    E) 326 mOsm/L

36. What is the approximate extracellular fluid volume in this patient after administration of the NaCl solution and after osmotic equilibrium?

    A) 15.1 Liters
    B) 17.2 Liters
    C) 19.1 Liters
    D) 19.8 Liters
    E) 21.2 Liters

37. Which changes would you expect to find after administering a vasodilator drug that caused a 50% decrease in afferent arteriolar resistance and no change in arterial pressure?

    A) Decreased renal blood flow, decreased GFR, and decreased peritubular capillary hydrostatic pressure
    B) Decreased renal blood flow, decreased GFR, and increased peritubular capillary hydrostatic pressure
    C) Increased renal blood flow, increased GFR, and increased peritubular capillary hydrostatic pressure
    D) Increased renal blood flow, increased GFR, and no change in peritubular capillary hydrostatic pressure
    E) Increased renal blood flow, increased GFR, and decreased peritubular capillary hydrostatic pressure

38. If the average hydrostatic pressure in the glomerular capillaries is 50 mm Hg, the hydrostatic pressure in the Bowman's space is 12 mm Hg, the average colloid osmotic pressure in the glomerular capillaries is 30 mm Hg, and there is no protein in the glomerular ultrafiltrate, what is the net pressure driving glomerular filtration?

    A) 8 mm Hg
    B) 32 mm Hg
    C) 48 mm Hg
    D) 60 mm Hg
    E) 92 mm Hg

39. In a patient who has chronic, uncontrolled diabetes mellitus, which set of conditions would you expect to find, compared with normal?

	Titratable Acid Excretion	NH$^+$ Excretion	HCO$_3^-$ Excretion	Plasma P$_{CO_2}$
A)	↔	↑	↓	↔
B)	↓	↑	↔	↓
C)	↑	↑	↔	↑
D)	↑	↑	↓	↓
E)	↓	↓	↓	↓
F)	↔	↑	↓	↔

40. Intravenous infusion of 1 liter of 0.45% NaCl solution (molecular weight of NaCl = 58.5) would cause which of the following changes, after osmotic equilibrium?

	Intracellular Fluid Volume	Intracellular Fluid Osmolarity	Extracellular Fluid Volume	Extracellular Fluid Osmolarity
A)	↑	↑	↑	↑
B)	↑	↓	↑	↓
C)	↔	↑	↑	↑
D)	↓	↑	↑	↑
E)	↓	↓	↓	↓

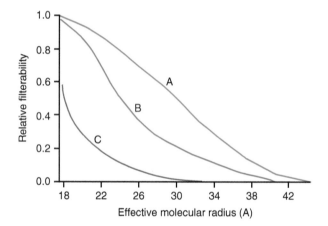

41. Lines A, B, and C on the figure above show the relative filterability by the glomerular capillaries of dextran molecules as a function of their molecular radius and electrical charges. Which lines on the graph best describe the electrical charges of the dextrans?

A) A = polycationic; B = neutral; C= polyanionic
B) A = polycationic; B = polyanionic; C = neutral
C) A = polyanionic; B = neutral; C = polycationic
D) A = polyanionic; B = polycationic; C = polycationic
E) A = neutral; B = polycationic; C = polyanionic
F) A = neutral; B = polyanionic; C = polycationic

42. If distal tubule fluid creatinine concentration is 5 mg/100 ml and plasma creatinine concentration is 1.0 mg/100 ml, what is the approximate percentage of the water filtered by the glomerular capillaries that remains in the distal tubule?

A) 5%
B) 10%
C) 20%
D) 50%
E) 80%
F) 95%

43. Which change tends to increase peritubular capillary fluid reabsorption?

A) Increased blood pressure
B) Decreased filtration fraction
C) Increased efferent arteriolar resistance
D) Decreased angiotensin II
E) Increased renal blood flow

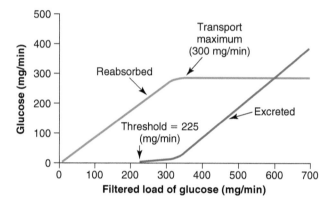

44. A 32-year-old man reports frequent urination. He is overweight (280 pounds [127 kilograms], 5 feet 10 inches [178 cm] tall). After measuring the 24-hour creatinine clearance, you estimate his GFR to be 150 ml/min. His plasma glucose level is 300 mg/dl. Assuming that his renal transport maximum for glucose is normal, as shown in the figure above, what would be this patient's approximate rate of urinary glucose excretion?

A) 0 mg/min
B) 100 mg/min
C) 150 mg/min
D) 225 mg/min
E) 300 mg/min
F) Information provided is inadequate to estimate the glucose excretion rate

45. An adrenal tumor that causes excess aldosterone secretion would tend to _____ plasma K$^+$ concentration, _____ plasma pH, _____ renin secretion, and _____ blood pressure.

A) Decrease, decrease, decrease, decrease
B) Decrease, increase, decrease, increase
C) Decrease, decrease, decrease, increase
D) Decrease, increase, increase, increase
E) Increase, increase, decrease, increase
F) Increase, decrease, decrease, increase

46. Which of the following tends to increase potassium secretion by the cortical collecting tubule?

    A) A diuretic that inhibits the action of aldosterone (e.g., spironolactone)
    B) A diuretic that decreases loop of Henle sodium reabsorption (e.g., furosemide)
    C) Decreased plasma potassium concentration
    D) Acute metabolic acidosis
    E) Low sodium intake

47. A diabetic patient has chronic renal disease and is referred to your nephrology clinic. According to his family physician, his creatinine clearance has decreased from 100 ml/min to 40 ml/min during the past 4 years. His glucose level has not been well controlled, and his plasma pH is 7.14. Which changes, compared with before the development of renal disease, would you expect to find, assuming steady-state conditions and no change in electrolyte intake?

	Sodium Excretion Rate	Creatinine Excretion Rate	Plasma Creatinine Concentration	Plasma HCO_3^- Concentration	NH_4^+ Excretion Rate
A)	↓	↓	↑	↑	↑
B)	↔	↔	↑	↓	↑
C)	↔	↔	↑	↓	↔
D)	↔	↓	↑	↓	↔
E)	↓	↓	↓	↓	↑
F)	↓	↓	↓	↓	↓

48. A 62-year-old woman has previously had a unilateral nephrectomy after diagnosis of renal carcinoma. Her GFR (estimated from creatinine clearance) is 50 ml/min, her urine flow rate is 2.0 ml/min, and her plasma glucose concentration is 200 mg/100 ml. If she has a kidney transport maximum for glucose of 150 mg/min, what would be her approximate rate of glucose excretion?

    A) 0 mg/min
    B) 50 mg/min
    C) 100 mg/min
    D) 150 mg/min
    E) 200 mg/min
    F) 300 mg/min
    G) Glucose excretion rate cannot be estimated from these data

49. A 20-year-old woman comes to your office because of rapid weight gain and marked fluid retention. Her blood pressure is 105/65 mm Hg, her plasma protein concentration is 3.6 g/dl (normal = 7.0), and she has no detectable protein in her urine. Which changes would you expect to find, compared with normal?

	Thoracic Lymph Flow	Interstitial Fluid Protein Concentration	Capillary Filtration	Interstitial Fluid Pressure
A)	↓	↓	↓	↓
B)	↓	↑	↔	↔
C)	↑	↓	↑	↑
D)	↑	↓	↑	↔
E)	↑	↑	↑	↑

50. A 48-year-old woman reports severe polyuria (producing about 0.5 liter of urine each hour) and polydipsia (drinking two to three glasses of water every hour). Her urine contains no glucose, and she is placed on overnight water restriction for further evaluation. The next morning, she is weak and confused, her sodium concentration is 160 mEq/L, and her urine osmolarity is 80 mOsm/L. Which of the following is the most likely diagnosis?

    A) Diabetes mellitus
    B) Diabetes insipidus
    C) Primary aldosteronism
    D) Renin-secreting tumor
    E) Syndrome of inappropriate ADH

51. Which substance is filtered most readily by the glomerular capillaries?

    A) Albumin in plasma
    B) Neutral dextran with a molecular weight of 25,000
    C) Polycationic dextran with a molecular weight of 25,000
    D) Polyanionic dextran with a molecular weight of 25,000
    E) Red blood cells

52. A 22-year-old woman runs a 10-kilometer race on a hot day and becomes dehydrated. Assuming that her ADH levels are very high and that her kidneys are functioning normally, in which part of the renal tubule is the most water reabsorbed?

    A) Proximal tubule
    B) Loop of Henle
    C) Distal tubule
    D) Cortical collecting tubule
    E) Medullary collecting duct

53. Furosemide (Lasix) is a diuretic that also produces natriuresis. Which of the following is an undesirable side effect of furosemide due to its site of action on the renal tubule?

    A) Edema
    B) Hyperkalemia
    C) Hypercalcemia
    D) Decreased ability to concentrate the urine
    E) Heart failure

54. A female patient has unexplained severe hypernatremia (plasma Na^+ = 167 mmol/L) and reports frequent urination and large urine volumes. A urine specimen reveals that the Na^+ concentration is 15 mmol/L (very low) and the osmolarity is 155 mOsm/L (very low). Laboratory tests reveal the following data: plasma renin activity = 3 ng angiotensin I/ml/h (normal = 1.0), plasma ADH = 30 pg/ml (normal = 3 pg/ml), and plasma aldosterone = 20 ng/dl (normal = 6 ng/dl). Which of the following is the most likely reason for her hypernatremia?

    A) Simple dehydration due to decreased water intake
    B) Nephrogenic diabetes insipidus
    C) Central diabetes insipidus
    D) Syndrome of inappropriate ADH
    E) Primary aldosteronism
    F) Renin-secreting tumor

55. Which change would you expect to find in a dehydrated person deprived of water for 24 hours?

    A) Decreased plasma renin activity
    B) Decreased plasma antidiuretic hormone concentration
    C) Increased plasma atrial natriuretic peptide concentration
    D) Increased water permeability of the collecting duct

56. Juvenile (type 1) diabetes mellitus is often diagnosed because of polyuria (high urine flow) and polydipsia (frequent drinking) that occur because of which of the following?

    A) Increased delivery of glucose to the collecting duct interferes with the action of antidiuretic hormone
    B) Increased glomerular filtration of glucose increases Na^+ reabsorption via the sodium-glucose co-transporter
    C) When the filtered load of glucose exceeds the renal threshold, a rising glucose concentration in the proximal tubule decreases the osmotic driving force for water reabsorption
    D) High plasma glucose concentration decreases thirst
    E) High plasma glucose concentration stimulates ADH release from the posterior pituitary

57. Which of the following would cause the most serious hypokalemia?

    A) A decrease in potassium intake from 150 mEq/day to 60 mEq/day
    B) An increase in sodium intake from 100 to 200 mEq/day
    C) Excessive aldosterone secretion plus high sodium intake
    D) Excessive aldosterone secretion plus low sodium intake
    E) A patient with Addison's disease
    F) Treatment with a β-adrenergic blocker
    G) Treatment with spironolactone

58. A 26-year-old woman reports that she has had a severe migraine and has taken six times more than the recommended dose of aspirin for the past 3 days to relieve her headaches. Her plasma pH is 7.24. Which of the following would you expect to find (compared with normal)?

	Plasma HCO_3^- Concentration	Plasma P_{CO_2}	Urine HCO_3^- Excretion	Urine NH_4^+ Excretion	Plasma Anion Gap
A)	↑	↓	↑	↑	↑
B)	↑	↑	↑	↓	↑
C)	↓	↓	↓	↓	↓
D)	↓	↓	↓	↑	↑
E)	↓	↓	↓	↑	↓
F)	↓	↔	↓	↓	↔

59. Under conditions of normal renal function, what is true of the concentration of urea in tubular fluid at the end of the proximal tubule?

    A) It is higher than the concentration of urea in tubular fluid at the tip of the loop of Henle
    B) It is higher than the concentration of urea in the plasma
    C) It is higher than the concentration of urea in the final urine in antidiuresis
    D) It is lower than plasma urea concentration because of active urea reabsorption along the proximal tubule

60. You begin treating a hypertensive patient with a powerful loop diuretic (e.g., furosemide). Which changes would you expect to find, compared with pretreatment values, when he returns for a follow-up examination 2 weeks later?

	Urine Sodium Excretion	Extracellular Fluid Volume	Blood Pressure	Plasma Potassium Concentration
A)	↑	↓	↓	↓
B)	↑	↓	↔	↔
C)	↔	↓	↓	↓
D)	↔	↓	↔	↔
E)	↑	↔	↓	↑

61. Which change, compared with normal, would be expected to occur, under steady-state conditions, in a patient whose severe renal disease has reduced the number of functional nephrons to 25% of normal?

    A) Increased GFR of the surviving nephrons
    B) Decreased urinary creatinine excretion rate
    C) Decreased urine flow rate in the surviving nephrons
    D) Decreased urinary excretion of sodium
    E) Increased urine-concentrating ability

62. Which of the following would likely lead to hyponatremia?

    A) Excessive ADH secretion
    B) Restriction of fluid intake
    C) Excess aldosterone secretion
    D) Administration of 2 liters of 3% NaCl solution
    E) Administration of 2 liters of 0.9% NaCl solution

63. Assuming steady-state conditions and that water and electrolyte intake remained constant, a 75% loss of nephrons and a 75% decrease in GFR due to chronic kidney disease would cause all of the following changes *except* what?

    A) A large increase in plasma sodium concentration
    B) An increase in plasma creatinine to four times normal
    C) An increase in average volume excreted per remaining nephron to four times normal
    D) A significant increase in plasma phosphate concentration
    E) Reduced ability of the kidney to maximally concentrate the urine

64. Which statement is correct?

    A) Urea reabsorption in the medullary collecting tubule is less than in the distal convoluted tubule during antidiuresis
    B) Urea concentration in the interstitial fluid of the renal cortex is greater than in the interstitial fluid of the renal medulla during antidiuresis
    C) The thick ascending limb of the loop of Henle reabsorbs more urea than the inner medullary collecting tubule during antidiuresis
    D) Urea reabsorption in the proximal tubule is greater than in the cortical collecting tubule

65. A patient's urine is collected for 2 hours, and the total volume is 600 milliliters during this time. Her urine osmolarity is 150 mOsm/L, and her plasma osmolarity is 300 mOsm/L. What is her "free water clearance"?

    A) +5.0 ml/min
    B) +2.5 ml/min
    C) 0.0 ml/min
    D) –2.5 ml/min
    E) –5.0 ml/min

Questions 66–69

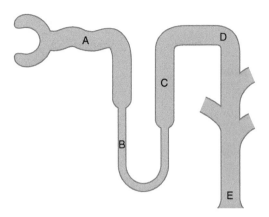

For Questions 66–69, choose the appropriate nephron site in the above figure.

66. In a patient with severe central diabetes insipidus caused by a lack of ADH secretion, which part of the tubule would have the lowest tubular fluid osmolarity?

    A) A
    B) B
    C) C
    D) D
    E) E

67. In a person on a very low potassium diet, which part of the nephron would be expected to reabsorb the most potassium?

    A) A
    B) B
    C) C
    D) D
    E) E

68. Which part of the nephron normally reabsorbs the most water?

    A) A
    B) B
    C) C
    D) D
    E) E

69. In a normally functioning kidney, which part of the tubule has the lowest permeability to water during antidiuresis?

    A) A
    B) B
    C) C
    D) D
    E) E

70. Which substances are best suited to measure interstitial fluid volume?

    A) Inulin and heavy water
    B) Inulin and ^{22}Na
    C) Heavy water and ^{125}I-albumin
    D) Inulin and ^{125}I-albumin
    E) ^{51}Cr red blood cells and ^{125}I-albumin

71. Long-term administration of furosemide (Lasix) would do what?

    A) Inhibit the Na$^+$-Cl$^-$ co-transporter in the renal distal tubules
    B) Inhibit the Na$^+$-Cl$^-$-K$^+$ co-transporter in the renal tubules
    C) Tend to reduce renal concentrating ability
    D) Tend to cause hyperkalemia
    E) A and C
    F) B and C
    G) B, C, and D

72. A patient with normal lungs who has uncontrolled type 1 diabetes and a plasma glucose concentration of 400 mg/100 ml (normal ~100 mg/100 ml) would be expected to have which set of blood values?

	pH	HCO$_3^-$ (mmol/L)	P$_{CO_2}$ (mm Hg)	Na$^+$ (mmol/L)	Cl$^-$ (mmol/L)
A)	7.66	22	20	143	111
B)	7.52	38	48	146	100
C)	7.29	14	30	143	117
D)	7.25	12	28	142	102
E)	7.07	14	50	144	102

73. Which of the following would be expected to cause a decrease in extracellular fluid potassium concentration (hypokalemia) at least in part by stimulating potassium uptake into the cells?

    A) α-adrenergic blockade
    B) Insulin deficiency
    C) Strenuous exercise
    D) Aldosterone deficiency (Addison's disease)
    E) Metabolic alkalosis

74. If a person has a kidney transport maximum for glucose of 350 mg/min, a GFR of 100 ml/min, a plasma glucose level of 150 mg/dl, a urine flow rate of 2 ml/min, and no detectable glucose in the urine, what would be the approximate rate of glucose reabsorption, assuming normal kidneys?

    A) Glucose reabsorption cannot be estimated from these data
    B) 0 mg/min
    C) 50 mg/min
    D) 150 mg/min
    E) 350 mg/min

75. Which diuretic inhibits Na$^+$-2Cl$^-$-K$^+$ co-transport in the loop of Henle as its primary action?

    A) Thiazide diuretic
    B) Furosemide
    C) Carbonic anhydrase inhibitor
    D) Osmotic diuretic
    E) Amiloride
    F) Spironolactone

76. A selective decrease in *efferent* arteriolar resistance would _____ glomerular hydrostatic pressure, _____ GFR, and _____ renal blood flow.

    A) Increase, increase, increase
    B) Increase, decrease, increase
    C) Increase, decrease, decrease
    D) Decrease, increase, decrease
    E) Decrease, decrease, increase
    F) Decrease, increase, increase

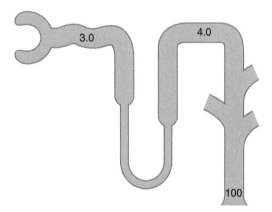

77. The above figure shows the concentration of inulin at different points along the renal tubule, expressed as the tubular fluid/plasma ratio of inulin concentration. If inulin is not reabsorbed, what is the approximate percentage of the filtered water that has been reabsorbed prior to the distal convoluted tubule?

    A) 25%
    B) 33%
    C) 66%
    D) 75%
    E) 99%
    F) 100%

78. A patient with renal tubular acidosis would be expected to have which set of blood values?

	pH	HCO$_3^-$ (mmol/L)	P$_{CO_2}$ (mm Hg)	Na$^+$ (mmol/L)	Cl$^-$ (mmol/L)
A)	7.66	22	20	143	111
B)	7.52	38	48	146	100
C)	7.07	14	50	144	102
D)	7.25	12	28	142	102
E)	7.29	14	30	143	117

79. A patient reports that he is always thirsty, and his breath has an acetone smell. You suspect that he has diabetes mellitus, and that diagnosis is confirmed by a urine sample that tests positive for glucose and a blood sample that shows a fasting blood glucose concentration of 400 mg/dl. Compared with normal, you would expect to find which changes in his urine?

	Urine pH	NH_4^+ Excretion	Urine volume (ml/24 h)	Renal HCO_3^- Production
A)	↓	↓	↓	↓
B)	↓	↑	↓	↓
C)	↑	↓	↓	↓
D)	↓	↑	↑	↑
E)	↑	↑	↑	↑

Questions 80–82

A person with normal body fluid volumes weighs 60 kg and has an extracellular fluid volume of approximately 12.8 L, a blood volume of 4.3 L, and a hematocrit of 0.4; 57% of his body weight is water. Use this information to answer Questions 80–82.

80. What is the approximate intracellular fluid volume?

    A) 17.1 liters
    B) 19.6 liters
    C) 21.4 liters
    D) 23.5 liters
    E) 25.6 liters

81. What is the approximate plasma volume?

    A) 2.0 liters
    B) 2.3 liters
    C) 2.6 liters
    D) 3.0 liters
    E) 3.3 liters

82. What is the approximate interstitial fluid volume?

    A) 6.4 liters
    B) 8.4 liters
    C) 10.2 liters
    D) 11.3 liters
    E) 12.0 liters

83. Which nephron segment is the primary site of magnesium reabsorption under normal conditions?

    A) Proximal tubule
    B) Descending limb of the loop of Henle
    C) Ascending limb of the loop of Henle
    D) Distal convoluted tubule
    E) Collecting ducts

84. The principal cells in the cortical collecting tubules

    A) Are the main site of action of the thiazide diuretics
    B) Have sodium-chloride-potassium co-transporters
    C) Are highly permeable to urea during antidiuresis
    D) Are an important site of action of amiloride
    E) Are the main site of action of furosemide

85. A patient has a GFR of 100 ml/min, her urine flow rate is 2.0 ml/min, and her plasma glucose concentration is 200 mg/100 ml. If the kidney transport maximum for glucose is 250 mg/min, what would be her approximate rate of glucose excretion?

    A) 0 mg/min
    B) 50 mg/min
    C) 100 mg/min
    D) 150 mg/min
    E) 200 mg/min
    F) 300 mg/min
    G) Glucose excretion rate cannot be estimated from these data

86. Which changes would you expect to find in a newly diagnosed 10-year-old patient with type 1 diabetes and uncontrolled hyperglycemia (plasma glucose = 300 mg/dl)?

	Thirst (Water Intake)	Urine Volume	Glomerular Filtration Rate	Afferent Arteriolar Resistance
A)	↑	↓	↑	↓
B)	↑	↑	↓	↑
C)	↑	↑	↑	↓
D)	↓	↑	↑	↑
E)	↓	↓	↓	↓

Questions 87 and 88

To evaluate kidney function in a 45-year-old woman with type 2 diabetes, you ask her to collect her urine for a 24-hour period. She collects 3600 milliliters of urine in that period. The clinical laboratory returns the following results after analyzing the patient's urine and plasma samples: plasma creatinine = 4 mg/dl, urine creatinine = 32 mg/dl, plasma potassium = 5 mmol/L, and urine potassium = 10 mmol/L.

87. What is this patient's approximate GFR, assuming that she collected all her urine in the 24-hour period?

    A) 10 ml/min
    B) 20 ml/min
    C) 30 ml/min
    D) 40 ml/min
    E) 80 ml/min

88. What is the net renal tubular reabsorption rate of potassium in this patient?

    A) 1.050 mmol/min
    B) 0.100 mmol/min
    C) 0.037 mmol/min
    D) 0.075 mmol/min
    E) Potassium is not reabsorbed in this example

Questions 89–93

Match each of the patients described in Questions 89–93 with the correct set of blood values in the following table (the same values may be used for more than one patient).

	pH	HCO_3^- (mEq/L)	P_{CO_2} (mm Hg)	Na^+ (mEq/L)	Cl^- (mEq/L)
A)	7.66	22	20	143	111
B)	7.28	30	65	142	102
C)	7.24	12	29	144	102
D)	7.29	14	30	143	117
E)	7.52	38	48	146	100
F)	7.07	14	50	144	102

89. A patient with severe diarrhea

90. A patient with primary aldosteronism

91. A patient with proximal renal tubular acidosis

92. A patient with diabetic ketoacidosis and emphysema

93. A patient treated chronically with a carbonic anhydrase inhibitor

94. Which change would you expect to find in a patient who developed acute renal failure after ingesting poisonous mushrooms that caused renal tubular necrosis?

    A) Increased plasma bicarbonate concentration
    B) Metabolic acidosis
    C) Decreased plasma potassium concentration
    D) Decreased blood urea nitrogen concentration
    E) Decreased hydrostatic pressure in Bowman's capsule

95. The type A intercalated cells in the collecting tubules

    A) Are highly permeable to urea during antidiuresis
    B) Secrete K^+
    C) Secrete H^+
    D) Are the main site of action of furosemide
    E) Are the main site of action of thiazide diuretics

96. Which of the following would be the most likely cause of hypernatremia associated with a small volume of highly concentrated urine (osmolarity = 1400 mOsm/L) in a person with normal kidneys?

    A) Primary aldosteronism
    B) Diabetes mellitus
    C) Diabetes insipidus
    D) Dehydration due to insufficient water intake and heavy exercise
    E) Bartter's syndrome
    F) Liddle's syndrome

97. The most serious hypokalemia would occur in which condition?

    A) Decrease in potassium intake from 150 to 60 mEq/day
    B) Increase in sodium intake from 100 to 200 mEq/day
    C) Fourfold increase in aldosterone secretion plus high sodium intake
    D) Fourfold increase in aldosterone secretion plus low sodium intake
    E) Addison's disease

98. Which of the following has similar values for both intracellular and interstitial body fluids?

    A) Potassium ion concentration
    B) Colloid osmotic pressure
    C) Sodium ion concentration
    D) Chloride ion concentration
    E) Total osmolarity

99. Which of the following is true of the tubular fluid that passes through the lumen of the early distal tubule in the region of the macula densa?

    A) It is usually isotonic
    B) It is usually hypotonic
    C) It is usually hypertonic
    D) It is hypertonic in antidiuresis
    E) It is hypertonic when the filtration rate of its own nephron decreases to 50% below normal

100. In a person with normal kidneys and normal lungs who has chronic metabolic acidosis, you would expect to find all of the following, compared with normal, *except*:

    A) Increased renal excretion of NH_4Cl
    B) Decreased urine pH
    C) Decreased urine HCO_3^- excretion
    D) Increased plasma HCO_3^- concentration
    E) Decreased plasma P_{CO_2}

101. In a patient with very high levels of aldosterone and otherwise normal kidney function, approximately what percentage of the filtered load of sodium would be reabsorbed by the distal convoluted tubule and collecting duct?

    A) >66%
    B) 40% to 60%
    C) 20% to 40%
    D) 10% to 20%
    E) <10%

Questions 102–104

The following test results were obtained: urine flow rate = 2.0 ml/min; urine inulin concentration = 60 mg/ml; plasma inulin concentration = 2 mg/ml; urine potassium concentration = 20 μmol/ml; plasma potassium concentration = 4.0 μmol/ml; urine osmolarity = 150 mOsm/L; and plasma osmolarity = 300 mOsm/L.

102. What is the approximate GFR?

    A) 20 ml/min
    B) 25 ml/min
    C) 30 ml/min
    D) 60 ml/min
    E) 75 ml/min
    F) 150 ml/min

103. What is the net potassium reabsorption rate?

    A) 0 μmol/min
    B) 20 μmol/min
    C) 60 μmol/min
    D) 200 μmol/min
    E) 240 μmol/min
    F) 300 μmol/min
    G) Potassium is not reabsorbed in this case

104. What is the free water clearance rate?

    A) +1.0 ml/min
    B) +1.5 ml/min
    C) +2.0 ml/min
    D) −1.0 ml/min
    E) −1.5 ml/min
    F) −2.0 ml/min

105. Assume that you have a patient who needs fluid therapy and you decide to administer by intravenous infusion 2.0 liters of 0.45% NaCl solution (molecular weight NaCl = 58.5). After osmotic equilibrium, which changes would you expect, compared with before infusion of the NaCl?

	Intracellular Volume	Intracellular Osmolarity	Extracellular Volume	Extracellular Osmolarity
A)	↑	↑	↑	↑
B)	↑	↓	↑	↓
C)	↔	↑	↑	↑
D)	↓	↑	↑	↑
E)	↓	↓	↓	↓

106. If the renal clearance of substance X is 300 ml/min and the glomerular filtration rate is 100 ml/min, it is most likely that substance X is

    A) Filtered freely but not secreted or reabsorbed
    B) Bound to plasma proteins
    C) Secreted
    D) Reabsorbed
    E) Bound to tubular proteins
    F) Clearance of a substance cannot be greater than the GFR

107. Which change tends to increase urinary calcium (Ca^{++}) excretion?

    A) Extracellular fluid volume expansion
    B) Increased plasma parathyroid hormone concentration
    C) Decreased blood pressure
    D) Increased plasma phosphate concentration
    E) Metabolic alkalosis

108. Which change would you expect to find in a patient consuming a high-sodium diet (200 mEq/day) compared with the same patient on a normal-sodium diet (100 mEq/day), assuming steady-state conditions?

    A) Increased plasma aldosterone concentration
    B) Increased urinary potassium excretion
    C) Decreased plasma renin activity
    D) Decreased plasma atrial natriuretic peptide
    E) An increase in plasma sodium concentration of at least 5 mmol/L

109. What would tend to decrease GFR by more than 10% in a normal kidney?

    A) Decrease in renal arterial pressure from 100 to 85 mm Hg
    B) 50% decrease in afferent arteriolar resistance
    C) 50% decrease in efferent arteriolar resistance
    D) 50% increase in the glomerular capillary filtration coefficient
    E) Decrease in plasma colloid osmotic pressure from 28 to 20 mm Hg

110. Acute metabolic acidosis tends to _____ intracellular K^+ concentration and _____ K^+ secretion by the cortical collecting tubules.

    A) Increase, increase
    B) Increase, decrease
    C) Decrease, increase
    D) Decrease, decrease
    E) Cause no change in, increase
    F) Cause no change in, cause no change in

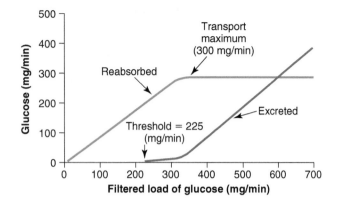

	Sodium Excretion Rate	Cr Excretion Rate	Cr Clearance	Filtered Load Cr	Plasma Cr Concentration
A)	↓	↓	↔	↔	↑
B)	↓	↓	↓	↓	↑
C)	↔	↔	↓	↓	↑
D)	↔	↔	↓	↓	↔
E)	↔	↔	↓	↔	↑
F)	↔	↔	↔	↔	↑

111. A 55-year-old overweight male patient reports frequent urination, and his blood pressure is 165/98 mm Hg. Based on 24-hour creatinine clearance, you estimate his GFR to be 150 ml/min. His plasma glucose is 400 mg/100 ml. Assuming that his renal transport maximum for glucose is normal, as shown in the above figure, what would be the approximate rate of urinary glucose excretion for this patient?

A) 0 mg/min
B) 100 mg/min
C) 150 mg/min
D) 225 mg/min
E) 300 mg/min
F) The information provided is inadequate to estimate the glucose excretion rate

112. Which statement is true?

A) ADH increases water reabsorption from the ascending loop of Henle
B) Water reabsorption from the descending loop of Henle is normally less than that from the ascending loop of Henle
C) Sodium reabsorption from the ascending loop of Henle is normally less than that from the descending loop of Henle
D) Osmolarity of fluid in the early distal tubule would be less than 300 mOsm/L in a dehydrated person with normal kidneys and increased ADH levels
E) ADH decreases the urea permeability in the medullary collecting tubules

113. You have been monitoring a patient with type 2 diabetes and chronic renal disease whose GFR has decreased from 80 ml/min to 40 ml/min during the past 4 years. Which of the following changes in sodium and creatinine (Cr) would you expect to find compared with 4 years ago, before the decline in GFR, assuming steady-state conditions and no change in electrolyte intake or protein metabolism?

114. In a person on a high-potassium (200 mmol/day) diet, which part of the nephron would be expected to secrete the most potassium?

A) Proximal tubule
B) Descending loop of Henle
C) Ascending loop of Henle
D) Early distal tubule
E) Collecting tubules

115. Which of the following would you expect to find in a patient who has chronic diabetic ketoacidosis?

A) Decreased renal HCO_3^- excretion, increased NH_4^+ excretion, increased plasma anion gap
B) Increased respiration rate, decreased arterial P_{CO_2}, decreased plasma anion gap
C) Increased NH_4^+ excretion, increased plasma anion gap, increased urine pH
D) Increased renal HCO_3^- production, increased NH_4^+ excretion, decreased plasma anion gap
E) Decreased urine pH, decreased renal HCO_3^- excretion, increased arterial P_{CO_2}

116. A patient has a creatinine clearance of 100 ml/min, a plasma K^+ concentration of 4.0 mmol/L, a urine flow rate of 2.0 ml/min, and a urine K^+ concentration of 60 mmol/L. What is his approximate rate of potassium excretion?

A) 0.12 mmol/min
B) 0.16 mmol/min
C) 0.32 mmol/min
D) 8.0 mmol/min
E) 120 mmol/min
F) 400 mmol/min

117. Using the indicator dilution method to assess body fluid volumes in a 40-year-old man weighing 70 kg, the inulin space is calculated to be 16 liters and ^{125}I-albumin space is 4 liters. If 60% of his total body weight is water, what is his approximate interstitial fluid volume?

A) 4 liters
B) 12 liters
C) 16 liters
D) 26 liters
E) 38 liters
F) 42 liters

118. What would tend to decrease plasma potassium concentration by causing a shift of potassium from the extracellular fluid into the cells?

A) Strenuous exercise
B) Aldosterone deficiency
C) Acidosis
D) β-adrenergic blockade
E) Insulin excess

119. A 26-year-old construction worker is brought to the emergency department with a change in mental status after working a 10-hour shift on a hot summer day (average outside temperature was 97°F [36°C]). The man had been sweating profusely during the day but did not drink fluids. He has a fever of 102°F [39°C], a heart rate of 140 beats/min, and a blood pressure of 100/55 mm Hg in the supine position. Upon examination, he has no perspiration, appears to have dry mucous membranes, and is poorly oriented to person, place, and time. Assuming that his kidneys were normal yesterday, which set of hormone levels describes his condition, compared with normal?

A) High ADH, high renin, low angiotensin II, low aldosterone
B) Low ADH, low renin, low angiotensin II, low aldosterone
C) High ADH, low renin, high angiotensin II, low aldosterone
D) High ADH, high renin, high angiotensin II, high aldosterone
E) Low ADH, high renin, low angiotensin II, high aldosterone

120. A 23-year-old man runs a 10-kilometer race in July and loses 2 liters of fluid by sweating. He also drinks 2 liters of water during the race. Which changes would you expect, compared with normal, after he absorbs the water and assuming osmotic equilibrium and no excretion of water or electrolytes?

	Intracellular Volume	Intracellular Osmolarity	Extracellular Volume	Extracellular Osmolarity
A)	↓	↑	↓	↑
B)	↓	↓	↓	↓
C)	↔	↓	↔	↓
D)	↔	↑	↓	↑
E)	↑	↓	↓	↓
F)	↑	↓	↑	↓

121. Which change would tend to increase Ca^{2+} reabsorption in the renal tubule?

A) Extracellular fluid volume expansion
B) Increased plasma parathyroid hormone concentration
C) Increased blood pressure
D) Decreased plasma phosphate concentration
E) Metabolic acidosis

122. A patient has the following laboratory values: arterial pH = 7.04, plasma $HCO_3^- $ = 13 mEq/L, plasma chloride concentration = 120 mEq/L, arterial P_{CO_2} = 30 mm Hg, and plasma sodium = 141 mEq/L. What is the most likely cause of his acidosis?

A) Emphysema
B) Methanol poisoning
C) Salicylic acid poisoning
D) Diarrhea
E) Diabetes mellitus

123. A young man is found comatose, having taken an unknown number of sleeping pills an unknown time before. An arterial blood sample yields the following values: pH = 7.02, HCO_3^- = 14 mEq/L, and P_{CO_2} = 68 mm Hg. Which of the following describes this patient's acid-base status most accurately?

A) Uncompensated metabolic acidosis
B) Uncompensated respiratory acidosis
C) Simultaneous respiratory and metabolic acidosis
D) Respiratory acidosis with partial renal compensation
E) Respiratory acidosis with complete renal compensation

124. If the GFR suddenly decreases from 150 ml/min to 75 ml/min and tubular fluid reabsorption simultaneously decreases from 149 ml/min to 75 ml/min, which change will occur (assuming that the changes in GFR and tubular fluid reabsorption are maintained)?

A) Urine flow rate will decrease to 0
B) Urine flow rate will decrease by 50%
C) Urine flow rate will not change
D) Urine flow rate will increase by 50%

125. In a person with chronic respiratory acidosis who has partial renal compensation, you would expect to find which changes, compared with normal: _____ urinary excretion of NH_4^+; _____ plasma HCO_3^- concentration; and _____ urine pH.

A) Increased, increased, decreased
B) Increased, decreased, decreased
C) No change in, increased, decreased
D) No change in, no change in, decreased
E) Increased, no change in, increased

126. At which renal tubular sites would the concentration of creatinine be expected to be highest in a normally hydrated person?

A) The concentration would be the same in all renal tubular segments because creatinine is neither secreted nor reabsorbed
B) Glomerular filtrate
C) End of the proximal tubule
D) End of the loop of Henle
E) Distal tubule
F) Collecting duct

Questions 127 and 128

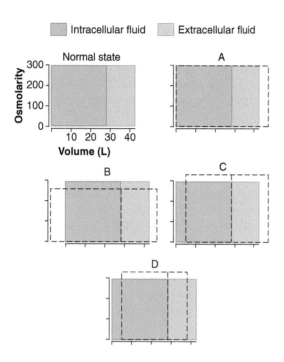

The figure above represents various states of abnormal hydration. In each diagram, the normal state (orange and lavender) is superimposed on the abnormal state (dashed lines) to illustrate the shifts in the volume (width of rectangles) and total osmolarity (height of rectangles) of the extracellular fluid and intracellular fluid compartments.

127. Which diagram represents the changes (after osmotic equilibrium) in extracellular and intracellular fluid volume and osmolarity after infusion of 2 liters of 3.0% dextrose?

    A) A
    B) B
    C) C
    D) D

128. Which diagram represents the changes (after osmotic equilibrium) in extracellular and intracellular fluid volume and osmolarity in a patient with severe "central" diabetes insipidus?

    A) A
    B) B
    C) C
    D) D

129. Increases in both renal blood flow and GFR are caused by which mechanism?

    A) Dilation of the afferent arterioles
    B) Increased glomerular capillary filtration coefficient
    C) Increased plasma colloid osmotic pressure
    D) Dilation of the efferent arterioles

130. If the cortical collecting tubule tubular fluid inulin concentration is 40 mg/100 ml and plasma concentration of inulin is 2.0 mg/100 ml, what is the approximate percentage of the filtered water that remains in the tubule at that point?

    A) 0%
    B) 2%
    C) 5%
    D) 10%
    E) 20%
    F) 100%

131. A 55-year-old male patient with hypertension has had his blood pressure reasonably well controlled by administration of a thiazide diuretic. At his last visit (6 months ago), his blood pressure was 130/75 mm Hg and his serum creatinine was 1 mg/100 ml. He has been exercising regularly for the past 2 years but recently has reported knee pain and began taking large amounts of a nonsteroidal anti-inflammatory drug. When he arrives at your office, his blood pressure is 155/85 mm Hg and his serum creatinine is 2.5 mg/100 ml. What best explains his increased serum creatinine level?

    A) Increased efferent arteriolar resistance that reduced GFR
    B) Increased afferent arteriolar resistance that reduced GFR
    C) Increased glomerular capillary filtration coefficient that reduced GFR
    D) Increased angiotensin II formation that decreased GFR
    E) Increased muscle mass due to the exercise

132. An elderly patient reports muscle weakness and lethargy. A urine specimen reveals a Na^+ concentration of 600 mmol/L and an osmolarity of 1200 mOsm/L. Additional laboratory tests provide the following information: plasma Na^+ concentration = 167 mmol/L, plasma renin activity = 4 ng angiotensin I/ml/h (normal = 1), plasma ADH = 60 pg/ml (normal = 3 pg/ml), and plasma aldosterone = 15 ng/dl (normal = 6 ng/dl). What is the most likely reason for this patient's hypernatremia?

    A) Dehydration caused by decreased fluid intake
    B) Syndrome of inappropriate ADH
    C) Nephrogenic diabetes insipidus
    D) Primary aldosteronism
    E) Renin-secreting tumor

1. C) A 3% NaCl solution is hypertonic, and when infused intravenously, it would increase extracellular fluid volume and osmolarity, thereby causing water to flow out of the cell. This action would decrease intracellular fluid volume and further increase extracellular fluid volume. The 0.9% NaCl solution and 5% dextrose solution are isotonic and therefore would not reduce intracellular fluid volume. Pure water and the 0.45% NaCl solution are hypotonic, and when infused, they would increase both intracellular and extracellular fluid volumes.

TMP13 pp. 311-314

2. B) Partial obstruction of a major vein draining a tissue would increase capillary hydrostatic pressure in the tissue, which, in turn, would raise capillary fluid filtration and cause increases interstitial fluid volume, interstitial fluid hydrostatic pressure, and lymph flow. The increased lymph flow would "wash out" proteins from the interstitial fluid, decreasing interstitial fluid protein concentration.

TMP 13 p. 317

3. C) The hypernatremia (plasma Na^+ = 165 mmol/L) associated with a low blood pressure (88/44 mm Hg) suggests dehydration. The frequent urination and low urine specific gravity (1.003, which implies a urine osmolarity of about 100-120 mOsm/L) despite hypernatremia and dehydration suggests diabetes insipidus due to either insufficient secretion of ADH (central diabetes insipidus) or failure of the kidneys to respond to ADH (nephrogenic diabetes insipidus).

TMP 13 pp. 315-316, 378-379, 438-439

4. D) A severe renal artery stenosis that reduces GFR to 25% of normal would also decrease renal blood flow but would cause only a transient decrease in urinary creatinine excretion. The transient decrease in creatinine excretion would increase serum creatinine (to about four times normal), which would restore the filtered creatinine load to normal and therefore return urinary creatinine excretion to normal levels under steady-state conditions. Urinary sodium secretion would also decrease transiently but would be restored to normal so that intake and excretion of sodium are balanced. Plasma sodium concentration would not change significantly because it is carefully regulated by the ADH–thirst mechanism.

TMP13 pp. 366, 435-436

5. B) A 1% solution of dextrose is hypotonic, and when infused, it would increase both intracellular and extracellular fluid volumes while decreasing the osmolarity of these compartments.

TMP13 pp. 311-313

6. B) Excessive secretion of ADH would increase renal tubular reabsorption of water, thereby increasing extracellular fluid volume and reducing extracellular fluid osmolarity. The reduced osmolarity, in turn, would cause water to flow into the cells and raise intracellular fluid volume. In the steady state, both extracellular and intracellular fluid volumes would increase, and osmolarity of both compartments would decrease.

TMP13 pp. 314, 381-382

7. C) A 3% solution of NaCl is hypertonic, and when infused into the extracellular fluid, it would raise osmolarity, thereby causing water to flow out of the cells into the extracellular fluid until osmotic equilibrium is achieved. In the steady state, extracellular fluid volume would increase, intracellular fluid volume would decrease, and osmolarity of both compartments would increase.

TMP13 pp. 311-312

8. C) Aldosterone stimulates potassium secretion by the principal cells of the collecting tubules. Therefore, blockade of the action of aldosterone with spironolactone would inhibit potassium secretion. Other factors that stimulate potassium secretion by the cortical collecting tubule include increased potassium concentration, increased cortical collecting tubule flow rate (as would occur with high sodium intake or a diuretic that reduces proximal tubular sodium reabsorption), and acute alkalosis.

TMP13 pp. 392-396

9. C) Phosphate excretion by the kidneys is controlled by an overflow mechanism. When the transport maximum for reabsorbing phosphate is exceeded, the remaining phosphate in the renal tubules is excreted in the urine and can be used to buffer hydrogen ions and form titratable acid. Phosphate normally begins to spill into the urine when the concentration of extracellular fluid rises above a threshold of 0.8 mmol/L, which is usually exceeded.

TMP13 pp. 397-398

10. B) GFR is equal to inulin clearance, which is calculated as the urine inulin concentration (100 mg/ml) × urine flow rate (1 ml/min)/plasma inulin concentration (2 mg/ml), which is equal to 50 ml/min.

TMP13 p. 365

11. **D)** The net urea reabsorption rate is equal to the filtered load of urea (GFR [50 ml/min] × plasma urea concentration [2.5 mg/ml]) − urinary excretion rate of urea (urine urea concentration [50 mg/ml] × urine flow rate [1 ml/min]). Therefore, net urea reabsorption = (50 ml/min × 2.5 mg/ml) − (50 mg/ml × 1 ml/min) = 75 mg/min.
    TMP13 p. 365

12. **A)** K^+ excretion rate = urine K^+ concentration (60 mEq/L) × urine flow rate (0.001 L/min) = 0.06 mEq/min.
    TMP13 p. 365

13. **E)** Filtration fraction (FF) = GFR ÷ Renal plasma flow (RPF).

    GFR= K_f × $(P_G − P_B − \pi_G)$ = 10 × (70 − 20 − 35) = 150 ml/min

    FF = 150 ml/min ÷ 428 ml/min = 0.35
    TMP13 pp. 337-338

14. **B)** As water flows up the ascending limb of the loop of Henle, solutes are reabsorbed, but this segment is relatively impermeable to water; progressive dilution of the tubular fluid occurs so that the osmolarity decreases to approximately 100 mOsm/L by the time the fluid reaches the early distal tubule. Even during maximal antidiuresis, this portion of the renal tubule is relatively impermeable to water and is therefore called the diluting segment of the renal tubule.
    TMP13 pp. 378-379

15. **C)** In the absence of ADH secretion, a marked increase in urine volume occurs because the late distal and collecting tubules are relatively impermeable to water. As a result of increased urine volume, there is dehydration and increased plasma osmolarity and high plasma sodium concentration. The resulting decrease in extracellular fluid volume stimulates renin secretion, resulting in an increase in plasma renin concentration.
    TMP13 p. 380

16. **C)** When potassium intake is doubled (from 80 to 160 mmol/day), potassium excretion also approximately doubles within a few days, and the plasma potassium concentration increases only slightly. Increased potassium excretion is achieved largely by increased secretion of potassium in the cortical collecting tubule. Increased aldosterone concentration plays a significant role in increasing potassium secretion and in maintaining a relatively constant plasma potassium concentration during increases in potassium intake. Sodium excretion does not change markedly during chronic increases in potassium intake.
    TMP13 pp. 392-396

17. **D)** Most of the daily variation in potassium excretion is caused by changes in potassium secretion in the late distal tubules and collecting tubules. Therefore, when the dietary intake of potassium increases, the total body balance of potassium is maintained primarily by an increase in potassium secretion in these tubular segments. Increased potassium intake has little effect on GFR or on reabsorption of potassium in the proximal tubule and loop of Henle. Although high potassium intake may cause a slight shift of potassium into the intracellular compartment, a balance between intake and output must be achieved by increasing the excretion of potassium during high potassium intake.
    TMP13 pp. 390-391

18. **E)** A 50% decrease in efferent arteriolar resistance would cause a substantial decrease in GFR. A decrease in renal arterial pressure from 100 to 80 mm Hg in a normal kidney would cause only a slight reduction in GFR in a normal kidney because of autoregulation. All of the other changes would tend to increase GFR.
    TMP13 pp. 337-339

19. **A)** The patient described has protein in the urine (proteinuria) and reduced plasma protein concentration as a result of glomerulonephritis caused by an untreated streptococcal infection ("strep throat"). The reduced plasma protein concentration, in turn, decreased the plasma colloid osmotic pressure and resulted in leakage from the plasma to the interstitium. The extracellular fluid edema raised interstitial fluid pressure and interstitial fluid volume, causing increased lymph flow and decreased interstitial fluid protein concentration. Increasing lymph flow causes a "washout" of the interstitial fluid protein as a safety factor against edema. The decreased blood volume would tend to lower blood pressure and stimulate the secretion of renin by the kidneys, raising the plasma renin concentration.
    TMP13 pp. 317-320

20. **C)** In a patient with a very high rate of renin secretion, there would also be increased formation of angiotensin II, which in turn would stimulate aldosterone secretion. The increased levels of angiotensin II and aldosterone would cause a transient decrease in sodium excretion, which would cause expansion of the extracellular fluid volume and increased arterial pressure. The increased arterial pressure, as well as other compensations, would return sodium excretion to normal so that intake and output are balanced. Therefore, under steady-state conditions, sodium excretion would be normal and equal to sodium intake. The increased aldosterone concentration would cause hypokalemia (decreased plasma potassium concentration), whereas the high level of angiotensin II would cause renal vasoconstriction and decreased renal blood flow.
    TMP13 pp. 399-401

21. **B)** This patient has respiratory acidosis because the plasma pH is lower than the normal level of 7.4 and the plasma P_{CO_2} is higher than the normal level of 40 mm Hg (see table below). The elevation in plasma bicarbonate concentration above normal (~24 mEq/L) is due to partial renal compensation for the respiratory acidosis. Therefore, this patient has respiratory acidosis with partial renal compensation.

   TMP12 pp. 421-422

Characteristics of Primary Acid-Base Disturbances

	pH	H+	P_{CO_2}	HCO_3^-
Normal	7.4	40 mEq/L	40 mm Hg	24 mEq/L
Respiratory acidosis	↓	↑	↑↑	↑
Respiratory alkalosis	↑	↓	↓↓	↓
Metabolic acidosis	↓	↑	↓	↓↓
Metabolic alkalosis	↑	↓	↑	↑↑

The primary event is indicated by the double arrows (↑↑ or ↓↓). Note that respiratory acid-base disorders are initiated by an increase or decrease in P_{CO_2}, whereas metabolic disorders are initiated by an increase or decrease in HCO_3^-.

22. **D)** GFR is approximately equal to creatinine clearance, which is calculated as the urine creatinine concentration (50 mg/100 ml) × urine flow rate (3 ml/min)/plasma creatinine concentration (3 mg/100 ml), which is equal to 50 ml/min. Urine flow rate = 4320 ml/24 h = 4320 ml/1440 min = 3 ml/min.

   TMP12, pp. 366-367

23. **D)** An important compensation for respiratory acidosis is increased renal production of NH_4^+ and increased NH_4^+ excretion. In acidosis, urinary excretion of HCO_3^- would be reduced, as would urine pH, and urinary titratable acid would be slightly increased as a compensatory response to the acidosis.

   TMP13 pp. 418-419

24. **C)** Because the patient has a low plasma pH (normal = 7.4), he has acidosis. The fact that his plasma bicarbonate concentration is also low (normal = 24 mEq/L) indicates that he has metabolic acidosis. However, he also appears to have respiratory acidosis because his plasma P_{CO_2} is high (normal = 40 mm Hg). The rise in P_{CO_2} is due to his impaired breathing as a result of cardiopulmonary arrest. Therefore, the patient has a mixed acidosis with combined metabolic and respiratory acidosis.

   TMP13 pp. 422-426

25. **B)** Inhibition of aldosterone causes hyperkalemia by two mechanisms: (1) shifting potassium out of the cells into the extracellular fluid, and (2) decreasing cortical collecting tubular secretion of potassium. Increasing potassium intake from 60 to 180 mmol/day would cause only a very small increase in plasma potassium concentration in a person with normal kidneys and normal aldosterone feedback mechanisms (see TMP13 **Figs. 30-7 and 30-8**). A reduction in sodium intake also has very little effect on plasma potassium concentration. Chronic treatment with a diuretic that inhibits loop of Henle Na^+-$2Cl^-$-K^+ cotransport would tend to cause potassium loss in the urine and hypokalemia. However, chronic treatment with a diuretic that inhibits sodium reabsorption in the collecting ducts, such as amiloride, would have little effect on plasma potassium concentration.

   TMP13 pp. 393-394

26. **D)** Excessive activity of the amiloride-sensitive sodium channel in the collecting tubules would cause a transient decrease in sodium excretion and expansion of extracellular fluid volume, which in turn would increase arterial pressure and decrease renin secretion, leading to decreased aldosterone secretion. Under steady-state conditions, sodium excretion would return to normal so that intake and renal excretion of sodium are balanced. One of the mechanisms that re-establishes this balance between intake and output of sodium is the rise in arterial pressure that induces a "pressure natriuresis."

   TMP13 pp. 399-401, 439-440

27. **A)** Primary excessive secretion of aldosterone (Conn's syndrome) would be associated with marked hypokalemia and metabolic alkalosis (increased plasma pH). Because aldosterone stimulates sodium reabsorption and potassium secretion by the cortical collecting tubule, there could be a transient decrease in sodium excretion and an increase in potassium excretion, but under steady-state conditions, both urinary sodium and potassium excretion would return to normal to match the intake of these electrolytes. However, the sodium retention and the hypertension associated with aldosterone excess would tend to reduce renin secretion.

   TMP13 pp. 392, 404

28. **B)** A doubling of plasma creatinine implies that the creatinine clearance and GFR have been reduced by approximately 50%. Although the reduction in creatinine clearance would initially cause a transient decrease in filtered load of creatinine, creatinine excretion rate, and sodium excretion rate, the plasma concentration of creatinine would increase until the filtered load of creatinine and the creatinine excretion rate returned to normal. However, creatinine clearance would remain reduced because creatinine clearance is

the urinary excretion rate of creatinine divided by the plasma creatinine concentration. Urinary sodium excretion would also return to normal and would equal the sodium intake, under steady-state conditions, as a result of compensatory mechanisms that reduce renal tubular reabsorption of sodium.

TMP13 pp. 366, 435-436

29. **C)** The glomerular capillary filtration coefficient is the product of the hydraulic conductivity and surface area of the glomerular capillaries. Therefore, increasing the glomerular capillary filtration coefficient tends to increase GFR. Increased afferent arteriolar resistance, decreased efferent arteriolar resistance, increased Bowman's capsule hydrostatic pressure, and decreased glomerular hydrostatic pressure tend to decrease GFR.

TMP13 pp. 337-340

30. **D)** Impairment of proximal tubular NaCl reabsorption would increase NaCl delivery to the macula densa, which in turn would cause a tubuloglomerular feedback–mediated increase in afferent arteriolar resistance. The increased afferent arteriolar resistance would decrease the GFR. Initially there would be a transient increase in sodium excretion, but after 3 weeks, steady-state conditions would be achieved. Sodium excretion would equal sodium intake, and no significant change would occur in urinary sodium excretion.

TMP13 pp. 343-345

31. **D)** The net potassium reabsorption rate is equal to the filtered load of urea (GFR [50 ml/min] × plasma potassium concentration [4 mmol/L]) – urinary excretion rate of potassium (urine potassium concentration [30 mmol/L] × urine flow rate [3 ml/min]). Therefore, net potassium reabsorption = (0.050 L/min × 4 mmol/L) – (30 mmol/L × 0.003 L/min) = 0.110 mmol/min. In this example the flow terms for GFR and urine flow rate are converted to L/min because the concentrations of potassium are in mmol/L.

TMP13 pp. 365-367

32. **D)** If a substance is completely cleared from the plasma, the clearance rate of that substance would equal the total renal plasma flow. In other words, the total amount of substance delivered to the kidneys in the blood (renal plasma flow × concentration of substance in the blood) would equal the amount of that substance excreted in the urine. Complete renal clearance of a substance would require both glomerular filtration and tubular secretion of that substance.

TMP13 pp. 365-368

33. **C)** The patient has a lower than normal pH and is therefore acidotic. Because the plasma bicarbonate concentration is also lower than normal, the patient has metabolic acidosis with respiratory compensation (i.e., P_{CO_2} is lower than normal). The plasma anion gap (Na^+-Cl^--HCO_3^- = 10 mEq/L) is in the normal range, suggesting

that the metabolic acidosis is not caused by excess nonvolatile acids such as salicylic acid or ketoacids caused by diabetes mellitus. Therefore, the most likely cause of the metabolic acidosis is diarrhea, which would cause a loss of HCO_3^- in the feces and would be associated with a normal anion gap and a hyperchloremic (increased chloride concentration) metabolic acidosis.

TMP13 pp. 422, 426

34. **A)** A 50% reduction of GFR would approximately double the plasma creatinine concentration because creatinine is not reabsorbed or secreted and its excretion depends largely on glomerular filtration. Therefore, when GFR decreases, the plasma concentration of creatinine increases until the renal excretion of creatinine returns to normal. Plasma concentrations of glucose, potassium, sodium, and hydrogen ions are closely regulated by multiple mechanisms that keep them relatively constant even when GFR falls to very low levels. Plasma phosphate concentration is also maintained near normal until GFR falls to below 20% to 30% of normal.

TMP13 pp. 366, 435-436

35. **C)** Calculation of fluid shifts and osmolarities after infusion of hypertonic saline solution is discussed in Chapter 25 of TMP13 (pp. 312-314). The tables shown above represent the initial conditions and the final conditions after infusion of 2 liters of 3% NaCl and osmotic equilibrium. Three percent NaCl is equal to 30 grams of NaCl/L, or 0.513 mol/L (513 mmol/L). Because NaCl has two osmotically active particles per mole, the net effect is to add a total of 2052 millimoles in 2 liters of solution. As an approximation, one can assume that cell membranes are impermeable to the NaCl and that the NaCl infused remains in the extracellular fluid compartment.

TMP13 pp. 311-314

36. **B)** Extracellular fluid volume is calculated by dividing the total milliosmoles in the extracellular compartment (5172 mOsm) by the concentration after osmotic equilibrium (300 mOsm/L) to give 17.2 liters.

TMP13 pp. 311-314

37. **C)** A 50% reduction in afferent arteriolar resistance with no change in arterial pressure would increase renal blood flow and glomerular hydrostatic pressure, thereby increasing GFR. At the same time, the reduction in afferent arteriolar resistance would raise peritubular capillary hydrostatic pressure.

TMP13 pp. 338-340

38. **A)** The net filtration pressure at the glomerular capillaries is equal to the sum of the forces favoring filtration (glomerular capillary hydrostatic pressure) minus the forces that oppose filtration (hydrostatic pressure in Bowman's space and glomerular colloid osmotic pressure). Therefore, the net pressure driving glomerular filtration is 50 – 12 – 30 = 8 mm Hg.

TMP13 p. 337

39. D) Uncontrolled diabetes mellitus results in increased blood acetoacetic acid levels, which in turn cause metabolic acidosis and decreased plasma HCO_3^- and pH. The acidosis causes several compensatory responses, including increased respiratory rate, which reduces plasma P_{CO_2}; increased renal NH^+ production, which leads to increased NH^+ excretion; and increased phosphate buffering of hydrogen ions secreted by the renal tubules, which increases titratable acid excretion.

TMP13 p. 422

40. B) Infusion of a hypotonic solution of NaCl would initially increase extracellular fluid volume and decrease extracellular fluid osmolarity. The reduction in extracellular fluid osmolarity would cause osmotic flow of fluid into the cells, thereby increasing intracellular fluid volume and decreasing intracellular fluid osmolarity after osmotic equilibrium.

TMP13 pp. 312-314

41. A) For any given molecular radius, positively charged molecules (cations) are filtered more readily than negatively charged molecules (anions) because negative charges on the proteins of the basement membrane and podocytes of the glomerular capillaries tend to repel large negatively changed molecules (e.g., polycationic dextrans, curve C). Large positively charged molecules (curve A) are filtered more readily.

TMP 13 p. 336

42. C) Because water is reabsorbed by the renal tubules whereas creatinine is not reabsorbed, the concentration of creatinine in the renal tubular fluid will increase as fluid flows from the proximal to the distal tubule. An increase in the concentration from 1.0 mg/100 ml in the proximal tubule to 5.0 mg/100 ml in the distal tubule means that only about one fifth (20%) of the water that was in the proximal tubules remains in the distal tubule.

TMP 13 p. 354

43. C) Peritubular capillary fluid reabsorption is determined by the balance of hydrostatic and colloid osmotic forces in the peritubular capillaries. Increased efferent arteriolar resistance reduces peritubular capillary hydrostatic pressure and therefore increases the net force favoring fluid reabsorption. Increased blood pressure tends to raise peritubular capillary hydrostatic pressure and reduce fluid reabsorption. Decreased filtration fraction increases the peritubular capillary colloid osmotic pressure and tends to reduce peritubular capillary reabsorption. Decreased angiotensin II causes vasodilatation of efferent arterioles, raising peritubular capillary hydrostatic pressure, decreasing reabsorption, and decreasing tubular transport of water and electrolytes. Increased renal blood flow also tends to raise peritubular capillary hydrostatic pressure and decrease fluid reabsorption.

TMP13 pp. 360-362

44. C) The filtered load of glucose in this example is determined as follows: GFR (150 ml/min) × plasma glucose (300 mg/dl) = 450 mg/min. The transport maximum for glucose in this example is 300 mg/min. Therefore, the maximum rate of glucose reabsorption is 300 mg/min. The urinary glucose excretion is equal to the filtered load (450 mg/min) minus the tubular reabsorption of glucose (300 mg/min), or 150 mg/min.

TMP13 pp. 350-351, 365

45. B) Excess aldosterone increases sodium reabsorption and potassium secretion by the principal cells of the collecting tubules, causing sodium retention, increased blood pressure, and decreased renin secretion while increasing excretion of potassium and tending to decrease plasma potassium concentration. Excess aldosterone also causes a shift of potassium from the extracellular fluid into the cells, further reducing plasma potassium concentration. Aldosterone excess also stimulates hydrogen ion secretion and bicarbonate reabsorption by the intercalated cells and tends to increase plasma pH (alkalosis). Therefore the classic manifestations of excess aldosterone secretion are hypokalemia, hypertension, alkalosis, and low renin levels.

TMP 13 pp. 356-357, 390

46. B) Potassium secretion by the cortical collecting ducts is stimulated by (1) aldosterone, (2) increased plasma potassium concentration, (3) increased flow rate in the cortical collecting tubules, and (4) alkalosis. Therefore, a diuretic that inhibits aldosterone, decreased plasma potassium concentration, acute acidosis, and low sodium intake would all tend to decrease potassium secretion by the cortical collecting tubules. A diuretic that decreases loop of Henle sodium reabsorption, however, would tend to increase the flow rate in the cortical collecting tubule and therefore stimulate potassium secretion.

TMP13 pp. 392, 396

47. B) This patient with diabetes mellitus and chronic renal disease has a reduction in creatinine clearance to 40% of normal, implying a marked reduction in GFR. He also has acidosis, as evidenced by a plasma pH of 7.14. The decrease in creatinine clearance would cause only a transient reduction in sodium excretion and creatinine excretion rate. As the plasma creatinine concentration increased, the urinary creatinine excretion rate would return to normal, despite the sustained decrease in creatinine clearance (creatinine excretion rate/plasma concentration of creatinine). Diabetes is associated with increased production of acetoacetic acid, which would cause metabolic acidosis and decreased plasma HCO_3^- concentration, as well as a compensatory increase in renal NH_4^+ production and increased NH_4^+ excretion rate.

TMP13 pp. 422, 435-436

48. A) The filtration rate of glucose in this example is GFR (50 ml/min) × plasma glucose concentration (200 mg/100 ml, or 2 mg/ml) = 100 mg/min. Because the transport maximum for glucose in this example is 150 mg/min, all of the filtered glucose would be reabsorbed and the renal excretion rate for glucose would be zero.
TMP 13 pp. 350-351

49. C) A reduction in plasma protein concentration to 3.6 g/dl would increase the capillary filtration rate, thereby raising interstitial fluid volume and interstitial fluid hydrostatic pressure. The increased interstitial fluid pressure would, in turn, increase the lymph flow rate and reduce the interstitial fluid protein concentration ("washout" of interstitial fluid protein).
TMP13 pp. 316-318

50. B) The most likely diagnosis for this patient is diabetes insipidus, which can account for the polyuria and the fact that her urine osmolarity is very low (80 mOsm/L) despite overnight water restriction. In many patients with diabetes insipidus, the plasma sodium concentration can be maintained relatively close to normal by increasing fluid intake (polydipsia). When water intake is restricted, however, the high urine flow rate leads to rapid depletion of extracellular fluid volume and severe hypernatremia, as occurred in this patient. The fact that she has no glucose in her urine rules out diabetes mellitus. Neither primary aldosteronism nor a renin-secreting tumor would lead to an inability to concentrate the urine after overnight water restriction. Syndrome of inappropriate ADH would cause excessive fluid retention and increased urine osmolarity.
TMP13 pp. 380-381, 385

51. C) The filterability of solutes in the plasma is inversely related to the size of the solute (molecular weight). Also, positively charged molecules are filtered more readily than are neutral molecules or negatively charged molecules of equal molecular weight. Therefore, the positively charged polycationic dextran with a molecular weight of 25,000 would be the most readily filtered substance of the choices provided. Red blood cells are not filtered at all by the glomerular capillaries under normal conditions.
TMP13 pp. 336-337

52. A) In normally functioning kidneys, approximately two thirds of the water filtered by the glomerular capillaries is reabsorbed in the proximal tubule. Although dehydration increases ADH levels and water reabsorption by the distal tubules, collecting tubules, and collecting ducts, and this action contributes importantly to decreased water excretion in dehydration, the total amount of water that remains in these tubular segments is small compared with the amount of water in the proximal tubules (see the figure below).
TMP 13 pp. 378-379

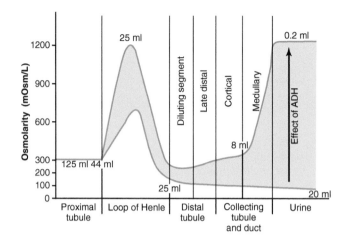

53. D) Furosemide (Lasix) inhibits the Na$^+$-2Cl$^-$-K$^+$ co-transporter in the ascending limb of the loop of Henle. This action not only causes marked natriuresis and diuresis but also reduces the urine-concentrating ability. Furosemide does not cause edema; in fact, it is often used to treat severe edema and heart failure. Furosemide also increases the renal excretion of potassium and calcium and therefore tends to cause hypokalemia and hypocalcemia rather than increasing the plasma concentrations of potassium and calcium.
TMP13 pp. 355, 394-397, 427-428

54. B) Hypernatremia can be caused by excessive sodium retention or water loss. The fact that the patient has large volumes of dilute urine suggests excessive urinary water excretion. Of the two possible disturbances listed that could cause excessive urinary water excretion (nephrogenic diabetes insipidus and central diabetes insipidus), nephrogenic diabetes insipidus is the most likely cause. Central diabetes insipidus (decreased ADH secretion) is not the correct answer because plasma ADH levels are markedly elevated. Simple dehydration due to decreased water intake is unlikely because the patient is excreting large volumes of dilute urine.
TMP13 pp. 314-315, 380-381

55. D) Dehydration due to water deprivation decreases extracellular fluid volume, which in turn increases renin secretion and decreases plasma atrial natriuretic peptide. Dehydration also increases the plasma sodium concentration, which stimulates the secretion of ADH. The increased ADH increases water permeability in the collecting ducts. The ascending limb of the loop of Henle is relatively impermeable to water, and this low permeability is not altered by water deprivation or increased levels of ADH.
TMP13 pp. 375-376

56. C) High urine flow occurs in type 1 diabetes because the filtered load of glucose exceeds the renal threshold, resulting in an increase in glucose concentration in the tubule, which decreases the osmotic driving force for water reabsorption. Increased urine flow reduces extracellular fluid volume and stimulates the release of ADH.
   TMP13 pp. 350-351, 381-382

57. C) Excess aldosterone and a high-salt diet could cause serious hypokalemia because aldosterone stimulates potassium secretion by the renal tubules (and therefore tends to increase potassium excretion), as well as causing a shift of potassium from the extracellular fluid into the cells. A high-salt diet would exacerbate the hypokalemia because this would increase collecting tubular flow rate, which would tend to further increase renal potassium secretion. Treatment with spironolactone or a β-adrenergic blocker or Addison's disease (adrenal insufficiency) would tend to increase plasma potassium concentration. Changes in sodium and potassium intakes over the ranges indicated would have minimal effects on plasma potassium concentration.
   TMP 13 pp. 390-395

58. D) Ingestion of excess aspirin (acetylsalicylic acid) would tend to cause metabolic acidosis, which would lead to decreases in plasma HCO_3^-, decreased Pco_2 (due to respiratory compensation), decreased urine HCO_3^- excretion and increased NH_4^+ excretion (renal compensation), and increased anion gap due to increased unmeasured anions.
   TMP 13 pp. 424-426

59. B) Approximately 30% to 40% of the filtered urea is reabsorbed in the proximal tubule. However, the tubular fluid urea concentration increases because urea is not nearly as permeant as water in this nephron segment. Urea concentration increases further in the tip of the loop of Henle because water is reabsorbed in the descending limb of the loop of Henle. Under conditions of antidiuresis, urea is further concentrated as water is reabsorbed and as fluid flows along the collecting ducts. Therefore, the final urine concentration of urea is substantially greater than the concentration in the proximal tubule or in the plasma.
   TMP13 pp. 376-377

60. C) Diuretics that inhibit loop of Henle sodium reabsorption are used to treat conditions associated with excessive fluid volume (e.g., hypertension and heart failure). These diuretics initially cause an increase in sodium excretion that reduces extracellular fluid volume and blood pressure, but under steady-state conditions, the urinary sodium excretion returns to normal, due in part to the fall in blood pressure. One of the important adverse effects of loop diuretics is hypokalemia that is caused by the inhibition of Na^+-$2Cl^-$-K^+ co-transport in the loop of Henle and by the increased tubular flow rate in the cortical collecting tubules, which stimulates potassium secretion.
   TMP13 pp. 394-395, 427-428

61. A) A reduction in the number of functional nephrons to 25% of normal would cause a compensatory increase in GFR and urine flow rate of the surviving nephrons and decreased urine concentrating ability. Under steady-state conditions, the urinary creatinine excretion rate and sodium excretion rate would be maintained at normal levels. (For further information, see TMP13, **Table 32-6.**)
   TMP13 pp. 435-436

62. A) Excessive secretion of ADH increases water reabsorption by the renal collecting tubules, which reduces extracellular fluid sodium concentration (hyponatremia). Restriction of fluid intake, excessive aldosterone secretion, or administration of hypertonic 3% NaCl solution would all cause increased plasma sodium concentration (hypernatremia), whereas administration of 0.9% NaCl (an isotonic solution) would cause no major changes in plasma osmolarity.
   TMP13 pp. 312-314

63. A) A 75% loss of nephrons would *not* cause a large increase in plasma sodium concentration because tubular reabsorption of sodium is reduced in proportion to the reduction in filtered load of sodium cause by nephron loss, and because the ADH–thirst mechanisms help maintain extracellular sodium concentration at a fairly constant level. Plasma creatinine is inversely related to GFR and would increase to approximately four times normal as GFR is reduced to one fourth normal. If fluid intake remains constant, the average volume excreted by the surviving nephrons would need to increase to four times normal to maintain fluid balance, and this high flow rate in the nephrons would reduce urine-concentrating ability. Plasma phosphate concentration is maintained at a nearly normal level until GFR falls below about 30% of normal, and then the plasma concentration rises progressively as GFR decreases further (see figure below).
   TMP 13 pp. 435-436

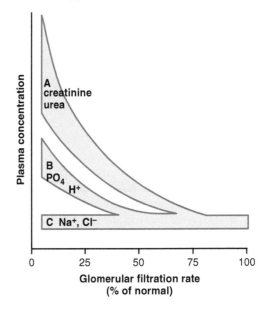

64. **D)** Approximately 40% to 50% of the filtered urea is reabsorbed in the proximal tubule. The distal convoluted tubule and the cortical collecting tubules are relatively impermeable to urea, even under conditions of antidiuresis; therefore, little urea reabsorption takes place in these segments. Likewise, very little urea reabsorption takes place in the thick ascending limb of the loop of Henle. Under conditions of antidiuresis, the concentration of urea in the renal medullary interstitial fluid is markedly increased because of reabsorption of urea from the collecting ducts, which contributes to the hyperosmotic renal medulla.
    TMP13 pp. 376-377

65. **B)** Free water clearance is calculated as urine flow rate (600 ml/2 h, or 5 ml/min) − osmolar clearance (urine osmolarity × urine flow rate/plasma osmolarity). Therefore, free water clearance is equal to +2.5 ml/min.
    TMP13 p. 380

66. **E)** In the absence of ADH, the late distal tubule and collecting tubules are not permeable to water (see above). Therefore, the tubular fluid, which is already dilute when it leaves the loop of Henle (about 100 mOsm/L), becomes further diluted as it flows through the late distal tubule and collecting tubules as electrolytes are reabsorbed. Therefore, the final urine osmolarity in the complete absence of ADH is less than 100 mOsm/L.
    TMP13 p. 378, Fig. 29-8

67. **A)** About 65% of the filtered potassium is reabsorbed in the proximal tubule, and another 20% to 30% is reabsorbed in the loop of Henle. Although most of the daily variation in potassium excretion is caused by changes in potassium secretion in the distal and collecting tubules, only a small percentage of the filtered potassium load can be reabsorbed in these nephron segments. (For further information, see TMP13, **Fig. 30-2.**)
    TMP13 pp. 390-391

68. **A)** The proximal tubule normally absorbs approximately 65% of the filtered water, with much smaller percentages being reabsorbed in the descending loop of Henle and in the distal and collecting tubules. The ascending limb of the loop of Henle is relatively impermeable to water and therefore reabsorbs very little water.
    TMP13 pp. 353, 378-379

69. **C)** The thick ascending limb of the loop of Henle is relatively impermeable to water even under conditions of maximal antidiuresis. The proximal tubule and descending limb of the loop of Henle are highly permeable to water under normal conditions, as well as during antidiuresis. Water permeability of the late distal and collecting tubules increases markedly during antidiuresis because of the effects of increased levels of ADH.
    TMP13 pp. 378-379

70. **D)** Interstitial fluid volume is equal to extracellular fluid volume minus plasma volume. Extracellular fluid volume can be estimated from the distribution of inulin or ^{22}Na, whereas plasma volume can be estimated from ^{125}I-albumin distribution. Therefore, interstitial fluid volume is calculated from the difference between the inulin distribution space and the ^{125}I-albumin distribution space.
    TMP13 pp. 309-310, Table 25-3

71. **F)** Furosemide (Lasix) is a "loop" diuretic that inhibits the Na^+-Cl^--K^+ co-transporter in the thick ascending loop of Henle, thus reducing urine-concentrating ability, increasing renal excretion of Na^+, Cl^-, and K^+, and tending to cause hypokalemia.
    TMP 13 pp. 427-428

72. **D)** Uncontrolled type 1 diabetes would tend to cause metabolic acidosis (decreases in plasma pH and HCO_3^-) due to increased metabolisms of fat and production of acetoacetic acid, which, in turn, would be associated with increased anion gap. The normal respiratory compensation would decrease plasma Pco_2.
    TMP 13 p. 426

73. **E)** Metabolic alkalosis is associated with hypokalemia due to a shift of potassium from the extracellular fluid into the cells (see table below). β-adrenergic blockade, insulin deficiency, strenuous exercise, and aldosterone deficiency all cause hyperkalemia due to a shift of potassium out of the cells into the extracellular fluid.
    TMP13 pp. 389-390, Table 30-1

Factors That Can Alter Potassium Distribution Between the Intracellular and Extracellular Fluid

Factors That Shift K$^+$ Into Cells (Decrease Extracellular K$^+$)	Factors That Shift K$^+$ Out of Cells (Increase Extracellular K$^+$)
Insulin	Insulin deficiency (diabetes mellitus)
Aldosterone	Aldosterone deficiency (Addison's disease)
β-Adrenergic stimulation	β-Adrenergic blockade
Alkalosis	Acidosis
	Cell lysis
	Strenuous exercise
	Increased extracellular fluid osmolarity

74. **D)** In this example, the filtered load of glucose is equal to GFR (100 ml/min) × plasma glucose (150 mg/dl), or 150 mg/min. If there is no detectable glucose in the urine, the reabsorption rate is equal to the filtered load of glucose, or 150 mg/min.
    TMP13 p. 365

75. **B)** Furosemide is a powerful inhibitor of the Na^+-$2Cl^-$-K^+ co-transporter in the loop of Henle. Thiazide diuretics primarily inhibit NaCl reabsorption into the distal tubule, whereas carbonic anhydrase inhibitors decrease bicarbonate reabsorption in the tubules. Amiloride inhibits sodium channel activity, whereas spironolactone inhibits the action of mineralocorticoids in the renal tubules. Osmotic diuretics inhibit water and solute reabsorption by increasing osmolarity of the tubular fluid.
TMP13 p. 428

76. **E)** Decreased efferent arteriolar resistance would increase renal blood flow while reducing glomerular hydrostatic pressure, which, in turn, would tend to decrease the GFR.
TMP 13 pp. 338-339

77. **D)** The tubular fluid–plasma ratio of inulin concentration is 4 in the early distal tubule, as shown in the figure. Because inulin is not reabsorbed from the tubule, this means that water reabsorption must have concentrated the inulin to four times the level in the plasma that was filtered. Therefore, the amount of water remaining in the tubule is only one fourth of what was filtered, indicating that 75% of the water has been reabsorbed prior to the distal convoluted tubule.
TMP13 p. 359

78. **E)** Renal tubular acidosis results from a defect of renal secretion or H^+, a defect in reabsorption of HCO_3^-, or both. This defect causes metabolic acidosis associated with decreases in plasma pH and HCO_3^- and a normal anion gap associated with hyperchloremia (increased plasma chloride concentration). Plasma Pco_2 is reduced because of respiratory compensation for the acidosis.
TMP 13 p. 423

79. **D)** The patient has classic symptoms of diabetes mellitus: increased thirst, breath smelling of acetone (due to increased acetoacetic acids in the blood), high fasting blood glucose concentration, and glucose in the urine. The acetoacetic acids in the blood cause metabolic acidosis that leads to a compensatory decrease in renal HCO_3^- excretion, decreased urine pH, and increased renal production of ammonium and HCO_3^-. The high level of blood glucose increases the filtered load of glucose, which exceeds the transport maximum for glucose, causing an osmotic diuresis (increased urine volume) due to the unreabsorbed glucose in the renal tubules acts as an osmotic diuretic.
TMP13 pp. 350-351, 422

80. **C)** Intracellular fluid volume is calculated as the difference between total body fluid (0.57×60 kilograms = 34.2 kilograms, or approximately 34.2 liters) and extracellular fluid volume (12.8 liters), which equals 21.4 liters.
TMP13 pp. 309-310

81. **C)** Plasma volume is calculated as blood volume (4.3 liters) $\times$ (1.0 – hematocrit), which is $4.3 \times 0.6 = 2.58$ liters (rounded up to 2.6).
TMP13 pp. 309-310

82. **C)** Interstitial fluid volume is calculated as the difference between extracellular fluid volume (12.8 liters) and plasma volume (2.6 liters), which is equal to 10.2 liters.
TMP13 pp. 309-310

83. **C)** The primary site of reabsorption of magnesium is in the loop of Henle, where about 65% of the filtered load of magnesium is reabsorbed. The proximal tubule normally reabsorbs only about 25% of filtered magnesium, and the distal and collecting tubules reabsorb less than 5%.
TMP13 p. 398

84. **D)** The principal cells of the collecting tubules are an important site of action of amiloride, which blocks entry of sodium into sodium channels. Thiazide diuretics inhibit Na^+-Cl^- co-transport in the early distal tubule. The collecting tubule cells are not very permeable to urea. Furosemide inhibits the Na^+-Cl^--K^+ co-transporter in the thick ascending loop of Henle.
TMP 13 pp. 358, 377, 428

85. **A)** The filtration rate of glucose in this example is GFR (100 ml/min) $\times$ plasma glucose concentration (200 mg/100 ml, or 2 mg/ml) = 100 mg/min. Because the transport maximum for glucose in this example is 250 mg/min, all of the filtered glucose would be reabsorbed and the renal excretion rate for glucose would be zero.
TMP 13 pp. 350-351

86. **C)** A plasma glucose concentration of 300 mg/dl would increase the filtered load of glucose above the renal tubular transport maximum and therefore increase urinary glucose excretion. The unreabsorbed glucose in the renal tubules would also cause an osmotic diuresis, increased urine volume, and decreased extracellular fluid volume, which would stimulate thirst. Increased glucose also causes vasodilatation of afferent arterioles, which increases GFR.
TMP13 pp. 345-346, 351, 384-385

87. **B)** GFR is approximately equal to the clearance of creatinine. Creatinine clearance = urine creatinine concentration (32 mg/dl) $\times$ urine flow rate (3600 ml/24 h, or 2.5 ml/min) $\div$ plasma creatinine concentration (4 mg/dL) = 20 ml/min.
TMP13 pp. 365-366

88. **D)** The net renal tubular reabsorption rate is the difference between the filtered load of potassium (GFR $\times$ plasma potassium concentration) and the urinary excretion of potassium (urine potassium concentration $\times$ urine flow rate). Therefore, the net tubular reabsorption of potassium is 0.075 mmol/min.
TMP13 pp. 365-366

89. D) Severe diarrhea would result in loss of HCO_3^- in the stool, thereby causing metabolic acidosis that is characterized by low plasma HCO_3^- and low pH. Respiratory compensation would reduce P_{CO_2}. The plasma anion gap would be normal, and the plasma chloride concentration would be elevated (hyperchloremic metabolic acidosis) in metabolic acidosis caused by HCO_3^- loss in the stool.

TMP13 pp. 421-426

90. E) Primary excessive secretion of aldosterone causes metabolic alkalosis due to increased secretion of hydrogen ions and HCO_3^- reabsorption by the intercalated cells of the collecting tubules. Therefore, the metabolic alkalosis would be associated with increases in plasma pH and HCO_3^-, with a compensatory reduction in respiration rate and increased P_{CO_2}. The plasma anion gap would be normal, with a slight reduction in plasma chloride concentration.

TMP13 pp. 424-426

91. D) Proximal tubular acidosis results from a defect of renal secretion of hydrogen ions, reabsorption of bicarbonate, or both. This defect leads to increased renal excretion of HCO_3^- and metabolic acidosis characterized by low plasma HCO_3^- concentration, low plasma pH, a compensatory increase in respiration rate and low P_{CO_2}, and a normal anion gap with an increased plasma chloride concentration.

TMP13 pp. 421-426

92. F) A patient with diabetic ketoacidosis and emphysema would be expected to have metabolic acidosis (due to excess ketoacids in the blood caused by diabetes), as well as increased plasma P_{CO_2} due to impaired pulmonary function. Therefore, the patient would be expected to have decreased plasma pH, decreased HCO_3^-, increased P_{CO_2}, and an increased anion gap (Na^+-Cl^--HCO_3^- > 10-12 mEq/L) due to the addition of ketoacids to the blood.

TMP13 pp. 422-426

93. D) Secretion of hydrogen ions and reabsorption of HCO_3^- depend critically on the presence of carbonic anhydrase in the renal tubules. After inhibition of carbonic anhydrase, renal tubular secretion of hydrogen ions and reabsorption of HCO_3^- would decrease, leading to increased renal excretion of HCO_3^-, reduced plasma HCO_3^- concentration, and metabolic acidosis. The metabolic acidosis, in turn, would stimulate the respiration rate, leading to decreased P_{CO_2}. The plasma anion gap would be within the normal range.

TMP13 pp. 416-417, 425-426

94. B) Acute renal failure caused by tubular necrosis would cause the rapid development of metabolic acidosis due to the kidneys' failure to rid the body of the acid waste products of metabolism. The metabolic acidosis would lead to decreased plasma HCO_3^- concentration. Acute renal failure would also lead to a rapid increase in blood urea nitrogen concentration and a significant increase in plasma potassium concentration due to the kidneys' failure to excrete electrolytes or nitrogenous waste products. Necrosis of the renal epithelial cells causes them to slough away from the basement membrane and plug up the renal tubules, thereby increasing hydrostatic pressure in Bowman's capsule and decreasing GFR.

TMP13 pp. 431, 438

95. C) The type A intercalated cells of the collecting tubules are important sites for H^+ secretion and K^+ *reabsorption*, but the collecting tubules are not highly permeable to urea. Furosemide acts mainly in the thick ascending loop of Henle, and thiazide diuretics act mainly in the early distal tubule.

TMP13 pp. 356-357

96. D) Dehydration due to insufficient water intake and heavy exercise would increase plasma sodium concentration, which would then stimulate release of ADH. This would increase water reabsorption in the distal and collecting tubules/ducts, causing a small volume of highly concentrated urine. Primary aldosteronism would be associated with sodium and water retention but normal renal excretion (equal to intake) of sodium and water after a few days. Uncontrolled diabetes mellitus is typically associated with large volumes of urine due to the osmotic diuresis associated with the hyperglycemia. Diabetes insipidus is associated with large volumes of dilute urine. Bartter's syndrome is defective Na^+-Cl^--K^+ co-transport in the thick ascending loop of Henle and is associated with increased urine volume. Liddle's syndrome is caused by increased sodium reabsorption and, like primary aldosteronism, is associated with sodium and water retention but normal renal excretion (equal to intake) of sodium and water after a few days.

TMP13 pp. 439-440

97. C) A large increase in aldosterone secretion combined with a high sodium intake would cause severe hypokalemia. Aldosterone stimulates potassium secretion and causes a shift of potassium from the extracellular fluid into the cells, and a high sodium intake increases the collecting tubular flow rate, which also enhances potassium secretion. In normal persons, potassium intake can be reduced to as low as one fourth of normal with only a mild decrease in plasma potassium concentration (for further information, see TMP13, **Fig. 30-8**). A low sodium intake would tend to oppose aldosterone's hypokalemic effect because a low sodium intake would reduce the collecting tubular flow rate and thus tend to reduce potassium secretion. Patients with Addison's disease have a deficiency of aldosterone secretion and therefore tend to have hyperkalemia.

TMP13 pp. 389, 392-395

98. E) Intracellular and extracellular body fluids have the same total osmolarity under steady-state conditions because the cell membrane is highly permeable to water. Therefore, water flows rapidly across the cell membrane until osmotic equilibrium is achieved. The colloid osmotic pressure is determined by the protein concentration, which is considerably higher inside the cell. The cell membrane is also relatively impermeable to potassium, sodium, and chloride, and active transport mechanisms maintain low intracellular concentrations of sodium and chloride and a high intracellular concentration of potassium.
TMP13 pp. 310-312

99. B) Fluid entering the early distal tubule is almost always hypotonic because sodium and other ions are actively transported out of the thick ascending loop of Henle, whereas this portion of the nephron is virtually impermeable to water. For this reason, the thick ascending limb of the loop of Henle and the early part of the distal tubule are often called the diluting segment.
TMP13 pp. 354-355

100. D) Chronic metabolic acidosis is, by definition, associated with decreased HCO_3^-. Decreased excretion of NH_4Cl and HCO_3^- occurs with renal compensation for the acidosis, and respiratory compensation for the acidosis increases the ventilation rate, resulting in decreased plasma P_{CO_2}.
TMP13 pp. 419-420

101. E) Although aldosterone is one of the body's most potent sodium-retaining hormones, it stimulates sodium reabsorption only in the late distal tubule and collecting tubules, which together reabsorb much less than 10% of the filtered load of sodium. Therefore, the maximum percentage of the filtered load of sodium that could be reabsorbed in the distal convoluted tubule and collecting duct, even in the presence of high levels of aldosterone, would be less than 10%.
TMP13 pp. 355, 357-359

102. D) GFR is equal to the clearance of inulin. Inulin clearance = urine inulin concentration (60 mg/ml) × urine flow rate (2 ml/min)/plasma inulin concentration (2 mg/ml) = 60 ml/min.
TMP13 pp. 365-368

103. D) The net renal tubular potassium reabsorption rate is the difference between the filtered load of potassium (GFR × plasma potassium concentration) and the urinary excretion rate of potassium (urine potassium concentration × urine flow rate). Therefore, the net tubular reabsorption rate of potassium is 200 μmol/min.
TMP13 pp. 365-368

104. A) Free water clearance is calculated as urine flow rate (2.0 ml/min) – osmolar clearance (urine osmolarity × urine flow rate/plasma osmolarity). Therefore, free water clearance is equal to +1.0 ml/min.
TMP13 p. 380

105. B) A 0.45% NaCl solution is *hypotonic*. Therefore, administration of 2.0 liters of this solution would reduce intracellular and extracellular fluid osmolarity and cause increases in intracellular and extracellular volumes.
TMP13 pp. 312-313

106. C) If the renal clearance is greater than the GFR, this implies that there must be secretion of that substance into the renal tubules. A substance that is freely filtered and not secreted or reabsorbed would have a renal clearance equal to the GFR.
TMP13 p. 368

107. A) In the proximal tubule, calcium reabsorption usually parallels sodium and water reabsorption. With extracellular volume expansion or increased blood pressure, proximal sodium and water reabsorption is reduced, and a reduction in calcium reabsorption also occurs, causing increased urinary excretion of calcium. Increased parathyroid hormone, increased plasma phosphate concentration, and metabolic alkalosis all tend to decrease the renal excretion of calcium.
TMP13 pp. 396-398

108. C) Increasing sodium intake would decrease renin secretion and plasma renin activity, as well as reduce plasma aldosterone concentration and increase plasma atrial natriuretic peptide because of a modest expansion of extracellular fluid volume. Although a high sodium intake would initially increase distal NaCl delivery, which would tend to increase potassium excretion, the decrease in aldosterone concentration would offset this effect, resulting in no change in potassium excretion under steady-state conditions. Even very large increases in sodium intake cause only minimal changes in plasma sodium concentration as long as the ADH–thirst mechanisms are fully operative.
TMP13 pp. 394-395

109. C) A 50% reduction in efferent arteriolar resistance would cause a large decrease in GFR—greater than 10%. A decrease in renal artery pressure from 100 to 85 mm Hg would cause only a slight decrease in GFR in a normal, autoregulating kidney. A decrease in afferent arteriole resistance, a decrease in plasma colloid osmotic pressure, or an increase in the glomerular capillary filtration coefficient would all tend to increase GFR.
TMP13 pp. 337-340, 343, Figs. 27-7 and 27-9

110. D) Acute metabolic acidosis reduces intracellular potassium concentration, which, in turn, decreases potassium secretion by the principal cells of the collecting tubules. The primary mechanism by which increased hydrogen ion concentration inhibits potassium secretion is by reducing the activity of the sodium-potassium adenosine triphosphatase pump. This action then reduces intracellular potassium concentration, which, in turn, decreases the rate of passive diffusion of potassium across the luminal membrane into the tubule.

TMP13 p. 395

111. E) The kidneys excrete little or no glucose as long as the filtered load of glucose (the product of the GFR and the plasma glucose concentration) does not exceed the tubular transport maximum for glucose. Once the filtered load of glucose rises above the transport maximum, the excess glucose filtered is not reabsorbed and passes into the urine. Therefore, the urinary excretion rate of glucose can be calculated as the filtered load of glucose minus the transport maximum. In this example, the filtered load of glucose is the GFR (150 ml/min) multiplied by the plasma glucose concentration (400 mg/100 ml, or 4 mg/ml), which is equal to 600 mg/min. Because the transport maximum is only 300 mg/min, the rate of glucose excretion would be 600 minus 300 mg/min, or 300 mg/min.

TMP13 pp. 350-351, 365-368

112. D) In a dehydrated person, osmolarity in the early distal tubule is usually less than 300 mOsm/L because the ascending limb of the loop of Henle and the early distal tubule are relatively impermeable to water, even in the presence of ADH. Therefore, the tubular fluid becomes progressively more dilute in these segments compared with plasma. ADH does not influence water reabsorption in the ascending limb of the loop of Henle. The ascending limb, however, reabsorbs sodium to a much greater extent than does the descending limb. Another important action of ADH is to increase the urea permeability in the medullary collecting ducts, which contributes to the hyperosmotic renal medullary interstitium in antidiuresis.

TMP13 pp. 378-379

113. E) A 50% reduction in GFR (from 80 to 40 ml/min) would result in an approximate 50% reduction in creatinine clearance rate because creatinine clearance is approximately equal to the GFR. This reduction would, in turn, lead to doubling of the plasma creatinine concentration. This rise in plasma creatinine concentration results from an initial decrease in creatinine excretion rate, but as the plasma creatinine concentration increases, the filtered load of creatinine (the product of GFR × plasma creatinine concentration) returns to normal and creatinine excretion rate returns to normal under steady-state conditions.

Thus, under the steady state conditions, a 50% reduction in GFR is associated with a doubling of plasma creatinine concentration, a 50% decrease in creatinine clearance, and a normal filtered load of creatinine, as well as no change in load of filtered creatinine and no change in the creatinine excretion rate as long as the person's protein metabolism is not altered. Likewise, the sodium excretion rate returns to normal even when the GFR is reduced because of multiple feedback systems that eventually re-establish sodium balance. Under steady-state conditions, sodium excretion must equal sodium intake to maintain life.

TMP13 pp. 366-367, 399

114. E) Most potassium secretion occurs in the collecting tubules. A high-potassium diet stimulates potassium secretion by the collecting tubules through multiple mechanisms, including small increases in extracellular potassium concentration, as well as increased levels of aldosterone.

TMP13 pp. 392-393

115. A) Diabetic ketoacidosis results in a metabolic acidosis that is characterized by a decrease in plasma bicarbonate concentration, increased anion gap (due to the addition of unmeasured anions to the extracellular fluid along with the ketoacids), and a renal compensatory response that includes increased secretion of NH_4^+. There is also an increased respiratory rate with a reduction in arterial P_{CO_2}, as well as decreased urine pH and decreased renal HCO_3^- excretion.

TMP13 pp. 421-426

116. A) Potassium excretion rate is calculated as urine K^+ concentration multiplied by urine flow rate, which in this case = 60 mmol/L × 0.002 L/min = 0.12 mmol/min.

TMP13 pp. 365-368

117. B) Interstitial fluid volume cannot be measured directly, but it can be calculated as the difference between extracellular fluid volume (inulin space = 16 liters) and plasma volume (^{125}I-albumin space = 4 liters). Therefore, interstitial fluid volume is approximately 12 liters.

TMP13 pp. 309-310

118. E) Increased levels of insulin cause a shift of potassium from the extracellular fluid into the cells. All the other conditions have the reverse effect of shifting potassium out of the cells into the extracellular fluid.

TMP13 pp. 389-390

119. D) This patient is severely dehydrated as a result of sweating and lack of adequate fluid intake. The dehydration markedly stimulates the release of ADH and renin secretion, which in turn stimulates the formation of angiotensin II and aldosterone secretion.

TMP13 pp. 363, 382

120. E) After running the race and losing both fluid and electrolytes, this person replaces his fluid volume by drinking 2 liters of water. However, he did not replace the electrolytes. Therefore, he would be expected to experience a decrease in plasma sodium concentration, resulting in a decrease in both intracellular and extracellular fluid osmolarity. The decrease in extracellular fluid osmolarity would lead to an increase in intracellular volume as fluid diffused into the cells from the extracellular compartment. Therefore, after drinking the water and absorbing it, the total body volume would be normal but intracellular volume would be increased and extracellular volume would be reduced.
TMP13 pp. 311-313

121. B) Increased levels of parathyroid hormone stimulate calcium reabsorption in the thick ascending loops of Henle and distal tubules. Extracellular fluid volume expansion, increased blood pressure, decreased plasma phosphate concentration, and metabolic acidosis are all associated with decreased calcium reabsorption by the renal tubules.
TMP13 pp. 396-397

122. D) The patient has metabolic acidosis as evidenced by the reduced plasma HCO_3^- concentration (normal = 24 mEq/L) and decreased arterial PCO_2 (normal is approximately 40 mm Hg). Because the plasma anion gap (plasma sodium – HCO_3^- – chloride) is normal (approximately 10 mEq/L), the acidosis is not caused by excess nonvolatile acids caused by salicylic acid poisoning, diabetes, or methanol poisoning. Therefore, the most likely cause of the metabolic acidosis is diarrhea, which leads to loss of bicarbonate in the feces. With emphysema, the acidosis would be associated with the increase in PCO_2.
TMP13 pp. 421-422, 426

123. C) In this example, the acidosis is associated with a reduced plasma bicarbonate concentration, signifying metabolic acidosis. In addition, the patient also has an elevated PCO_2, signifying respiratory acidosis. Therefore, the patient has simultaneous respiratory and metabolic acidosis.
TMP13 pp. 422-426

124. A) Urine flow rate is calculated as the difference between GFR and tubular fluid reabsorption rate. If GFR decreases from 150 to 75 ml/min and tubular fluid reabsorption rate simultaneously decreases from 149 to 75 ml/min, the urine flow rate would be the GFR minus the tubular reabsorption rate, or 75 – 75 ml/min, which would equal 0 ml/min.
TMP13 pp. 347, 365-366

125. A) Chronic respiratory acidosis is caused by insufficient pulmonary ventilation, resulting in an increase in PCO_2. Acidosis, in turn, stimulates the secretion of hydrogen ions into the tubular fluid and increased

renal tubular production of NH_4^+, which further contributes to the excretion of hydrogen ions and the renal production of HCO_3^-, thereby increasing plasma bicarbonate concentration. The increased tubular secretion of hydrogen ions also reduces urine pH.
TMP13 p. 422

126. F) Because creatinine is not reabsorbed significantly in the renal tubules, the concentration of creatinine progressively increases as water is reabsorbed along the renal tubular segments (see figure below). Therefore, in a normally hydrated person, the concentration of creatinine would be greatest in the collecting ducts.
TMP13 p. 359

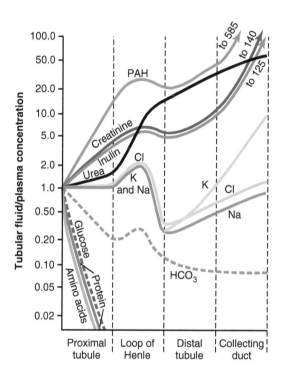

127. B) Three percent dextrose is a hypotonic solution. Therefore, infusing the 3% dextrose would decrease extracellular fluid osmolarity, which, in turn, would lead to diffusion of water into the cells. Under steady-state conditions, there would be a reduction in intracellular and extracellular osmolarity, as well as an increase in the fluid volume of both compartments.
TMP13 pp. 311-314

128. D) A patient with central diabetes insipidus would have deficient secretion of ADH, resulting in excretion of large volumes of water. This excretion, in turn, would cause dehydration and hypernatremia (increased plasma osmolarity). The hypernatremia would result in decreased intracellular volume. Therefore, the primary loss of water would lead to increases in both extracellular and intracellular fluid osmolarity, as well as decreases in intracellular and extracellular fluid volumes.
TMP13 pp. 313-316

129. **A)** Dilation of the afferent arterioles leads to an increase in the glomerular hydrostatic pressure and therefore an increase in GFR, as well as an increase in renal blood flow. Increased glomerular capillary filtration coefficient would also raise the GFR but would not be expected to alter renal blood flow. Increased plasma colloid osmotic pressure or dilation of the efferent arterioles would both tend to reduce the GFR. Increased blood viscosity would tend to reduce renal blood flow and GFR.

    TMP13 pp. 337-341

130. **C)** Because inulin is not reabsorbed or secreted by the renal tubules, increasing concentration of inulin in the renal tubules reflects water reabsorption. Thus, an increase of inulin concentration from a level of 2 mg/100 ml in the plasma to 40 mg/100 ml in the cortical collecting tubule implies that there has been a 20-fold increase in concentration of inulin. In other words, only 1/20th (5%) of the water that was filtered into the renal tubule remains in the collecting tubule.

    TMP13 p. 359

131. **B)** Nonsteroidal anti-inflammatory drugs inhibit the synthesis of prostaglandins, which, in turn, causes constriction of afferent arterioles that can reduce the GFR. The decrease in GFR, in turn, leads to an increase in serum creatinine. Increased efferent arteriole resistance and increased glomerular capillary filtration coefficient would both tend to increase rather than reduce GFR. Increasing muscle mass due to exercise would cause very little change in serum creatinine.

    TMP13 pp. 337-340, 342

132. **A)** In this example, the plasma sodium concentration is markedly increased but the urine sodium concentration is relatively normal, and urine osmolarity is almost maximally increased to 1200 mOsm/L. In addition, there are increases in plasma renin, ADH, and aldosterone, which is consistent with dehydration caused by decreased fluid intake. The syndrome of inappropriate ADH would result in a decrease in plasma sodium concentration, as well as suppression of renin and aldosterone secretion. Nephrogenic diabetes insipidus, caused by the kidneys' failure to respond to ADH, would also be associated with dehydration, but urine osmolarity would be reduced rather than increased. Primary aldosteronism would tend to cause sodium and water retention with only a modest change in plasma sodium concentration and a marked reduction in the secretion of renin. Likewise, a renin-secreting tumor would be associated with increases in plasma aldosterone concentration and plasma renin activity but only a modest change in plasma sodium concentration.

    TMP13 pp. 380-381, 385-386

Blood Cells, Immunity, and Blood Coagulation

The following table of normal test values can be referenced throughout Unit VI.

Test	Normal Values
Bleeding time (template)	2-7 minutes
Erythrocyte count	Male: 4.3-5.9 million/μl^3
	Female: 3.5-5.5 million/μl^3
Hematocrit	Male: 41%-53%
	Female: 36%-46%
Hemoglobin, blood	Male: 13.5-17.5 g/dl
	Female: 12.0-16.0 g/dl
Mean corpuscular hemoglobin	25.4-34.6 pg/cell
Mean corpuscular hemoglobin concentration	31%-36% hemoglobin/cell
Mean corpuscular volume	80-100 fl
Reticulocyte count	0.5%-1.5% of red blood cells
Platelet count	150,000-400,000/μl^3
Leukocyte count and differential	
Leukocyte count	4500-11,000/μl^3
Neutrophils	54%-62%
Eosinophils	1%-3%
Basophils	0-0.75%
Lymphocytes	25%-33%
Monocytes	3%-7%
Partial thromboplastin time (activated)	25-40 seconds
Prothrombin time	11-15 seconds
Bleeding time	2-7 minutes

1. A 40-year-old woman visits the clinic complaining of fatigue. She had recently been treated for an infection. Her laboratory values are as follows: red blood cell (RBC) count, $1.8 \times 10^6/\mu l$; hemoglobin (Hb), 5.2 g/dl; hematocrit (Hct), 15; white blood cell (WBC) count, $7.6 \times 10^3/\mu l$; platelet count, 320,000/μl; mean corpuscular volume (MCV), 92 fL; and reticulocyte count, 24%. What is the most likely explanation for this presentation?

A) Aplastic anemia
B) Hemolytic anemia
C) Hereditary spherocytosis
D) B_{12} deficiency

2. What RBC enzyme facilitates transport of carbon dioxide (CO_2)?

A) Myeloperoxidase
B) Carbonic anhydrase
C) Superoxide dismutase
D) Globin reductase

Questions 3–6

Which points in the figure below most closely define the following conditions? Normal erythropoietin (EPO) levels are approximately 10.

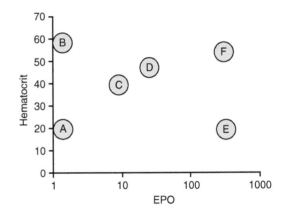

3. Olympic marathoner

4. Aplastic anemia

5. End-stage renal disease

6. Polycythemia vera

7. How many oxygen *atoms* can be transported by each hemoglobin molecule?

A) 2
B) 4
C) 8
D) 16

8. During the second trimester of pregnancy, where is the predominant site of RBC production?

   A) Yolk sac
   B) Bone marrow
   C) Lymph nodes
   D) Liver

9. What function do vitamin B_{12} and folic acid perform that is critical to hematopoiesis?

   A) Support porphyrin production
   B) Serve as cofactors for iron uptake
   C) Support terminal differentiation of erythroid and myeloid cells
   D) Support production of thymidine triphosphate

10. A 62-year-old man complains of headaches, visual difficulties, and chest pains. Physical examination reveals a red complexion and a large spleen. His complete blood cell count (CBC) is as follows: Hct, 58%; WBC, 13,300/μl; and platelets, 600,000/μl. His arterial oxygen saturation is 97% on room air. Which treatment would you recommend?

    A) Chemotherapy
    B) Phlebotomy
    C) Iron supplement
    D) Inhaled oxygen therapy

11. A 38-year-old healthy woman comes to you for a routine visit. She has spent the past 2 months hiking through the Himalayas and climbed to the base camp of Mount Everest. Which results would you expect to see on her CBC?

	Hematocrit	RBC count	WBC count	MCV
A)	↑	↑	↑	↑
B)	↑	↑	↔	↑
C)	↑	↑	↔	↔
D)	↑	↔	↔	↔
E)	↔	↑	↑	↔
F)	↑	↔	↑	↑
G)	↔	↑	↔	↑

12. A 34-year-old man with schizophrenia has had chronic fatigue for 6 months. He has a good appetite but has refused to eat vegetables for 1 year because he hears voices saying that vegetables are poisoned. His physical and neurological examinations are normal. His hemoglobin level is 9.1 g/dl, his leukocyte count is 10,000/μl³, and his MCV is 122. What is the most likely diagnosis?

    A) Acute blood loss
    B) Sickle cell anemia
    C) Aplastic anemia
    D) Hemolytic anemia
    E) Folic acid deficiency

13. What immunologic signal causes mast cells to release their granular contents (e.g., heparin, histamine, bradykinin, serotonin, and leukotrienes)?

    A) Release of interleukin (IL)-1 by macrophages
    B) Cross-linking of cell surface–bound immunoglobulin E (IgE) by antigen
    C) Binding of antigen-antibody complexes to immunoglobulin G (IgG) receptors
    D) Binding of tissue factor to surface glycoproteins

14. A 24-year-old African American man comes to the emergency department 3 hours after the onset of severe back and chest pain. These problems started while he was skiing. He lives in Los Angeles and had a previous episode of these symptoms 5 years ago while visiting Wyoming. He is in obvious pain. Laboratory studies show the following values:

    Hemoglobin = 11 g/dl
    Leukocyte count = 22,000/μl³
    Reticulocyte count = 25%

    What is this patient's diagnosis?
    A) Acute blood loss
    B) Sickle cell anemia
    C) Anemia of chronic disease
    D) End-stage renal disease

15. After a person is placed in an atmosphere with low oxygen, how long does it take for increased numbers of reticulocytes to develop?

    A) 6 hours
    B) 12 hours
    C) 3 days
    D) 5 days
    E) 2 weeks

16. A patient presents to your office complaining of extreme fatigue and shortness of breath on exertion that has gradually worsened during the past 2 weeks. Physical examination reveals a well-nourished woman who appears comfortable but somewhat short of breath. Her vital signs include a pulse of 120, a respiratory rate of 20, and blood pressure of 120/70. When she stands up, her pulse increases to 150 and her blood pressure falls to 80/50. Her hematologic values are as follows: Hb, 7 g/dl; Hct, 20%; RBC count, 2 × 10⁶/μl; and platelet count, 400,000/μl. On a peripheral smear, her RBCs are microcytic and hypochromic. What is your diagnosis?

    A) Aplastic anemia
    B) Renal failure
    C) Iron deficiency anemia
    D) Sickle cell anemia
    E) Megaloblastic anemia

17. Which phagocytes can extrude digestion products and continue to survive and function for many months?

    A) Neutrophils
    B) Basophils
    C) Macrophages
    D) Eosinophils

18. During an inflammatory response, what is the correct order of cellular events?

    A) Filtration of monocytes from blood, increased production of neutrophils, activation of tissue macrophages, infiltration of neutrophils from the blood
    B) Activation of tissue macrophages, infiltration of neutrophils from the blood, infiltration of monocytes from blood, increased production of neutrophils
    C) Increased production of neutrophils, activation of tissue macrophages, infiltration of neutrophils from the blood, infiltration of monocytes from blood
    D) Infiltration of neutrophils from the blood, activation of tissue macrophages, infiltration of monocytes from blood, increased production of neutrophils

19. A 45-year-old man presents to the emergency department with a 2-week history of diarrhea that has gotten progressively worse during the past several days. He has minimal urine output and is admitted to the hospital for dehydration. His stool specimen is positive for parasitic eggs. Which type of WBC would have an elevated number?

    A) Eosinophils
    B) Neutrophils
    C) T lymphocytes
    D) B lymphocytes
    E) Monocytes

20. A 24-year-old man came to the emergency department with a broken leg. A blood test revealed his WBC count to be $22 \times 10^3/\mu l$. Five hours later, a second blood test revealed values of $7 \times 10^3/\mu l$. What is the cause of the increased WBC count in the first test?

    A) Increased production of WBCs by the bone marrow
    B) Release of pre-formed, mature WBCs into the circulation
    C) Decreased destruction of WBCs
    D) Increased production of selectins

21. A 62-year-old man who was known to have a normal blood cell count and differential count 3 months ago presents with pallor, bone pain, bruising, and a WBC count of 42,000. Eighty-five percent of cells in the circulation appear to be immature granulocytes. What is the diagnosis?

    A) Acute lymphocytic leukemia
    B) Acute myelocytic leukemia
    C) Chronic lymphocytic leukemia
    D) Chronic myelocytic leukemia

22. Adhesion of WBCs to the endothelium is

    A) Due to a decrease in selectins
    B) Dependent on activation of integrins
    C) Due to the inhibition of histamine release
    D) Greater on the arterial than on the venous side of the circulation

23. A 65-year-old alcoholic experienced chest pain and cough with an expectoration of sputum. A blood sample revealed that his WBC count was 21,000/μl. What is the origin of these WBCs?

    A) Pulmonary alveoli
    B) Bronchioles
    C) Bronchi
    D) Trachea
    E) Bone marrow

24. Where does the transmigration of WBCs occur in response to infectious agents?

    A) Arterioles
    B) Lymphatic ducts
    C) Venules
    D) Inflamed arteries

25. An 8-year-old boy frequently comes to the clinic for persistent skin infections that do not heal within a normal time frame. He had a normal recovery from the measles. A check of his antibodies after immunizations yielded normal antibody responses. A defect in which of the following cells would most likely be the cause of the continual infections?

    A) B lymphocytes
    B) Plasma cells
    C) Neutrophils
    D) Macrophages
    E) CD4 T lymphocytes

26. Which cell type migrates into inflammatory sites to clean up necrotic tissue and direct tissue remodeling?

    A) Neutrophil
    B) Macrophage
    C) Dendritic cell
    D) Eosinophil

27. A 3-year-old child who has had frequent ear infections is found to have reduced immunoglobulin levels and is unresponsive to vaccination with tetanus toxoid. However, the child has normal skin test reactivity (delayed redness and induration) to a common environmental antigen. Which cell lineage is not functioning normally?

    A) Macrophages
    B) Helper T cells
    C) Cytotoxic T cells
    D) B cells

28. Patients with human immunodeficiency virus (HIV) exhibit abnormal functioning of which of the following mechanisms?

    A) Antibody production only
    B) T cell–mediated cytotoxicity only
    C) Degranulation of appropriately stimulated mast cells
    D) Both antibody production and T cell–mediated cytotoxicity

29. What is the term for binding of IgG and complement to an invading microbe to facilitate recognition?

    A) Chemokinesis
    B) Opsonization
    C) Phagolysosome fusion
    D) Signal transduction

30. Presentation of antigen on major histocompatibility complex (MHC)-I by a cell will result in which of the following?

    A) Generation of antibodies
    B) Activation of cytotoxic T cells
    C) Increase in phagocytosis
    D) Release of histamine by mast cells

31. Which of the following applies to patients with acquired immunodeficiency virus (AIDS)?

    A) Able to generate a normal antibody response
    B) Increased helper T cells
    C) Increased secretion of interleukins
    D) Decrease in helper T cells

32. Fluid exudation into the tissue in an acute inflammatory reaction is due to which of the following?

    A) Decreased blood pressure
    B) Decreased protein in the interstitium
    C) Obstruction of the lymph vessels
    D) Increased clotting factors
    E) Increased vascular permeability

33. What will occur after presentation of antigen by a macrophage?

    A) Direct generation of antibodies
    B) Activation of cytotoxic T cells
    C) Increase in phagocytosis
    D) Activation of helper T cells

34. CD4 is a marker of which of the following?

    A) B cells
    B) Cytotoxic T cells
    C) Helper T cells
    D) An activated macrophage
    E) A neutrophil precursor

35. What is the function of IL-2 in the immune response?

    A) Binds to and presents antigen
    B) Stimulates proliferation of T cells
    C) Kills virus-infected cells
    D) Is required for an anaphylactic response

36. Which of the following is true about helper T cells?

    A) They are activated by the presentation of antigen by an infected cell
    B) They require the presence of a competent B-cell system
    C) They destroy bacteria by phagocytosis
    D) They are activated by the presentation of antigen by macrophage or dendritic cells

37. Which of the following applies to cytotoxic T cells?

    A) They require the presence of a competent B-lymphocyte system
    B) They require the presence of a competent suppressor T-lymphocyte system
    C) They are activated by the presentation of antigen by an infected cell
    D) They destroy bacteria by initiating macrophage phagocytosis

38. A 9-year-old girl has nasal discharge and itching of the eyes in the spring every year. An allergist performs a skin test using a mixture of grass pollens. Within a few minutes the girl exhibits a focal redness and swelling at the test site. This response is most likely due to

    A) Antigen–antibody complexes being formed in blood vessels in the skin
    B) Activation of neutrophils due to injected antigens
    C) Activation of CD4 helper cells and the resultant generation of specific antibodies
    D) Activation of cytotoxic T lymphocytes to destroy antigens

39. Activation of the complement system results in which action?

    A) Binding of the invading microbe with IgG
    B) Inactivation of eosinophils
    C) Decreased tissue levels of complement
    D) Generation of chemotactic substances

40. Which statement is true concerning erythroblastosis fetalis (hemolytic disease of the newborn [HDN])?

    A) HDN occurs when an Rh-positive mother has an Rh-negative child
    B) HDN is prevented by giving the mother a blood transfusion
    C) A complete blood transfusion after the first birth will prevent HDN
    D) The father of the child must be Rh positive

41. Which statement is true?

    A) In a transfusion reaction, agglutination of the recipient blood occurs
    B) Shutdown of the kidneys after a transfusion reaction occurs slowly
    C) Blood transfusion of Rh-positive blood into any Rh-negative recipient will result in an immediate transfusion reaction
    D) A person with type AB Rh-positive blood is considered a universal recipient

42. A woman whose blood type is A, Rh positive, and a man whose blood type is B, Rh positive, come to the clinic with a 3-year-old girl whose blood type is O, Rh negative. What can be said about the relationship of these two adults to this child?

    A) The woman can be the child's natural mother, but the man cannot be the natural father
    B) The man can be the child's natural father, but the woman cannot be the natural mother
    C) Neither adult can be the natural parent of this child
    D) This couple can be the natural parents of this child

43. What is the appropriate treatment for an infant born with severe HDN (erythroblastosis fetalis)?

    A) Passive immunization with anti-Rh(D) immuno-globulin
    B) Immunization with Rh(D) antigen
    C) Exchange transfusion with Rh(D)-positive blood
    D) Exchange transfusion with Rh(D)-negative blood

44. Chronic allograft rejection results primarily from the actions of what effector cell type?

    A) Activated macrophages
    B) Helper T lymphocytes
    C) Cytotoxic T lymphocytes
    D) Dendritic cells

45. Which of the following transfusions will result in an immediate transfusion reaction?

    A) O Rh-negative whole blood to an O Rh-positive patient
    B) A Rh-negative whole blood to a B Rh-negative patient
    C) AB Rh-negative whole blood to an AB Rh-positive patient
    D) B Rh-negative whole blood to a B Rh-negative patient

46. Which blood unit carries the least risks for inducing an immediate transfusion reaction into a B-positive (B, rhesus positive) recipient?

    A) Whole blood A positive
    B) Whole blood O positive
    C) Whole blood AB positive
    D) Packed red blood cells O positive
    E) Packed red blood cells AB negative

47. What condition leads to a deficiency in factor IX that can be corrected by an intravenous injection of vitamin K?

    A) Classic hemophilia
    B) Hepatitis B
    C) Bile duct obstruction
    D) Genetic deficiency in antithrombin III

48. Which transfusion will result in a transfusion reaction? Assume that the patient has never had a transfusion.

    A) Type O Rh-negative packed cells to an AB Rh-positive patient
    B) Type A Rh-positive packed cells to an A Rh-negative patient
    C) Type AB Rh-positive packed cells to an AB Rh-positive patient
    D) Type A Rh-positive packed cells to an O Rh-positive patient

49. Which antigens must be matched optimally between donors and recipients of solid organ transplants?

    A) Class I human leukocyte antigen (HLA) antigens only
    B) Class II HLA antigens only
    C) Class I and Class II HLA antigens only
    D) Class I and Class II HLA antigens and ABO antigens

50. A 55-year-old man who has been undergoing stable and successful anticoagulation with warfarin for recurrent deep vein thrombosis is treated for pneumonia, and 8 days later he presents with lower intestinal bleeding. His prothrombin time is quite prolonged. What is the appropriate therapy?

    A) Treatment with tissue plasminogen activator
    B) Infusion of calcium citrate
    C) Treatment with fresh frozen plasma and vitamin K
    D) Rapid infusion of protamine

51. A woman whose blood type is A positive and who has always been healthy just delivered her second child. The father's blood type is O negative. Because the child's blood type is O negative (O, Rh negative), what would you expect to find in this child?

    A) Erythroblastosis fetalis due to rhesus incompatibility
    B) Erythroblastosis fetalis due to ABO blood group incompatibility
    C) Both A and B
    D) The child would not be expected to have HDN

52. A 2-year-old boy bleeds excessively from minor injuries and has previously had bleeding gums. The maternal grandfather has a bleeding disorder. The child's physical examination shows slight tenderness of his knee with fluid accumulation in the knee joint. You suspect this patient is deficient in which coagulation factor?

    A) Prothrombin activator
    B) Factor II
    C) Factor VIII
    D) Factor X

53. A patient has a congenital deficiency in factor XIII (fibrin-stabilizing factor). What would analysis of his blood reveal?

    A) Prolonged prothrombin time
    B) Prolonged whole blood clotting time
    C) Prolonged partial thromboplastin time
    D) Easily breakable clot

54. Which agent is not effective as an in vitro anticoagulant?

    A) Heparin
    B) Warfarin (Coumadin)
    C) Ethylenediamine tetraacetic acid (EDTA)
    D) Sodium citrate

55. What would most likely be used for prophylaxis of an ischemic heart attack?

    A) Heparin
    B) Warfarin
    C) Aspirin
    D) Streptokinase

56. A 63-year-old woman returned to work after a vacation in New Zealand. Several days after returning home, she awoke with swelling and pain in her right leg, which was blue. She immediately went to the emergency department, where examination showed an extensive deep vein thrombosis involving the femoral and iliac veins on the right side. After resolution of the clot, this patient will require which treatment in the future?

    A) Continual heparin infusion
    B) Warfarin
    C) Aspirin
    D) Vitamin K

57. Which coagulation pathway begins with tissue thromboplastin?

    A) Extrinsic pathway
    B) Intrinsic pathway
    C) Common pathway
    D) Fibrin stabilization

58. Which of the following causes some malnourished patients to bleed excessively when injured?

    A) Vitamin K deficiency
    B) Platelet sequestration by fatty liver
    C) Serum bilirubin that raises neutralizing thrombin
    D) Low serum protein levels that cause factor XIII problems

59. Which of the following would best explain a prolonged bleeding time test?

    A) Hemophilia A
    B) Hemophilia B
    C) Thrombocytopenia
    D) Coumadin use

60. Which of the following is appropriate therapy for a massive pulmonary embolism?

    A) Heparin
    B) Warfarin
    C) Aspirin
    D) Tissue plasminogen activator

61. What is the primary mechanism by which heparin prevents blood coagulation?

    A) Antithrombin III activation
    B) Binding and inhibition of tissue factor
    C) Binding available calcium
    D) Inhibition of platelet-activating factor

1. **B)** This patient has increased production of RBCs as indicated by a markedly increased reticulocyte count in the setting of significant anemia (low number, Hb, and Hct). The RBCs being produced have a normal size (MCV = 90), and thus the patient does not have spherocytosis (small RBCs) or vitamin B_{12} deficiency (large RBCs). The normal WBC count and the increased reticulocyte count suggest that the bone marrow is functioning. The increased reticulocyte count means that a large number of RBCs are being produced. These laboratory values support an anemia due to some type of blood loss—in this case an anemia due to hemolysis.
   TMP13 p. 452

2. **B)** Carbonic anhydrase catalyzes the reaction of CO_2 with water to allow large amounts of CO_2 to be transported in blood as soluble bicarbonate ion.
   TMP13 p. 445

3. **D)** A well-trained athlete will have a slightly elevated EPO level, and the hematocrit will be elevated up to a value of 50%. A hematocrit higher than 50% suggests EPO treatment.
   TMP13 p. 448

4. **E)** Aplastic anemia is a condition in which the bone marrow has a decreased production but does not respond to EPO. Therefore, a person with aplastic anemia would have a low hematocrit and an elevated EPO level.
   TMP13 p. 452

5. **A)** People with end-stage renal disease have a decrease in EPO level due to decreased release from the diseased kidneys. As a consequence of the decreased EPO level, the hematocrit will be decreased.
   TMP13 p. 448

6. **B)** In persons with polycythemia vera, the bone marrow produces RBCs without a stimulus from EPO. The hematocrit is very high, even up to 60%. With the elevated hematocrit there is a feedback suppression of EPO, and the EPO levels are very low.
   TMP13 p. 453

7. **C)** Each hemoglobin molecule has four globin chains (in hemoglobin A, the predominant form in adults, the hemoglobin molecule includes two alpha and two beta chains). Each globin chain is associated with one heme group, containing one atom of iron. Each of the four iron atoms can bind loosely with one molecule (two atoms) of oxygen. Thus each hemoglobin molecule can transport eight oxygen atoms.
   TMP13 p. 450

8. **D)** RBC production begins in the yolk sac for the first trimester. Production in the yolk sac decreases at the beginning of the second trimester, and the liver becomes the predominate source of RBC production. During the third trimester, RBC production increases from the bone marrow and continues throughout life.
   TMP13 p. 446

9. **D)** Cell proliferation requires DNA replication, which requires an adequate supply of thymidine triphosphate. Both vitamin B_{12} and folate are needed to make thymidine triphosphate.
   TMP13 p. 449

10. **B)** This patient has polycythemia vera: increased RBCs, WBCs, and platelets. His increased hematocrit also increases the viscosity of the blood, resulting in increased afterload for the heart, which is probably the reason for his chest pain. Thus, a phlebotomy (bleeding) is needed to decrease his elevated blood cell count.
    TMP13 p. 453

11. **C)** Secondary polycythemia has developed because of exposure to low oxygen levels. She will have an increased hematocrit level, and thus an increased RBC count, but a normal WBC count. The cells are normal, so the MCV will be normal.
    TMP13 p. 453

12. **E)** This patient is anemic; Hg levels are <14 g/dl. The WBC count is normal, suggesting normal bone marrow. His RBCs are considerably larger than normal (normal MCV = 90). His lack of vegetable consumption suggests either a vitamin B_{12} or folic acid deficiency. However, the body has sufficient stores of vitamin B_{12} to last 4 to 5 years, so he does not appear to have vitamin B_{12} deficiency. The body only stores folic acid for 3 to 6 months, so not eating vegetables for 1 year would result in a folic acid deficiency.
    TMP13 pp. 449, 452

13. **B)** Mast cells express large numbers of high-affinity IgE receptors that are "pre-loaded" with IgE molecules that have been bound from plasma. When multiple IgE molecules of the appropriate specificity encounter their cognate antigen, cross-linking of the cell-bound IgE and initiation of degranulation through signals generated by the IgE receptors result.
    TMP13 p. 463

14. **B)** This African American man has sickle cell anemia, as demonstrated by his decreased hemoglobin concentration and elevated reticulocyte count. He has some

infectious/inflammatory response, as illustrated by the elevated WBC count. The high altitude was the stimulus for a hypoxic episode that caused sickling of his RBCs.
TMP13 pp. 450, 452

15. **C)** EPO levels increase after a decreased arterial oxygen level, with the maximum EPO production occurring within 24 hours. It takes 3 days for new reticulocytes to appear in the circulation, and after a total of 5 days from the beginning of hypoxemia, these reticulocytes will be circulating as mature erythrocytes. Because it takes 1 to 2 days for a reticulocyte to become an erythrocyte, the correct answer is 3 days until the person has an increased number of reticulocytes.
TMP13 pp. 446-448

16. **C)** The blood cell count values show that the patient is anemic. Her bone marrow is functioning and she has a normal platelet count, but she is generating a decreased number of abnormal RBCs. The microcytic (small), hypochromic (decreased intracellular hemoglobin) RBCs are a classic finding of iron deficiency anemia. If she had renal failure, she would be anemic with normal RBCs. People with sickle cell anemia have misshapen RBCs. Megaloblastic anemia is characterized by macrocytic (large) RBCs.
TMP13 pp. 447, 450, 452

17. **C)** Basophils are not phagocytic, and eosinophils are weak phagocytes. Neutrophils respond rapidly to infection or inflammation and ingest from 3 to 20 bacteria or other particles before dying. Macrophages become activated and enlarged at sites of inflammation and can ingest up to 100 bacteria per macrophage. They can extrude digested material and remain viable and active for many months.
TMP13 p. 458

18. **B)** The first cellular event during an inflammatory state is activation of the tissue macrophages. Invasion of neutrophils and monocytes then occur in that order. Finally, production of WBCs is increased by the bone marrow.
TMP13 p. 461

19. **A)** Eosinophils constitute about 2% of the total WBC count, but they are produced in large numbers in people with parasitic infections.
TMP13 p. 462

20. **B)** The majority of WBCs are stored in the bone marrow, waiting for an increased level of cytokines to stimulate their release into the circulation. However, trauma to bone can result in a release of WBCs into the circulation. This increase in WBC count is not primarily due to any inflammatory response, but instead is attributed to mechanical trauma and associated stress responses.
TMP13 p. 456

21. **B)** The WBC count of 42,000 is higher than the range usually seen as a response to infection and suggests leukemia. The patient's florid clinical presentation suggests an acute process, and findings of a normal CBC 3 months previously confirm that this patient has an acute leukemia. Granulocytes are myeloid cells, and the fact that they are in the circulation while still being immature is wholly compatible with leukemia. Thus the patient has acute myelocytic (also referred to as "myelogenous" or "myeloid") leukemia.
TMP13 p. 463

22. **B)** Activation of selections or integrins results in adhesion of WBCs to endothelium.
TMP13 pp. 460, 461

23. **E)** All WBCs originate from the bone marrow from myelocytes or lymphocyte precursors.
TMP13 p. 456

24. **C)** Transmigration of WBCs occurs through parts of the vasculature that have very thin walls and minimal vascular smooth muscle layers. This includes capillaries and venules.
TMP13 pp. 457, 461

25. **C)** For the acquired immune response, T and B lymphocytes and plasma cells, along with macrophages, are needed. Neutrophils are needed for routine infections.
TMP13 pp. 460-461

26. **B)** Dendritic cells are resident antigen-presenting cells, whereas eosinophils are weakly phagocytic cells whose products (e.g., major basic protein) can kill parasites without the eosinophils ingesting them. Macrophages follow the initial influx of neutrophils into an inflammatory site. Whereas neutrophils ingest a modest number of bacteria per cell before dying, macrophages persist at the site, ingesting and digesting infectious organisms and necrotic material and producing cytokines that direct tissue remodeling by fibroblasts and other cell types.
TMP13 p. 461

27. **D)** The presence of normal skin test reactivity, which is T cell–mediated, indicates normal function of macrophages and other antigen-presenting cells, helper T cells, and cytotoxic T cells. This information, and the reduction in antibody production, localizes the defect to the B-cell lineage.
TMP13 pp. 466, 469, 473

28. **D)** Patients with HIV have specific loss of T-helper cells, resulting in a loss of T-cell help for both antibody production and activation/proliferation of cytotoxic T cells. Assuming that mast cells can be appropriately stimulated (i.e., bear sufficient residual surface-bound IgE and are exposed to relevant antigen), their processes for degranulation are intact.
TMP13 p. 473

29. B) Phagocytosis of bacteria is enhanced by the presence on their surfaces of both immunoglobulin and products of the complement cascade, which in turn bind to surface receptors on phagocytes. This "tagging" of bacteria and other particles for enhanced phagocytosis is called *opsonization.*
TMP13 p. 471

30. B) Presentation of an antigen on an infected cell will result in activation of the cytotoxic T cells to kill the infected cell. Presentation of an antigen by macrophages will activate helper T cells, which can promote antibody production and support proliferation of both helper and cytotoxic T cells.
TMP13 p. 472

31. D) Helper T cells are destroyed by the AIDS virus, leaving the patient unprotected against infectious diseases.
TMP13 p. 473

32. E) Fluid leaks into the tissue due to an increase in capillary permeability.
TMP13 p. 460

33. D) Presentation of an antigen on the surface of macrophages or dendritic cells results in the activation of helper T cells. Activation of helper T cells then initiates the release of lymphokines that stimulate proliferation and activation of helper and cytotoxic T cells and B cells and the generation of antibodies.
TMP13 pp. 472-473

34. C) CD4 helper T cells recognize the MHC class II + peptide on the presenting cell. CD8 T cells recognize the MHC class I + peptide on the infected cell.
TMP13 p. 472

35. B) IL-2 is secreted by helper T cells when the T cells are activated by specific antigens. IL-2 plays a specific role in the growth and proliferation of helper, cytotoxic, and suppressor T cells.
TMP13 pp. 472-473

36. D) Helper T cells are activated by the presentation of antigens on the surface of antigen-presenting cells. Helper T cells activate B cells to form antibodies, but B cells are not required for activation of helper T cells. Helper T cells help macrophages with phagocytosis but do not have the capability to phagocytize bacteria.
TMP13 pp. 472-473

37. C) Cytotoxic cells act on infected cells when the cells have the appropriate antigen located on the surface. The cytotoxic T cells are stimulated by lymphokines generated by activation of helper T cells. Cytotoxic T cells destroy an infected cell by releasing proteins that punch large holes in the membrane of the infected cells. There is no interaction between cytotoxic T cells and B cells.
TMP13 p. 473

38. A) Because the person has demonstrated allergic reactions, the initial reaction would be due to an antigen–antibody reaction and the activation of the complement system. Influx of neutrophils, activation of T-helper cells, and sensitized lymphocytes would take some time.
TMP13 p. 475

39. D) Activation of the complement system results in a series of actions, including opsonization and phagocytosis by neutrophils, lysis of bacteria, agglutination of organisms, activation of basophils and mast cells, and chemotaxis. Fragment C5a of the complement system causes chemotaxis of neutrophils and macrophages.
TMP13 p. 471

40. D) HDN occurs when an Rh-negative mother gives birth to a second Rh-positive child. Therefore, the father must be Rh positive. The mother becomes sensitized to the Rh antigens after the birth of the first Rh-positive child. HDN is prevented by treating the mother with antibodies against Rh antigen after the birth of each Rh-positive child. This treatment will destroy all fetal RBCs in the mother and prevent the mother from being sensitized to the Rh antigen. A transfusion of the first child after the birth will not accomplish anything because the mother has been exposed to the Rh-positive antigen during the birth process.
TMP13 pp. 479-480

41. D) The recipient blood has the larger amount of plasma and thus antibodies. These antibodies will act on the donor RBCs. The donor's plasma will be diluted and have minimal effect on the recipient's RBCs. With any antigen–antibody transfusion reaction a rapid breakdown of RBCs occurs, releasing hemoglobin into the plasma, which can cause rapid acute renal shutdown. Transfusion of Rh-positive blood will only result in a transfusion reaction if the Rh-negative person has previously undergone a transfusion or been exposed to Rh-positive antibodies. Type AB Rh-positive people have no antibodies to the A, B, or Rh(D) antigens in their plasma, so they can receive any blood type.
TMP13 p. 480

42. D) Each parent needs only a single allele for either the A or B antigen or the Rh(D) antigen to express these antigens on their blood cells and other cell types. Thus, if each parent also carries an allele for blood type O, as well as a null allele for the Rh(D) antigen, then the child can be homozygous for the recessive O allele and the Rh(D)-negative allele.
TMP13 pp. 478-479

43. D) The appropriate treatment is repetitive removal of Rh-positive blood, replacing it with Rh-negative blood (an exchange of about 400 milliliters over 90 minutes). This treatment may be performed several times over

a few weeks. Maternal antibodies disappear over 1 to 2 months, so the newborn's endogenous Rh-positive cells cease to be a target. Exchange transfusions can actually be initiated in utero when there is evidence of an active immune reaction against the fetus's blood cells.
TMP13 p. 480

44. C) Allograft rejection occurs primarily through the actions of cytotoxic T cells. T-helper cells promote this reaction but are not the effector cells. Both macrophages and dendritic cells may present antigen that promotes the immune response, but the key effector cells are cytotoxic T cells.
TMP13 pp. 473, 482

45. B) Transfusion of Rh-negative blood into an Rh-positive person with the same ABO type will not result in any reaction. Type A blood has A antigen on the surface and type B antibodies. Type B blood has B antigens and A antibodies. Therefore, transfusing A blood into a person with type B blood will cause the A antibodies in the type B person to react with the donor blood.
TMP13 pp. 477-480

46. D) In any patient, transfusion of O-type packed cells will minimize a transfusion reaction because the antibodies will be removed with the plasma removal. Matching the Rh factor will also minimize transfusion reaction. Therefore, in a patient with type B-positive blood, a B-positive transfusion or an O-positive transfusion will elicit no transfusion reaction.
TMP13 pp. 477-480

47. C) Hemophilia is due to a genetic loss of clotting factor VIII. Most clotting factors are formed in the liver. Correction of the problem with a vitamin K injection implies that the liver is working fine and that the patient does not have hepatitis. Vitamin K is a fat-soluble vitamin that is absorbed from the intestine along with fats. Bile secreted by the gallbladder is required for the absorption of fats. If the patient is deficient in vitamin K, then clotting deficiency can be corrected by an injection of vitamin K. Antithrombin III has no relationship to factor IX.
TMP13 p. 490

48. D) Type O RBCs are considered to be universal donor blood. Reactions occur between the recipient's antibody and donor antigen as shown in the following table.
TMP13 pp. 477-478

Donor	Donor Antigen	Recipient	Recipient Antibody	Reaction
O-negative	None	AB-positive	None	None
A-positive	A, Rh	A-negative	B	None
AB-positive	A, B, Rh	AB-positive	None	None
A-positive	A, Rh	O-positive	A, B	A (antigen) and A (antibody)

49. D) Unmatched donor HLA antigens of both classes are recognized as foreign by recipient T cells. In addition, blood group (ABO) antigens are expressed on the cells of solid organs and can lead to strong organ rejection.
TMP13 p. 481

50. C) Antibiotic treatment for pneumonia can kill flora in the gastrointestinal tract that are critical for the production of vitamin K. Production of several active clotting factors (prothrombin and factors VII, IX, and X) has been suppressed in this patient by warfarin inhibition of VKOR c1, which normally reduces vitamin K so that it can activate the listed clotting factors. Further reduction of vitamin K by the death of critical gut flora has produced excessive anticoagulation and resulted in bleeding in this patient. Fresh frozen plasma is infused to provide active clotting factors immediately, and vitamin K is provided to promote endogenous production of active clotting factors. Both are needed in the setting of acute bleeding.
TMP13 p. 490

51. D) HDN occurs when the mother is Rh negative and the father is Rh positive, resulting in an Rh-positive child. Because the child is O negative and the father is Rh negative, HDN would not be expected to develop.
TMP13 pp. 478-479

52. C) A young man with a bleeding disorder and a history of bleeding disorders in the males of his family would lead one to suspect hemophilia A, a deficiency of factor VIII. The physical examination suggests bleeding into the knee joint, which is frequently seen in hemophilia A.
TMP13 p. 490

53. D) Fibrin monomers polymerize to form a clot. Creation of a strong clot requires the presence of fibrin-stabilizing factor that is released from platelets within the clot. The other clotting tests determine the activation of extrinsic and intrinsic pathways or number of platelets.
TMP13 pp. 484, 486, 493

54. B) Warfarin interferes with endogenous production of active clotting factors but does not affect their function once they are present, as in normal plasma. Heparin activates antithrombin III to produce anticoagulation either in vitro or in vivo. Both EDTA and sodium citrate bind calcium, which is necessary for clotting to proceed.
TMP13 p. 492

55. C) Heparin is used for the prevention of a clot, but it must be infused. Heparin prevents formation of clots by binding to antithrombin III, resulting in the inactivation of thrombin. Warfarin is used to inhibit the formation of vitamin K clotting factors. Aspirin is used to prevent activation of platelets. Activation of plate-

lets after exposure to an atherosclerotic plaque and the formation of a platelet plug will impede blood flow and result in an ischemic heart attack. Streptokinase (or, alternatively, tissue plasminogen activator) is used to break down an already formed clot, which is appropriate therapy for a pulmonary embolus.
TMP13 pp. 491-492

56. **B)** This clot is due to stasis of blood flow in the patient's venous circulation. Heparin is used for the prevention of a clot, but it must be infused. This anticoagulation occurs by heparin binding to antithrombin III, with subsequent inactivation of thrombin. A continuous heparin drip is impractical. Warfarin is used to inhibit the formation of vitamin K clotting factors and would prevent the formation of any clot. Aspirin is used to prevent activation of platelets. The current clot is not due to activation of platelets. Vitamin K would be used to restore clotting factors that may be decreased after warfarin treatment. This patient has sufficient clotting factors, as evidenced by her venous clot.
TMP13 pp. 491-492

57. **A)** The extrinsic pathway begins with the release of tissue thromboplastin in response to vascular injury or contact between traumatized extravascular tissue and blood. Tissue thromboplastin is composed of phospholipids from the membranes of tissue.
TMP13 p. 487

58. **A)** Several clotting factors that are formed in the liver require vitamin K to be functional. Vitamin K is a fat-soluble vitamin, and absorption is dependent on adequate fat digestion and absorption. Therefore, any state of malnutrition could have decreased fat absorption and result in decreased vitamin K absorption and decreased synthesis of clotting factors.
TMP13 p. 490

59. **C)** Three major tests are used to determine coagulation defects. Prothrombin time is used to test the extrinsic pathway and is based on the time required for the formation of a clot after the addition of tissue thromboplastin. Bleeding time after a small cut is used to test for several clotting factors but is especially prolonged by a lack of platelets.
TMP13 pp. 492-493

60. **D)** Heparin is used for the prevention of a clot. Heparin binds to antithrombin III, resulting in the inactivation of thrombin. Warfarin is used to inhibit the formation of vitamin K clotting factors. Aspirin is used to prevent activation of platelets. Tissue plasminogen activator is used to break down an already formed clot, which is appropriate therapy for a pulmonary embolus.
TMP13 p. 491

61. **A)** The primary function of heparin is to bind to and activate antithrombin III.
TMP13 p. 489

Minute ventilation: ~~VT × VR~~

TV × RR

Respiration

1. What tends to decrease airway resistance?

   A) Asthma
   B) Stimulation by sympathetic fibers
   C) Treatment with acetylcholine
   D) Exhalation to residual volume

2. The pleural pressure of a normal 56-year-old woman is approximately –5 cm H_2O during resting conditions immediately before inspiration (i.e., at functional residual capacity [FRC]). What is the pleural pressure (in cm H_2O) during inspiration?

   A) +1
   B) +4
   C) 0
   D) –3
   E) –7

3. A healthy, 25-year-old medical student participates in a 10-kilometer charity run for the American Heart Association. Which muscles does the student use (contract) during expiration?

   A) Diaphragm and external intercostals
   B) Diaphragm and internal intercostals
   C) Diaphragm only
   D) Internal intercostals and abdominal recti
   E) Scaleni
   F) Sternocleidomastoid muscles

4. Which of the following would be expected to increase the measured airway resistance?

   A) Stimulation of parasympathetic nerves to the lungs
   B) Low lung volumes
   C) Release of histamine by mast cells
   D) Forced expirations
   E) All of the above

5. Several students are trying to see who can generate the highest expiratory flow. Which muscle is most effective at producing a maximal effort?

   A) Diaphragm
   B) Internal intercostals
   C) External intercostals
   D) Rectus abdominis
   E) Sternocleidomastoid

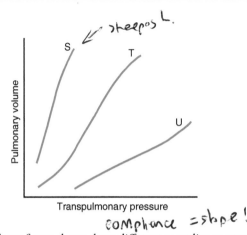

sleepos L.

compliance = slope!

6. The above figure shows three different compliance curves (S, T, and U) for isolated lungs subjected to various transpulmonary pressures. Which of the following best describes the relative compliances for the three curves?

   A) S < T < U
   B) S < T > U
   C) S – T – U
   D) S > T < U
   E) S > T > U

S > T > U

Questions 7 and 8
Use the figure below to answer Questions 7 and 8.

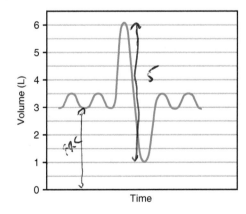

7. Assuming a respiratory rate of 12 breaths/min, calculate the minute ventilation.

   A) 1 L/min
   B) 2 L/min
   C) 4 L/min
   D) 5 L/min
   E) 6 L/min

minute ventilation

: TV × RR

8. A 22-year-old woman inhales as much air as possible and exhales as much air as she can, producing the spirogram shown in the figure. A residual volume of 1.0 liter was determined using the helium dilution technique. What is her FRC (in liters)?

A) 2.0
B) 2.5
C) 3.0
D) 3.5
E) 4.0
F) 5.0

FRC = RV + ERV

9. With a slow decrease in left heart function, which of the following will minimize the formation of pulmonary edema?

A) An increase in plasma protein concentration due to fluid loss
B) Increase in the negative interstitial hydrostatic pressure
C) Increased pumping of lymphatics
D) Increase in the concentration of interstitial proteins

10. A 22-year-old woman has a pulmonary compliance of 0.2 L/cm H_2O and a pleural pressure of –4 cm H_2O. What is the pleural pressure (in cm H_2O) when the woman inhales 1.0 liter of air?

A) –6
B) –7
C) –8
D) –9
E) –10

$\frac{G}{.2} = 5$ *decrease in pressure*

11. A preterm infant has a surfactant deficiency. Without surfactant, many of the alveoli collapse at the end of each expiration, which in turn leads to pulmonary failure. Which set of changes is present in the preterm infant compared with a normal infant?

	Alveolar Surface Tension	Pulmonary Compliance
A)	Decreased	Decreased
B)	Decreased	Increased
C)	Decreased	No change
D)	Increased ✓	Decreased ✓
E)	Increased	Increased
F)	Increased	No change
G)	No change	No change

12. A patient has a dead space of 150 milliliters, FRC of 3 liters, tidal volume (VT) of 650 milliliters, expiratory reserve volume (ERV) of 1.5 liters, total lung capacity (TLC) of 8 liters, and respiratory rate of 15 breaths/min. What is the residual volume (RV)?

A) 500 milliliters
B) 1000 milliliters
C) 1500 milliliters
D) 2500 milliliters
E) 6500 milliliters

FRC = RV + ERV

13. A patient has a dead space of 150 milliliters, FRC of 3 liters, VT of 650 milliliters, ERV of 1.5 liters, TLC of 8 liters, and respiratory rate of 15 breaths/min. What is the alveolar ventilation (VA)?

A) 5 L/min
B) 7.5 L/min
C) 6.0 L/min
D) 9.0 L/min

$V_A = $ *frequency* $\times (V_T - V_D)$
$15 - (650 - 150)$

14. The various lung volumes and capacities include the total lung capacity (TLC), vital capacity (VC), inspiratory capacity (IC), tidal volume (VT), expiratory capacity (EC), expiratory reserve volume (ERV), inspiratory reserve volume (IRV), functional residual capacity (FRC), and residual volume (RV). Which of the following lung volumes and capacities can be measured using direct spirometry without additional methods?

	TLC	VC	IC	VT	EC	ERV	IRV	FRC	RV
A)	No	No	Yes	No	Yes	No	Yes	No	No
B)	No	Yes	Yes	Yes	Yes	Yes	Yes	No	No
C)	No	Yes	Yes	Yes	Yes	Yes	Yes	Yes	No
D)	Yes	Yes	Yes	Yes	Yes	Yes	Yes	No	Yes
E)	Yes	Yes	Yes	Yes	Yes	Yes	Yes	Yes	Yes

15. What happens during exercise?

A) Blood flow is uniform throughout the lung
B) Lung-diffusing capacity increases because blood flow is continuous in all pulmonary capillaries
C) Pulmonary blood volume decreases
D) The transit time of blood in the pulmonary capillaries does not change from rest

16. A 34-year-old man sustains a bullet wound to the chest that causes a pneumothorax. What best describes the changes in lung volume and thoracic volume in this man compared with normal?

	Lung Volume	Thoracic Volume
A)	Decreased	Decreased
B)	Decreased	Increased
C)	Decreased	No change
D)	Increased	Decreased
E)	Increased	Increased
F)	No change	Decreased

17. A healthy 10-year-old boy breathes quietly under resting conditions. His tidal volume is 400 milliliters and his ventilation frequency is 12/min. Which of the following best describes the ventilation of the upper, middle, and lower lung zones in this boy?

	Upper Zone	Middle Zone	Lower Zone
A)	Highest	Lowest	Intermediate
B)	Highest	Intermediate	Lowest
C)	Intermediate	Lowest	Highest
D)	Lowest	Intermediate	Highest
E)	Same	Same	Same

18. An experiment is conducted in two persons (subjects T and V) with identical VTs (1000 milliliters), dead space volumes (200 milliliters), and ventilation frequencies (20 breaths per minute). Subject T doubles his VT and reduces his ventilation frequency by 50%. Subject V doubles his ventilation frequency and reduces his VT by 50%. What best describes the total ventilation (also called minute ventilation) and VA of subjects T and V?

	Total Ventilation	VA
A)	T < V	T – V
B)	T < V	T > V
C)	T – V	T < V
D)	T – V	T – V
E)	T – V	T > V
F)	T > V	T < V
G)	T > V	T – V

Alveolar Ventilation

19. A person with normal lungs has an oxygen (O_2) consumption of 750 ml O_2/min. The hemoglobin (Hb) concentration is 15 g/dl. The mixed venous saturation is 25%. What is the cardiac output?

A) 2500 ml/min
B) 5000 ml/min
C) 7500 ml/min
D) 10,000 ml/min
E) 20,000 ml/min

$15 \times 1.34 = 20$
$.25 \times 20 = 5$ mL/O_2
750 mL/O_2 = $(O \times (20-5))$
= 5000 mL/min
O_2 consumption = $CO \times (A - V)$

20. A cardiac catheterization is performed in a healthy adult. The blood sample withdrawn from the catheter shows 60% O_2 saturation, and the pressure recording shows oscillations from a maximum of 27 mm Hg to a minimum of 12 mm Hg. Where was the catheter tip located?

A) Ductus arteriosus — Connects Pulmonary artery to aorta
B) Foramen ovale
C) Left atrium ~7 - 5mm Hg
D) Pulmonary artery
E) Right atrium 0-2

21. If alveolar surface area is decreased 50% and pulmonary edema leads to a doubling of diffusion distance, how does diffusion of O_2 compare with normal?

A) 25% increase
B) 50% increase
C) 25% decrease
D) 50% decrease
E) 75% decrease

$Diffusion = \dfrac{\Delta P \times SA \times Solubility}{Distance \times \sqrt{MW}}$

22. Which of the following sets of differences best describes the hemodynamics of the pulmonary circulation when compared with the system circulation?

	Flow	Resistance	Arterial Pressure
A)	Higher	Higher	Higher
B)	Higher	Lower	Lower
C)	Lower	Higher	Lower
D)	Lower	Lower	Lower
E)	Same	Higher	Lower
F)	Same	Lower	Lower

23. A 67-year-old man is admitted emergently to the hospital because of severe chest pain. A Swan-Ganz catheter is floated into the pulmonary artery, the balloon is inflated, and the pulmonary wedge pressure is measured. The pulmonary wedge pressure is used clinically to monitor which pressure?

A) Left atrial pressure
B) Left ventricular pressure
C) Pulmonary artery diastolic pressure
D) Pulmonary artery systolic pressure
E) Pulmonary capillary pressure

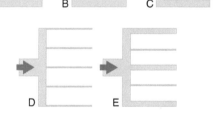

24. Which diagram in the above figure best illustrates the pulmonary vasculature when the cardiac output has increased to a maximum extent?

A) A
B) B
C) C
D) D
E) E

25. A 19-year-old man sustains a full-thickness burn over 60% of his body surface area. A systemic *Pseudomonas aeruginosa* infection occurs, and severe pulmonary edema follows 7 days later. The following data are collected from the patient: plasma colloid osmotic pressure, 19 mm Hg; pulmonary capillary hydrostatic pressure, 7 mm Hg; and interstitial fluid hydrostatic pressure, 1 mm Hg. Which set of changes has occurred in the lungs of this patient as a result of the burn and subsequent infection?

	Lymph Flow	Plasma Colloid Osmotic Pressure	Pulmonary Capillary Permeability
A)	Decrease	Decrease	Decrease
B)	Increase	Decrease	Decrease
C)	Increase	Decrease	Increase
D)	Increase	Increase	Decrease
E)	Increase	Increase	Increase

26. A human experiment is being performed in which forearm blood flow is being measured under a variety of conditions. The forearm is infused with a vasodilator, resulting in an increase in blood flow. Which of the following occurs?

A) Tissue interstitial partial pressure of oxygen (Po_2) will increase

B) Tissue interstitial partial pressure of carbon dioxide (Pco_2) will increase

C) Tissue pH will decrease

27. Blood gas measurements are obtained in a resting patient who is breathing room air. The patient has an arterial content of 19 ml O_2/min with a Po_2 of 95. The mixed venous O_2 content is 4 ml O_2/100 ml blood. Which condition does the patient have?

A) An increase in physiological dead space

B) Pulmonary edema

C) A low Hb concentration

D) A low cardiac output

28. A normal male subject has the following initial conditions (in the steady state):

Arterial Po_2 = 92 mm Hg
Arterial O_2 saturation = 97%
Venous O_2 saturation = 20%
Venous Po_2 = 30 mm Hg
Cardiac output = 5600 ml/min
O_2 consumption = 256 ml/min
Hb concentration = 12 gm/dl

If you ignore the contribution of dissolved O_2 to the O_2 content, what is the venous O_2 content?

A) 2.2 ml O_2/100 ml blood
B) 3.2 ml O_2/100 ml blood
C) 4 ml O_2/100 ml blood
D) 4.6 ml O_2/100 ml blood
E) 6.2 ml O_2/100 ml blood
F) 10.8 ml O_2/100 ml blood
G) 16 ml O_2/100 ml blood

Arterial content: 12 × 1.34 = 16

.20 × 16

29. A man fell asleep in his running car. He was unconscious when he was brought into the emergency department. With carbon monoxide (CO) poisoning, you would expect his alveolar O_2 partial pressure (Pao_2) would be _____, while his arterial O_2 content (Cao_2) would be _____.

A) Normal, decreased
B) Decreased, decreased
C) Increased, normal
D) Increased, normal

30. A 30-year-old woman performs a Valsalva maneuver about 30 minutes after eating lunch. Which option best describes the changes in pulmonary and systemic blood volumes that occur in this woman?

	Pulmonary Volume	Systemic Volume
A)	Decreases	Decreases
B)	Decreases	Increases
C)	Decreases	No change
D)	Increases	Decreases
E)	Increases	Increases
F)	Increases	No change
G)	No change	Decreases
H)	No change	Increases
I)	No change	No change

31. A child who is eating round candies approximately 1 and 1.5 cm in diameter inhales one down his airway, blocking his left bronchiole. Which of the following describes the changes that occur?

	Left Lung Alveolar Pco_2	Left Lung Alveolar Po_2	Systemic Arterial Po_2
A)	↑	↑	↔
B)	↑	↔	↑
C)	↓	↓	↓
D)	↑	↑	↑
E)	↑	↓	↓

32. A person with normal lungs at sea level (760 mm Hg) is breathing 50% O_2. What is the approximate alveolar Po_2?

A) 100
B) 159
C) 306
D) 330
E) 380

33. The forces governing the diffusion of a gas through a biological membrane include the pressure difference across the membrane (ΔP), the cross-sectional area of the membrane (A), the solubility of the gas (S), the distance of diffusion (d), and the molecular weight of the gas (MW). Which changes increase the diffusion of a gas through a biological membrane?

	ΔP	A	S	d	MW
A)	Increase	Increase	Increase	Increase	Increase
B)	Increase	Increase	Increase	Increase	Decrease
C)	Increase	Decrease	Increase	Decrease	Decrease
D)	Increase	Increase	Increase	Decrease	Increase
E)	Increase	Increase	Increase	Decrease	Decrease

34. A person's normal VT is 400 milliliters with a dead space of 100 milliliters. The respiratory rate is 12 breaths/min. The person undergoes ventilation during surgery, and the VT is 700 with a rate of 12. What is the approximate alveolar P_{CO_2} for this person?

A) 10
B) 20
C) 30
D) 40
E) 45

35. Arterial P_{O_2} is 100 mm Hg and arterial P_{CO_2} is 40 mm Hg. Total blood flow to a muscle is 700 ml/min. There is a sympathetic activation resulting in a decrease in blood flow of this muscle to 350 ml/min. There is no neuromuscular activation, and thus no contraction of the muscle. Which of the following will occur?

	Venous P_{O_2}	Venous P_{CO_2}
A)	↑	↓
B)	↓	↑
C)	↓	↔
D)	↔	↑
E)	↑	↑
F)	↓	↓
G)	↔	↔

36. A 45-year-old man at sea level has an inspired O_2 tension of 149 mm Hg, nitrogen tension of 563 mm Hg, and water vapor pressure of 47 mm Hg. A small tumor pushes against a pulmonary blood vessel, completely blocking the blood flow to a small group of alveoli. What are the O_2 and carbon dioxide (CO_2) tensions of the alveoli that are not perfused (in mm Hg)?

	CO_2	O_2
A)	0	0
B)	0	149
C)	40	104
D)	47	149
E)	45	149

37. In which conditions is alveolar P_{O_2} increased and alveolar P_{CO_2} decreased?

A) Increased VA and unchanged metabolism
B) Decreased VA and unchanged metabolism
C) Increased metabolism and unchanged VA
D) Proportional increase in metabolism and VA

38. The diffusing capacity of a gas is the volume of gas that will diffuse through a membrane each minute for a pressure difference of 1 mm Hg. Which gas is often used to estimate the O_2-diffusing capacity of the lungs?

A) CO_2
B) CO
C) Cyanide gas
D) Nitrogen
E) O_2

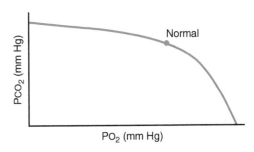

39. The O_2-CO_2 diagram above shows a ventilation-perfusion (V/Q) ratio line for the normal lung. Which of the following best describes the effect of decreasing V/Q ratio on the alveolar P_{O_2} and P_{CO_2}?

	CO_2 Tension	O_2 Tension
A)	Decrease	Decrease
B)	Decrease	Increase
C)	Decrease	No change
D)	Increase	Decrease
E)	Increase	Increase

40. A 23-year-old medical student has mixed venous O_2 and CO_2 tensions of 40 mm Hg and 45 mm Hg, respectively. A group of alveoli are not ventilated in this student because mucus blocks a local airway. What are the alveolar O_2 and CO_2 tensions distal to the mucus block (in mm Hg)?

	CO_2	O_2
A)	40	100
B)	40	40
C)	45	40
D)	50	50
E)	90	40

Questions 41 and 42

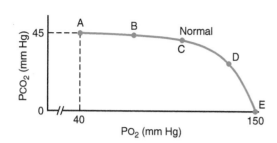

41. A 67-year-old man has a solid tumor that pushes against an airway, partially obstructing air flow to the distal alveoli. Which point on the V/Q line of the O_2-CO_2 diagram above corresponds to the alveolar gas of these distal alveoli?

    A) A
    B) B
    C) C
    D) D
    E) E

42. A 55-year-old man has a pulmonary embolism that completely blocks the blood flow to his right lung. Which point on the V/Q line of the O_2-CO_2 diagram above corresponds to the alveolar gas of his right lung?

    A) A
    B) B
    C) C
    D) D
    E) E

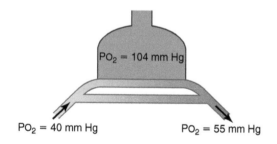

43. The figure above shows a lung with a large shunt in which mixed venous blood bypasses the O_2 exchange areas of the lung. Breathing room air produces the O_2 partial pressures shown on the diagram. What is the O_2 tension of the arterial blood (in mm Hg) when the person breathes 100% O_2 and the inspired O_2 tension is greater than 600 mm Hg?

    A) 40
    B) 55
    C) 60
    D) 175
    E) 200
    F) 400
    G) 600

44. The figure above shows two lung units (S and T) with their blood supplies. Lung unit S has an ideal relationship between blood flow and ventilation. Lung unit T has a compromised blood flow. What is the relationship between alveolar dead space (D_{ALV}), physiologic dead space (D_{PHY}) and anatomic dead space (D_{ANAT}) for these lung units?

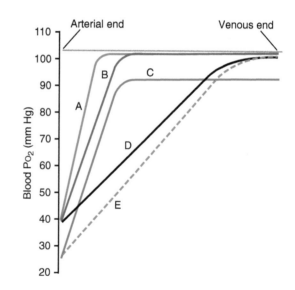

	Lung Unit S	Lung Unit T
A)	$D_{PHY} < D_{ANAT}$	$D_{PHY} = D_{ANAT}$
B)	$D_{PHY} = D_{ALV}$	$D_{PHY} > D_{ALV}$
C)	$D_{PHY} = D_{ANAT}$	$D_{PHY} < D_{ANAT}$
D)	$D_{PHY} = D_{ANAT}$	$D_{PHY} > D_{ANAT}$
E)	$D_{PHY} > D_{ANAT}$	$D_{PHY} < D_{ANAT}$

45. A 32-year-old medical student has a fourfold increase in cardiac output during strenuous exercise. Which curve on the above figure most likely represents the changes in O_2 tension that occur as blood flows from the arterial end to the venous end of the pulmonary capillaries in this student?

    A) A
    B) B
    C) C
    D) D
    E) E

A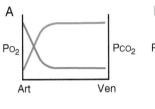

PO₂   PCO₂

Art   Ven

B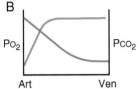

PO₂   PCO₂

Art   Ven

C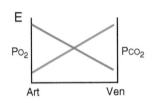

PO₂   PCO₂

Art   Ven

D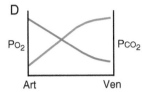

PO₂   PCO₂

Art   Ven

E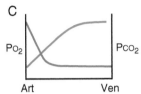

PO₂   PCO₂

Art   Ven

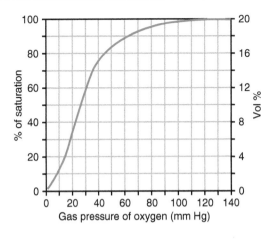

46. The above figure shows changes in the partial pressures of O_2 and CO_2 as blood flows from the arterial (Art) end to the venous (Ven) end of the pulmonary capillaries. Which diagram best depicts the normal relationship between Po_2 (red line) and Pco_2 (green line) during resting conditions?

A) A
B) B
C) C
D) D
E) E

47. Which of the following would be true if the blood lacked red blood cells and just had plasma and the lungs were functioning normally?

A) The arterial Po_2 would be normal
B) The O_2 content of arterial blood would be normal
C) Both A and B
D) Neither A nor B

48. The above figure shows a normal O_2-Hb dissociation curve. What are the approximate values of Hb saturation (% Hb-O_2), Po_2, and O_2 content for oxygenated blood leaving the lungs and reduced blood returning to the lungs from the tissues?

	Oxygenated Blood			Reduced Blood		
	% Hb-O_2	Po_2	O_2 Content	% Hb-O_2	Po_2	O_2 Content
A)	100	104	15	80	42	16
B)	100	104	20	30	20	6
C)	100	104	20	75	40	15
D)	90	100	16	60	30	12
E)	98	140	20	75	40	15

49. A person with anemia has an Hb concentration of 12 g/dl. He starts exercising and uses 12 ml O_2/dl. What is the mixed venous Po_2?

A) 0 mm Hg
B) 10 mm Hg
C) 20 mm Hg
D) 40 mm Hg
E) 100 mm Hg

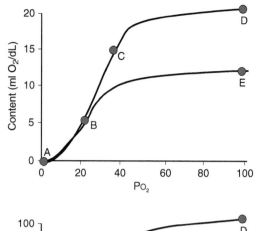

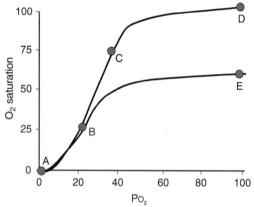

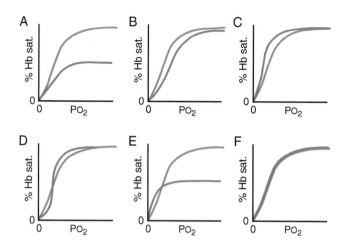

50. Which points on the above figure represent arterial blood in a severely anemic person?

	Top Graph	Bottom Graph
A)	D	D
B)	E	E
C)	D	E
D)	E	D

51. A stroke that destroys the respiratory area of the medulla would be expected to lead to which of the following?

A) Immediate cessation of breathing
B) Apneustic breathing
C) Ataxic breathing
D) Rapid breathing (hyperpnea)
E) None of the above (breathing would remain normal)

52. Which of the above O_2-Hb dissociation curves corresponds to normal blood (red line) and blood containing CO (green line)?

A) A
B) B
C) C
D) D
E) E
F) F

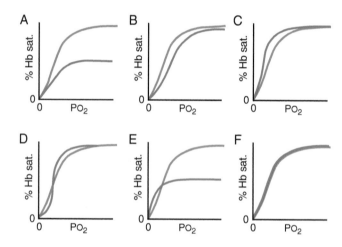

53. Which of the above O_2-Hb dissociation curves corresponds to blood during resting conditions (red line) and blood during exercise (green line)?

A) A
B) B
C) C
D) D
E) E
F) F

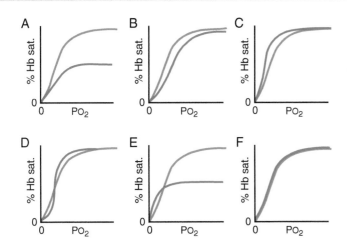

A

B

C

D

E

F

(y-axes: % Hb sat.; x-axes: PO₂)

54. Which of the above O₂-Hb dissociation curves corresponds to blood from an adult (red line) and blood from a fetus (green line)?

   A) A
   B) B
   C) C
   D) D
   E) E
   F) F

55. Arterial P_{O_2} is 100 mm Hg and arterial P_{CO_2} is 40 mm Hg. Total blood flow to all muscle is 700 ml/min. There is a sympathetic activation resulting in a decrease in blood flow to 350 ml/min. What will occur?

	Venous P_{O_2}	Venous P_{CO_2}
A)	↑	↓
B)	↓	↑
C)	↓	↔
D)	↔	↑
E)	↑	↑
F)	↓	↓
G)	↔	↔

56. What is the *most important* pathway for the respiratory response to systemic arterial CO₂ (P_{CO_2})?

   A) CO₂ activation of the carotid bodies
   B) Hydrogen ion (H⁺) activation of the carotid bodies
   C) CO₂ activation of the chemosensitive area of the medulla
   D) H⁺ activation of the chemosensitive area of the medulla
   E) CO₂ activation of receptors in the lungs

57. The basic rhythm of respiration is generated by neurons located in the medulla. What limits the duration of inspiration and increases respiratory rate?

   A) Apneustic center
   B) Dorsal respiratory group
   C) Nucleus of the tractus solitarius
   D) Pneumotaxic center
   E) Ventral respiratory group

58. When the respiratory drive for increased pulmonary ventilation becomes greater than normal, a special set of respiratory neurons that are inactive during normal quiet breathing then becomes active, contributing to the respiratory drive. These neurons are located in which structure?

   A) Apneustic center
   B) Dorsal respiratory group
   C) Nucleus of the tractus solitarius
   D) Pneumotaxic center
   E) Ventral respiratory group

59. A 26-year-old medical student on a normal diet has a respiratory exchange ratio of 0.8. How much O₂ and CO₂ are transported between the lungs and tissues of this student (in ml gas/100 ml blood)?

	O₂	CO₂
A)	4	4
B)	5	3
C)	5	4
D)	5	5
E)	6	3
F)	6	4

60. CO₂ is transported from the tissues to the lungs predominantly in the form of bicarbonate ion. Compared with arterial red blood cells, which of the following options best describes venous red blood cells?

	Intracellular Chloride Concentration	Cell Volume
A)	Decreased	Decreased
B)	Decreased	Increased
C)	Decreased	No change
D)	Increased	Decreased
E)	Increased	No change
F)	Increased	Increased
G)	No change	Decreased
H)	No change	Increased
I)	No change	No change

61. The afferent (sensory) endings for the Hering-Breuer reflex are mechanoreceptors located in the

   A) Carotid arteries
   B) Alveoli
   C) External intercostals
   D) Bronchi and bronchioles
   E) Diaphragm

62. An anesthetized man is breathing with no assistance. He then undergoes artificial ventilation for 10 minutes at his normal VT but at twice his normal frequency. He undergoes ventilation with a gas mixture of 60% O_2 and 40% nitrogen. The artificial ventilation is stopped and he fails to breathe for several minutes. This apneic episode is due to which of the following?

A) High arterial Po_2 suppressing the activity of the peripheral chemoreceptors

B) Decrease in arterial pH suppressing the activity of the peripheral chemoreceptors

C) Low arterial Pco_2 suppressing the activity of the medullary chemoreceptors

D) High arterial Pco_2 suppressing the activity of the medullary chemoreceptors

E) Low arterial Pco_2 suppressing the activity of the peripheral chemoreceptors

63. Which of the following describes a patient with constricted lungs compared with a normal patient?

	TLC	RV	Maximum Expiratory Flow
A)	Normal	Normal	Normal
B)	Normal	Normal	Reduced
C)	Normal	Reduced	Reduced
D)	Reduced	Normal	Normal
E)	Reduced	Reduced	Normal
F)	Reduced	Reduced	Reduced

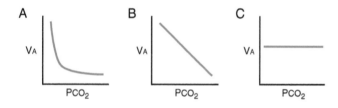

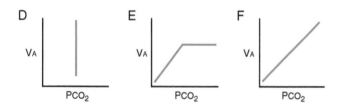

64. Which diagram in the above figure best describes the relationship between VA and arterial CO_2 tension (Pco_2) when the Pco_2 is changed acutely over a range of 35 to 75 mm Hg?

A) A
B) B
C) C
D) D
E) E
F) F

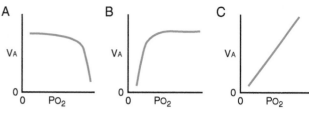

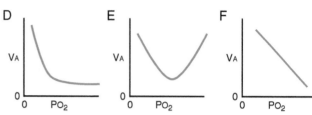

65. Which diagram in the above figure best describes the relationship between VA and arterial O_2 tension (Po_2) when the Po_2 is changed acutely over a range of 0 to 160 mm Hg and the arterial Pco_2 and H^+ concentration remain normal?

A) A
B) B
C) C
D) D
E) E
F) F

66. At a fraternity party a 17-year-old male places a paper bag over his mouth and breathes in and out of the bag. As he continues to breathe into this bag, his rate of breathing continues to increase. Which of the following is responsible for the increased ventilation?

A) Increased alveolar Po_2
B) Increased alveolar Pco_2
C) Decreased arterial Pco_2
D) Increased pH

67. VA increases severalfold during strenuous exercise. Which factor is most likely to stimulate ventilation during strenuous exercise?

A) Collateral impulses from higher brain centers
B) Decreased mean arterial pH
C) Decreased mean arterial Po_2
D) Decreased mean venous Po_2
E) Increased mean arterial Pco_2

68. During strenuous exercise, O_2 consumption and CO_2 formation can increase as much as 20-fold. VA increases almost exactly in step with the increase in O_2 consumption. Which option best describes what happens to the mean arterial O_2 tension (Po_2), CO_2 tension (Pco_2), and pH in a healthy athlete during strenuous exercise?

	Arterial Po_2	Arterial Pco_2	Arterial pH
A)	Decreases	Decreases	Decreases
B)	Decreases	Increases	Decreases
C)	Increases	Decreases	Increases
D)	Increases	Increases	Increases
E)	No change	No change	No change

69. A 54-year-old woman with advanced emphysema due to long-term cigarette smoking is admitted to the hospital for shortness of breath. She is diagnosed with pulmonary hypertension. Her arterial blood gases are

$P_{O_2} = 75$ mm Hg
$P_{CO_2} = 45$ mm Hg
pH = 7.35

What is the cause of the pulmonary hypertension in this woman?

A) Increased alveolar P_{CO_2}
B) Increased sympathetic tone
C) Decreased alveolar P_{O_2}
D) Decreased pulmonary capillary number

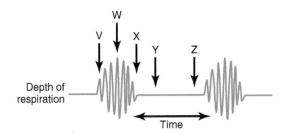

70. Cheyne-Stokes breathing is an abnormal breathing pattern characterized by a gradual increase in the depth of breathing, followed by a progressive decrease in the depth of breathing that occurs again and again approximately every minute. Which time points on the above figure (V-Z) are associated with the highest P_{CO_2} of lung blood and highest P_{CO_2} of the neurons in the respiratory center?

	Lung Blood	Respiratory Center
A)	V	V
B)	V	W
C)	W	W
D)	X	Z
E)	Y	Z

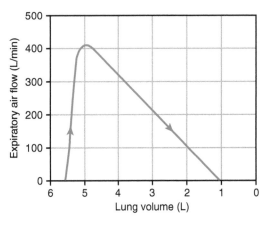

71. A 45-year-old man inhaled as much air as possible and then expired with a maximum effort until no more air could be expired. This action produced the maximum expiratory flow-volume (MEFV) curve shown in the above figure. What is the forced vital capacity (FVC) of this man (in liters)?

A) 1.5
B) 2.5
C) 3.5
D) 4.5
E) 5.5
F) 6.5

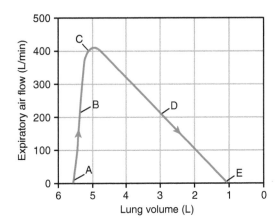

72. The MEFV curve shown in the above figure is used as a diagnostic tool for identifying obstructive and restrictive lung diseases. At which point on the curve does airway collapse limit maximum expiratory air flow?

A) A
B) B
C) C
D) D
E) E

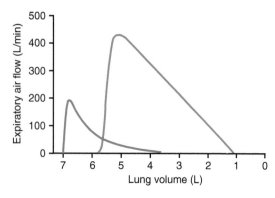

73. The MEFV curves shown in the above figure were obtained from a healthy person (red curve) and a 57-year-old man with shortness of breath (green curve). The man with shortness of breath likely has which disorder?

    A) Asbestosis
    B) Emphysema
    C) Kyphosis
    D) Scoliosis
    E) Silicosis
    F) Tuberculosis

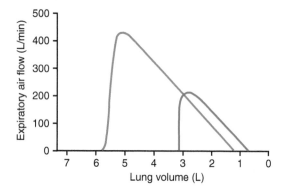

74. A 62-year-old man reports difficulty breathing. The above figure shows an MEFV curve from the patient (green line) and from a typical healthy individual (red curve). Which of the following best explains the MEFV curve of the patient?

    A) Asbestosis
    B) Asthma
    C) Bronchospasm
    D) Emphysema
    E) Old age

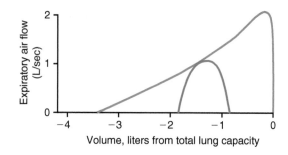

75. The MEFV curve shown in the above figure (red line) was obtained from a 75-year-old man who smoked 40 cigarettes per day for 60 years. The green flow-volume curve was obtained from the man during resting conditions. Which set of changes is most likely to apply to this man?

	Exercise Tolerance	TLC	RV
A)	Decreased	Decreased	Decreased
B)	Decreased	Increased	Increased
C)	Decreased	Normal	Normal
D)	Increased	Increased	Increased
E)	Normal	Decreased	Decreased

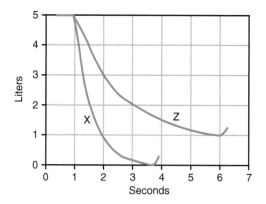

76. The above figure shows a forced expiration for a healthy person (curve X) and a person with a pulmonary disease (curve Z). What is the forced expiratory volume in the first second of expiration (FEV_1/FVC ratio (as a percent) in these persons?

	Person X	Person Z
A)	80	50
B)	80	40
C)	100	80
D)	100	60
E)	90	50
F)	90	60

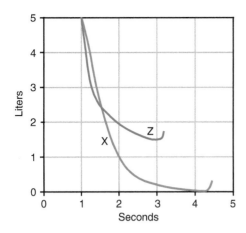

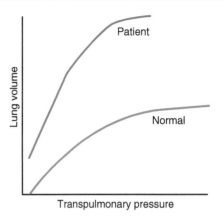

77. The above figure shows forced expirations from a person with healthy lungs (curve X) and from a patient (curve Z). The patient most likely has which condition?

A) Asthma
B) Bronchospasm
C) Emphysema
D) Old age
E) Silicosis

78. Which of the following describes blood gases during consolidated pneumonia?

	Arterial P_{O_2}	Arterial O_2 Content	Arterial P_{CO_2}
A)	Normal	Normal	Normal
B)	Normal	Normal	Increased
C)	Decreased	Normal	Normal
D)	Decreased	Decreased	Increased
E)	Decreased	Decreased	Decreased
F)	Decreased	Decreased	Normal

79. Which of the following occurs during atelectasis of one lung?

A) Increase in arterial P_{CO_2}
B) A 40% decrease in P_{O_2}
C) Normal blood flow in the lung with atelectasis
D) Slight decrease in arterial content

80. The volume–pressure curves in the above figure were obtained from a normal subject and a patient with a pulmonary disease. Which abnormality is most likely present in the patient?

A) Asbestosis
B) Emphysema
C) Mitral obstruction
D) Rheumatic heart disease
E) Silicosis
F) Tuberculosis

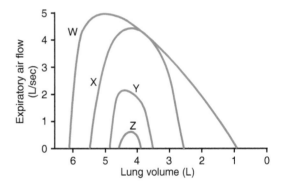

81. A 34-year-old medical student generates the flow-volume curves shown in the above figure. Curve W is a normal MEFV curve generated when the student was healthy. Which of the following best explains curve X?

A) Asthma attack
B) Aspiration of meat into the trachea
C) Heavy exercise
D) Light exercise
E) Normal breathing at rest
F) Pneumonia
G) Tuberculosis

129

82. Which of the following best describes comparison of the lung compliance and surfactant levels in a premature infant with respiratory distress syndrome versus a normal full-term infant?

	Lung Compliance (Premature vs. Full Term Infant)	Surfactant Levels (Premature vs. Full Term Infant)
A)	↑	↓
B)	↑	↑
C)	↓	↓
D)	↓	↑
E)	↔	↑
F)	↔	↓

83. Compared with a normal healthy person, how do TLC and maximum expiratory flow (MEF) change with restrictive lung disease?

	TLC	MEF
A)	↑	↓
B)	↓	↓
C)	↑	↑
D)	↓	↑

84. A 78-year-old man who smoked 60 cigarettes per day for 55 years reports shortness of breath. The patient is diagnosed with chronic pulmonary emphysema. Which set of changes is present in this man compared with a healthy nonsmoker?

	Pulmonary Compliance	Lung Elastic Recoil	TLC
A)	Decreased	Decreased	Decreased
B)	Decreased	Decreased	Increased
C)	Decreased	Increased	Increased
D)	Increased	Decreased	Decreased
E)	Increased	Decreased	Increased
F)	Increased	Increased	Increased

85. While breathing room air, a patient with chronic obstructive pulmonary disease, has a systemic arterial Pco_2 of 65 mm Hg and a Po_2 of 40 mm Hg. Supplemental oxygen is administered at a 40% fractional concentration of oxygen in inspired gas (Fio_2), which resulted in an increase of Po_2 to 55 mm Hg and Pco_2 to 70 mm Hg. Which of the following describes the supplemental O_2?

A) Restored arterial dissolved O_2 to normal
B) Did not change breathing
C) Reduced the hypoxic stimulation of breathing
D) Increased the pulmonary excretion of CO_2

86. Which of the following describes diffusing capacity of O_2 in the lung?

A) Does not change during exercise
B) Is greater than diffusing capacity for CO_2
C) Is greater in residents at sea level than in residents at 3000 meters altitude
D) Is directly related to alveolar capillary surface area

87. When he was in his early 40s, a 75-year-old man worked for 5 years in a factory where asbestos was used as an insulator. The man is diagnosed with asbestosis. Which set of changes is present in this man compared with a person with healthy lungs?

	Pulmonary Compliance	Lung Elastic Recoil	TLC
A)	Decreased	Decreased	Decreased
B)	Decreased	Increased	Increased
C)	Decreased	Increased	Decreased
D)	Increased	Decreased	Decreased
E)	Increased	Decreased	Increased
F)	Increased	Increased	Increased

1. **B)** A decrease in airway resistance is due to an increase in the diameter of the airway. Asthma causes bronchoconstriction, which is prevented by β-agonists. Sympathetic stimulation of the airways results in a relaxation of airways, decreasing resistance. Acetylcholine is a bronchoconstrictor, increasing resistance. With low lung volumes there is a collapse of the airways, leading to decreased diameter and increased resistance.
    TMP13 p. 505

2. **E)** The pleural pressure (sometimes called the intrapleural pressure) is the pressure of the fluid in the narrow space between the visceral pleura of the lungs and parietal pleura of the chest wall. The pleural pressure is normally about –5 cm H_2O immediately before inspiration (i.e., at FRC) when all of the respiratory muscles are relaxed. During inspiration, the volume of the chest cavity increases and the pleural pressure becomes more negative. The pleural pressure averages about –7.5 cm H_2O immediately before expiration when the lungs are fully expanded. The pleural pressure then returns to its resting value of –5 cm H_2O as the diaphragm relaxes and lung volume returns to FRC. Therefore, the intrapleural pressure is always subatmospheric under normal conditions, varying between –5 and –7.5 cm H_2O during quiet breathing.
    TMP13 pp. 498-499

3. **D)** Contraction of the internal intercostals and abdominal recti pull the rib cage downward during expiration. The abdominal recti and other abdominal muscles compress the abdominal contents upward toward the diaphragm, which also helps to eliminate air from the lungs. The diaphragm relaxes during expiration. The external intercostals, sternocleidomastoid muscles, and scaleni increase the diameter of the chest cavity during exercise and thus assist with inspiration, but only the diaphragm is necessary for inspiration during quiet breathing.
    TMP13 pp. 497-498

4. **E)** Stimulation of parasympathetic nerves results in a bronchoconstriction. With low lung volumes a collapse of the airways occurs, leading to decreased diameter and increased resistance. Histamine is a bronchoconstrictor. Forced exhalations will increase pleural pressure, decreasing airway diameter, and thus increasing resistance. All the responses are correct.
    TMP13 pp. 504, 505, 550

5. **D)** The diaphragm and external intercostals are used for inhalation. The sternocleidomastoid is a muscle in the neck and is not used for inhalation or exhalation. The rectus abdominis and internal intercostals are used for exhalation. The majority of the force for exhalation is generated by the rectus abdominis.
    TMP13 p. 497

6. **E)** Compliance (C) is the change in lung volume (ΔV) that occurs for a given change in the transpulmonary pressure (ΔP): that is, $C = \Delta V/\Delta P$. (The transpulmonary pressure is the difference between the alveolar pressure and pleural pressure.) Because compliance is equal to the slope of the volume–pressure relationship, it should be clear that curve S represents the highest compliance and that curve U represents the lowest compliance.
    TMP13 p. 499

7. **E)** Minute ventilation is VT × respiratory rate. VT from the graph is 500 milliliters. Therefore, minute ventilation = 500 × 12 = 6 L/min.
    TMP13 p. 503

8. **C)** A slow increase in left heart function will lead to a gradual increase in pulmonary capillary pressure, and thus greater fluid filtration. Over time there will be an increase in lymphatics and lymphatic pumping to remove the fluid from the interstitial space. With heart failure there is an increase in fluid retention, and thus no decrease in plasma protein concentration. An increase in interstitial hydrostatic pressure will result in an increase in edema (see Chapter 25, pp. 316-320). An increase in interstitial proteins will cause an increase in interstitial osmotic pressure, leading to an increase in net filtration pressure and increased filtration.
    TMP13 pp. 513-514

9. **C)** The FRC equals the ERV (2 liters) plus the RV (1.0 liter). This is the amount of air that remains in the lungs at the end of a normal expiration. FRC is considered to be the resting volume of the lungs because none of the respiratory muscles is contracted at FRC. This problem illustrates an important point: a spirogram can measure changes in lung volume but not absolute lung volumes. Thus, a spirogram alone cannot be used to determine RV, FRC, or TLC.
    TMP13 pp. 501-503

10. **D)** Because the compliance is 0.2 L/cm H_2O, it should be clear that a 1.0-liter increase in volume will cause a 5 cm H_2O decrease in pleural pressure (1.0 L/0.2 L/cm H_2O = 5.0 cm H_2O), and because the initial pleural pressure was –4 cm H_2O before inhalation,

$C = \dfrac{\Delta V}{P}$

the pressure is reduced by 5 cm H_2O (to −9 cm H_2O) when 1.0 liter of air is inhaled.
TMP13 pp. 498-499

11. **D)** Surfactant is formed relatively late in fetal life. Premature babies born without adequate amounts of surfactant can develop pulmonary failure and die. Surfactant is a surface active agent that greatly reduces the surface tension of the water lining the alveoli. Water is normally attracted to itself, which is why raindrops are round. By reducing the surface tension of the water lining the alveoli (and thus reducing the tendency of water molecules to coalesce), the surfactant reduces the work of breathing—that is, less transpulmonary pressure is required to inhale a given volume of air. Because compliance is equal to the change in lung volume for a given change in transpulmonary pressure, it should be clear that pulmonary compliance is decreased in the absence of surfactant.
TMP13 pp. 499-500

12. **C)** Residual volume = FRC − ERV = 3 L − 1.5 L = 1.5 L
TMP13 pp. 501-503

13. **B)** V_A = Frequency × (V_T − V_D) = 15/min × (650 − 150) = 7.5 L/min
TMP13 p. 504

14. **B)** A spirometer can be used to measure changes in lung volume, but it cannot determine absolute volume. It consists of a drum filled with air inverted over a chamber of water. When the person breathes in and out, the drum moves up and down, recording the changes in lung volume. The spirometer cannot be used to measure RV because the RV of air in the lungs cannot be exhaled into the spirometer. The FRC is the amount of air left in the lungs after a normal expiration. FRC cannot be measured using a spirometer because it contains the RV. The TLC is the total amount of air that the lungs can hold after a maximum inspiration. Because the TLC includes the RV, it cannot be measured using a spirometer. TLC, FRC, and RV can be determined using the helium dilution method or a body plethysmograph.
TMP13 pp. 501-503

15. **B)** Blood flow during exercise is still higher at the base of the lung compared with the apex due to gravity. During exercise there is an opening of more blood vessels in the lung, and thus better perfusion. With the opening of more blood vessels an increase in diffusing capacity occurs, allowing equilibration of the blood with O_2 in spite of the increase in flow. Due to the opening of unperfused vessels and vasodilation of existing vessels, there would be no decrease in lung blood volume. With an increase in cardiac output there will be a decrease in transit time; however, the blood is still equilibrated.
TMP13 pp. 511-513, 524-525

16. **B)** Both the lung and thoracic cage are elastic. Under normal conditions, the elastic tendency of the lungs to collapse is exactly balanced by the elastic tendency of the thoracic cage to expand. When air is introduced into the pleural space, the pleural pressure becomes equal to atmospheric pressure—the chest wall springs outward and the lungs collapse.
TMP13 pp. 498-499

17. **D)** The lower zones of the lung ventilate better than the upper zones, and the middle zones have intermediate ventilation. These differences in regional ventilation can be explained by regional differences in pleural pressure. The pleural pressure is typically about −10 cm H_2O in the upper regions and about −2.5 cm H_2O in the lower regions. A less negative pleural pressure in the lower regions of the chest cavity causes less expansion of the lower zones of the lung during resting conditions. Therefore, the bottom of the lung is relatively compressed during rest but expands better during inspiration compared with the apex.
TMP13 pp. 525-526

18. **E)** Total ventilation is equal to the tidal volume (V_T) times the ventilation frequency. V_A = (V_T − V_D) × Frequency, where V_D is the dead space volume. Both persons have the same total ventilation: subject T, 1000 × 10 = 10 L/min; subject V, 500 × 20 = 10 L/min. However, subject T has a V_A of 18 liters (i.e., (2000 − 200) × 10), whereas subject V has a V_A of only 12 liters (i.e., (500 − 200) × 40). This problem further illustrates that the most effective means of increasing V_A is to increase the V_T, not the respiratory frequency.
TMP13 p. 504

19. **B)** Arterial content = 15 g/dl × 1.34 ml O_2/gm Hb = 20 ml O_2/dl (1 dl = 100 ml)
Venous saturation is 25%, so venous content is 20 ml O_2/dl × 0.25 = 5 ml O_2/dl
Fick's principal is O_2 consumption = cardiac output (arterial content − venous content)
750 ml O_2/min = cardiac output × (20 ml O_2/dl − 5 ml O_2/dl)
Cardiac output = (750 ml O_2/min)/(15 ml O_2/dl) = 5000 ml/min
TMP13 pp. 257, 530-531

20. **D)** Ductus arteriosus is present in a fetus, not a healthy adult, in the segment that connects the pulmonary artery to the aorta. Either this is not present in an adult or the pressures would be higher than measured because this is connected to the aorta. The foramen ovale is a cardiac shunt in the fetal heart from right atrium to left atrium, so pressures would be very low. The left atrial pressure should be between 1 and 5 mm Hg. The pulmonary artery pressure ranges from 25 systolic to ~12 to 14 mm Hg diastolic. The right atrial pressure is ~0 to 2 mm Hg.
TMP13 p. 510

21. E) Fick's law of diffusion states that Diffusion = (Pressure gradient × Surface area × Solubility)/(Distance × MW$^{\frac{1}{2}}$). To simplify, make everything have a value of 1 so diffusion = 1. Now decrease surface area to 0.5 (50% decrease) and double distance to 2. Then diffusion = (1 × 0.5 × 1)/(2 × 1) = 0.25. Thus, the answer is 0.25, which is a 75% decrease from normal.
TMP13 p. 517

22. F) The pulmonary and systemic circulations both receive about the same amount of blood flow because the lungs receive the entire cardiac output. (However, the output of the left ventricle is actually 1% to 2% higher than that of the right ventricle because the bronchial arterial blood originates from the left ventricle and the bronchial venous blood empties into the pulmonary veins.) The pulmonary blood vessels have a relatively low resistance, allowing the entire cardiac output to pass through them without increasing the pressure to a great extent. The pulmonary artery pressure averages about 15 mm Hg, which is much lower than the systemic arterial pressure of about 100 mm Hg.
TMP13 pp. 509-511

23. A) It is usually not feasible to measure the left atrial pressure directly in a normal human being because it is difficult to pass a catheter through the heart chambers into the left atrium. The balloon-tipped, flow-directed catheter (Swan-Ganz catheter) was developed nearly 30 years ago to estimate left atrial pressure for the management of acute myocardial infarction. When the balloon is inflated on a Swan-Ganz catheter, the pressure measured through the catheter, called the wedge pressure, approximates the left atrial pressure for the following reason: blood flow distal to the catheter tip has been stopped all the way to the left atrium, which allows left atrial pressure to be estimated. The wedge pressure is actually a few mm Hg higher than the left atrial pressure, depending on where the catheter is wedged, but this still allows changes in left atrial pressure to be monitored in patients with left ventricular failure.
TMP13 p. 510

24. A) The pulmonary blood flow can increase severalfold without causing an excessive increase in pulmonary artery pressure for the following two reasons: previously closed vessels open up (recruitment), and the vessels enlarge (distension). Recruitment and distension of the pulmonary blood vessels both serve to lower the pulmonary vascular resistance (and thus to maintain low pulmonary blood pressures) when the cardiac output has increased.
TMP13 p. 512

25. C) A *P. aeruginosa* infection can increase the capillary permeability in the lungs and elsewhere in the body, which leads to excess loss of plasma proteins into the interstitial spaces. This leakage of plasma proteins from the vasculature caused the plasma colloid osmotic pressure to decrease from a normal value of about 28 mm Hg to 19 mm Hg. The capillary hydrostatic pressure remained at a normal value of 7 mm Hg, but it can sometimes increase to higher levels, exacerbating the formation of edema. The interstitial fluid hydrostatic pressure has increased from a normal value of about –5 mm Hg to 1 mm Hg, which tends to decrease fluid loss from the capillaries. Excess fluid in the interstitial spaces (edema) causes lymph flow to increase.
TMP13 pp. 513-515

26. A) With an increase in blood flow to a tissue, with no change in metabolism, there will be an increase in tissue P_{O_2} due to the increased delivery of O_2 with no change in metabolism. This increase in tissue P_{O_2} leads to a decreased P_{CO_2} due to increased washout of CO_2 and an increase in pH, due to the fall in P_{CO_2}.
TMP13 pp. 528-529

27. D) With a P_{O_2} of 95 and a content of 19 ml O_2/dl on room air, the patient has no issues with V/Q ratio or pulmonary edema. An arterial content of 19 ml O_2/dl and a P_{O_2} of 95 suggest a normal Hb concentration. A low cardiac output would require a greater extraction of O_2 from the blood to supply O_2 to the tissue, resulting in a decreased mixed venous content.
TMP13 pp. 522-523, 528

28. B) Arterial content = 12 g Hb/dl × 1.34 ml O_2/dl = 16 ml O_2/dl
Venous saturation = 20%, so venous content = 16 ml O_2/dl × 0.2 = 3.2 ml O_2/dl
TMP13 pp. 530-531

29. A) CO binds to the Hb, displacing the O_2 bound to Hb, leading to a decrease in content. The normal particle pressure of CO is a couple of mm Hg. However, arterial P_{O_2} is a measure of dissolved P_{O_2}; therefore, the P_{O_2} will be normal.
TMP13 pp. 528, 534

30. B) When a person performs the Valsalva maneuver (forcing air against a closed glottis), high pressure builds up in the lungs that can force as much as 250 milliliters of blood from the pulmonary circulation into the systemic circulation. The lungs have an important blood reservoir function, automatically shifting blood to the systemic circulation as a compensatory response to hemorrhage and other conditions in which the systemic blood volume is too low.
TMP13 p. 510

31. E) When an airway is blocked, no movement of fresh air occurs. Therefore, the air in the alveoli reaches an equilibration with pulmonary arterial blood. Therefore, P_{O_2} will decrease from 100 to 40, P_{CO_2} will increase from 40 to 45, and systemic P_{O_2} will decrease because there is a decrease in O_2 uptake from the alveoli and thus decreased O_2 diffusion from the alveoli.

   TMP13 pp. 524-525

32. C) To calculate inspired P_{O_2}, one must remember that the air is humidified when it enters the body. Therefore, the humidified air has an effective total pressure of atmospheric pressure (760) – water vapor pressure (47), which yields a pressure of (760 – 47) = 713 mm Hg. The O_2 is 50% of the total gas, so the P_{O_2} is 713 × 0.5 = 356 mm Hg. To correct for the CO_2 in the alveoli, one then must subtract the P_{CO_2} divided by the respiratory quotient (normally 0.8). Therefore, the alveolar P_{O_2} = P_{IO_2} – (P_{CO_2}/R) – 356 – (40/0.8) = 356 – 50 = 306 mm Hg.

   TMP13 pp. 519-521

33. E) Fick's law of diffusion states that the rate of diffusion (D) of a gas through a biological membrane is proportional to ΔP, A, and S, and inversely proportional to d and the square root of the MW of the gas (i.e., D α (ΔP × A × S) / (d × MW^{-2}). The greater the pressure gradient, the faster the diffusion. The larger the cross-sectional area of the membrane, the higher will be the total number of molecules that can diffuse through the membrane. The higher the solubility of the gas, the higher will be the number of gas molecules available to diffuse for a given difference in pressure. When the distance of the diffusion pathway is shorter, it will take less time for the molecules to diffuse the entire distance. When the MW of the gas molecule is decreased, the velocity of kinetic movement of the molecule will be higher, which also increases the rate of diffusion.

   TMP13 pp. 518-519

34. B) Normal alveolar P_{CO_2} is 40 mm Hg. Normal V_A for this person is 3.6 L/min. On the ventilator the V_A is 7.2 L/min. A doubling of V_A results in a decrease in alveolar P_{CO_2} by one-half. Thus, alveolar P_{CO_2} would be 20.

   TMP13 p. 520

35. B) Venous P_{O_2} and P_{CO_2} are measures of the balance between blood flow in and metabolism by the tissue. If metabolism does not change and blood flow decreases, then there will be greater diffusion of O_2 from the blood into the tissue to supply the same amount of O_2, leading to a decreased venous P_{O_2}. With a decrease in blood flow, there will be a decreased washout of CO_2, leading to an increase in venous P_{CO_2}.

   TMP13 pp. 528-529, 533

36. B) Alveolar air normally equilibrates with the mixed venous blood that perfuses them; thus, the gas composition of alveolar air and pulmonary capillary blood are identical. When a group of alveoli are not perfused, the composition of the alveolar air becomes equal to the inspired gas composition, which has an O_2 tension of 149 mm Hg and CO_2 tension of about 0 mm Hg.

   TMP13 pp. 524-526

37. A) Alveolar P_{O_2} depends on inspired gas and alveolar P_{CO_2}. Alveolar P_{CO_2} is a balance between V_A and CO_2 production. To decrease alveolar P_{CO_2}, there must be increased V_A in relation to metabolism. Low P_{O_2} will not directly affect P_{CO_2}, but it can stimulate respiration (if P_{O_2} is sufficiently low), which would then reduce P_{CO_2}. An increased metabolism with unchanged V_A will increase P_{CO_2}. A doubling in metabolism with a doubling in V_A will have no effect on P_{CO_2}.

   TMP13 pp. 520-521

38. B) It is not practical to measure the O_2-diffusing capacity directly because it is not possible to measure accurately the O_2 tension of the pulmonary capillary blood. However, the diffusing capacity for CO can be measured accurately because the CO tension in pulmonary capillary blood is zero under normal conditions. The CO diffusing capacity is then used to calculate the O_2-diffusing capacity by taking into account the differences in diffusion coefficient between O_2 and CO. Knowing the rate of transfer of CO across the respiratory membrane is often helpful for evaluating the presence of possible parenchymal lung disease when spirometry and/or lung volume determinations suggest a reduced VC, RV, and/or TLC.

   TMP13 p. 524

39. D) A decrease in the V_A/Q is depicted by moving to the left along the normal ventilation-perfusion line shown in the figure. Whenever the V_A/Q is below normal, there is inadequate ventilation to provide the O_2 needed to fully oxygenate the blood flowing through the alveolar capillaries (i.e., alveolar P_{O_2} is low). Therefore, a certain fraction of the venous blood passing through the pulmonary capillaries does not become oxygenated. Poorly ventilated areas of the lung also accumulate CO_2 diffusing into the alveoli from the mixed venous blood. The result of decreasing V_A/Q (moving to the left along the V_A/Q line) on alveolar P_{O_2} and P_{CO_2} is shown in the figure; that is, P_{O_2} decreases and P_{CO_2} increases.

   TMP13 pp. 524-526

40. C) Because the blood that perfuses the pulmonary capillaries is venous blood returning to the lungs (i.e., mixed venous blood) from the systemic circulation, it is the gases in this blood with which the alveolar gases equilibrate. Therefore, when an airway is blocked, the alveolar air equilibrates with the mixed venous blood and the partial pressures of the gases in both the blood and alveolar air become identical.

   TMP13 pp. 524-526

41. B) When the ventilation is reduced to zero (VA/Q = 0), alveolar air equilibrates with the mixed venous blood entering the lung, which causes the gas composition of the alveolar air to become identical to that of the blood. This occurs at point A, where the alveolar P_{O_2} is 40 mm Hg and the alveolar P_{CO_2} is 45 mm Hg, as shown in the figure. A reduction in VA/Q (caused by the partially obstructed airway in this problem) causes the alveolar P_{O_2} and P_{CO_2} to approach the values achieved when VA/Q = 0.

      TMP13 pp. 524-526

42. E) A pulmonary embolism decreases blood flow to the affected lung, causing ventilation to exceed blood flow. When the embolism completely blocks all blood flow to an area of the lung, the gas composition of the inspired air entering the alveoli equilibrates with blood trapped in the alveolar capillaries so that within a short time, the gas composition of the alveolar air is identical to that of inspired air. An increase in VA/Q caused by the partially obstructed blood flow in this problem causes the alveolar P_{O_2} and P_{CO_2} to approach the values achieved when VA/Q = ∞. The point at which VA/Q is equal to infinity corresponds to point E in the figure (inspired gas).

      TMP13 pp. 524-526

43. C) Breathing 100% O_2 has a limited effect on the arterial P_{O_2} when the cause of arterial hypoxemia is a vascular shunt. However, breathing 100% O_2 raises the arterial P_{O_2} to more than 600 mm Hg in a normal subject. With a vascular shunt, the arterial P_{O_2} is determined by (a) highly oxygenated end-capillary blood (P_{O_2} > 600 mm Hg) that has passed through ventilated portions of the lung, and (b) shunted blood that has bypassed the ventilated portions of the lungs and thus has an O_2 partial pressure equal to that of mixed venous blood (P_{O_2} = 40 mm Hg). A mixture of the two bloods causes a large fall in P_{O_2} because the O_2 dissociation curve is so flat in its upper range.

      TMP13 pp. 525-526

44. D) The anatomic dead space (D_{ANAT}) is the air that a person breathes in that fills the respiratory passageways but never reaches the alveoli. Alveolar dead space (D_{ALV}) is the air in the alveoli that are ventilated but not perfused. Physiologic dead space (D_{PHY}) is the sum of D_{ANAT} and D_{ALV} (i.e., $D_{PHY} = D_{ANAT} + D_{ALV}$). The D_{ALV} is zero in lung unit S (the ideal lung unit), and the D_{ANAT} and D_{PHY} are thus equal to each other. The figure shows a group of alveoli with a poor blood supply (lung unit T), which means that the D_{ALV} is substantial. Thus, D_{PHY} is greater than either D_{ANAT} or D_{ALV} in lung unit T.

      TMP13 pp. 521, 525-526

45. E) The P_{O_2} of mixed venous blood entering the pulmonary capillaries is normally about 40 mm Hg, and the P_{O_2} at the venous end of the capillaries is normally equal to that of the alveolar gas (104 mm Hg). The P_{O_2} of the pulmonary blood normally rises to equal that of the alveolar air by the time the blood has moved a third of the distance through the capillaries, becoming almost 104 mm Hg. Thus, curve B represents the normal resting state. During exercise, the cardiac output can increase severalfold, but the pulmonary capillary blood still becomes almost saturated with O_2 during its transit through the lungs. However, because of the faster flow of blood through the lungs during exercise, the O_2 has less time to diffuse into the pulmonary capillary blood, and therefore the P_{O_2} of the capillary blood does not reach its maximum value until it reaches the venous end of the pulmonary capillaries. Although curves D and E both show that O_2 saturation of blood occurs near the venous end, note that only curve E shows a low P_{O_2} of 25 mm Hg at the arterial end of the pulmonary capillaries, which is typical of mixed venous blood during strenuous exercise.

      TMP13 pp. 527-528

46. A) The P_{O_2} of mixed venous blood entering the pulmonary capillaries increases during its transit through the pulmonary capillaries (from 40 mm Hg to 104 mm Hg), and the P_{CO_2} decreases simultaneously from 45 mm Hg to 40 mm Hg. Thus, P_{O_2} is represented by the red lines and P_{CO_2} is represented by the green lines in the various diagrams. During resting conditions, O_2 has a 64 mm Hg pressure gradient (104 – 64 = 64 mm Hg), and CO_2 has a 5 mm Hg pressure gradient (45 – 40 = 5 mm Hg) between the blood at the arterial end of the capillaries and the alveolar air. Despite this large difference in pressure gradients between O_2 and CO_2, both gases equilibrate with the alveolar air by the time the blood has moved a third of the distance through the capillaries in the normal resting state (choice A). This is possible because CO_2 can diffuse about 20 times as rapidly as O_2.

      TMP13 pp. 528-529

47. A) O_2 diffuses from the lung into the blood and is both dissolved and bound to Hb. In spite of having no red blood cells, the P_{O_2} would be normal as the O_2 is dissolved in the plasma. The content would be minimal, just due to the dissolved O_2 in the plasma.

      TMP13 pp. 528, 530, 533

48. C) Pulmonary venous blood is nearly 100% saturated with O_2 and has a P_{O_2} of about 104 mm Hg, and each 100 milliliters of blood carries about 20 m/s of O_2 (i.e., O_2 content is about 20 vol%). Approximately 25% of the O_2 carried in the arterial blood is used by the tissues under resting conditions. Thus, reduced blood returning to the lungs is about 75% saturated with O_2, has a P_{O_2} of about 40 mm Hg, and has an O_2 content of about 15 vol%. Note that it necessary to know only one value for oxygenated and reduced blood and that the other two values requested in the question can be read from the O_2-Hb dissociation curve.

      TMP13 pp. 528, 530-531

49. C) Each gram of Hb can normally carry 1.34 milliliters of O_2. Hb = 12 g/dl. Arterial oxygen content = 12 × 1.34 = 16 ml O_2/dl. Using 12 ml O_2/dl yields a mixed venous saturation of 25%. With a saturation of 25%, the venous Po_2 should be close to 20 mm Hg.
TMP13 pp. 531-532

50. D) When a person is anemic, there is a decrease in O_2 content. The O_2 saturation of Hb in the arterial blood and the arterial O_2 partial pressure are not affected by the Hb concentration of the blood.
TMP13 pp. 530-531

51. A) The respiratory area of the medulla controls all aspects of respiration, so a destruction of this area would cause a cessation of breathing.
TMP13 pp. 539-540

52. E) CO combines with Hb at the same point on the Hb molecule as O_2 and therefore can displace O_2 from the Hb, reducing the O_2 saturation of Hb. Because CO binds with Hb (to form carboxyhemoglobin) with about 250 times as much tenacity as O_2, even small amounts of CO in the blood can severely limit the O_2-carrying capacity of the blood. The presence of carboxyhemoglobin also shifts the O_2 dissociation curve to the left (which means that O_2 binds more tightly to Hb), which further limits the transfer of O_2 to the tissues.
TMP13 pp. 531, 533

53. B) In exercise, several factors shift the O_2-Hb curve to the right, which serves to deliver extra amounts of O_2 to the exercising muscle fibers. These factors include increased quantities of CO_2 released from the muscle fibers, increased H^+ concentration in the muscle capillary blood, and increased temperature resulting from heat generated by the exercising muscle. The right shift of the O_2-Hb curve allows more O_2 to be released to the muscle at a given O_2 partial pressure in the blood.
TMP13 pp. 531-532

54. C) Structural differences between fetal Hb and adult Hb make fetal Hb unable to react with 2,3 diphosphoglycerate (2,3-DPG) and thus to have a higher affinity for O_2 at a given Po_2. The fetal dissociation curve is thus shifted to the left relative to the adult curve. Typically, fetal arterial O_2 pressures are low, and hence the leftward shift enhances the placental uptake of O_2.
TMP13 pp. 531-532

55. B) Tissue Po_2 is a balance between delivery and usages. When a decrease in blood flow occurs with no change in metabolism, there will be a decrease in venous Po_2 (less delivery but no change in metabolism) and an increase in venous Pco_2 (less washout).
TMP13 pp. 528-529

56. D) CO_2 is the major controller of respiration as a result of a direct effect of H^+ on the chemosensitive area of the medulla. H^+ do not cross the blood-brain barrier. Thus, CO_2 diffuses across the blood-brain barrier and then is converted to H^+, which acts on the chemosensitive area. CO_2 and H^+ activation of carotid bodies is minimal under normal conditions.
TMP13 pp. 541-542

57. D) The pneumotaxic center transmits signals to the dorsal respiratory group that "switch off" inspiratory signals, thus controlling the duration of the filling phase of the lung cycle. This has a secondary effect of increasing the rate of breathing because limitation of inspiration also shortens expiration and the entire period of respiration.
TMP13 pp. 539-540

58. E) The basic rhythm of respiration is generated in the dorsal respiratory group of neurons, which is located almost entirely within the nucleus of the tractus solitarius. When the respiratory drive for increased pulmonary ventilation becomes greater than normal, respiratory signals spill over into the ventral respiratory neurons, causing the ventral respiratory area to contribute to the respiratory drive. However, neurons of the ventral respiratory group remain almost totally inactive during normal quiet breathing.
TMP13 pp. 539-540

59. C) The respiratory exchange ratio (R) is equal to the rate of CO_2 output divided by the rate of O_2 uptake. A value of 0.8 therefore means that the amount of CO_2 produced by the tissues is 80% of the amount of O_2 used by the tissues, which also means that the amount of CO_2 transported from the tissues to the lungs in each 100 milliliters of blood is 80% of the amount of O_2 transported from the lungs to the tissues in each 100 milliliters of blood. Choice C is the only answer in which the ratio of CO_2 to O_2 is 0.8 (4/5 = 0.8). Although R changes under different metabolic conditions, ranging from 1.00 in those who consume carbohydrates exclusively to 0.7 in those who consume fats exclusively, the average value for R is close to 0.8.
TMP13 p. 535

60. F) Dissolved CO_2 combines with water in red blood cells to form carbonic acid, which dissociates to form bicarbonate and H^+ ions. Many of the bicarbonate ions diffuse out of the red blood cells, whereas chloride ions diffuse into the red blood cells to maintain electrical neutrality. The phenomenon, called the chloride shift, is made possible by a special bicarbonate-chloride carrier protein in the red blood cell membrane that shuttles the ions in opposite directions. Water moves into the red blood cells to maintain osmotic equilibrium, which results in a slight swelling of the red blood cells in the venous blood.
TMP13 pp. 534-535

61. D) The Hering-Breuer reflex mechanoreceptors are located in the bronchi and bronchioles and respond to increased stretch to limit respiration.

TMP13 p. 540

62. C) This patient would have increased V_A, therefore resulting in a decrease in arterial P_{CO_2}. The effect of this decrease in P_{CO_2} would be an inhibition of the chemosensitive area and a decrease in ventilation until P_{CO_2} was back to normal. Breathing high O_2 does not decrease nerve activity sufficient to decrease respiration. The response of peripheral chemoreceptors to CO_2 and pH is mild and does not play a major role in the control of respiration.

TMP13 pp. 541-543

63. F) A person with constricted lungs has a reduced TLC and RV. Because the lung cannot expand to a normal size, the MEF cannot equal normal values.

TMP13 p. 550

64. F) V_A can increase by more than eightfold when the arterial CO_2 tension is increased over a physiological range from about 35 to 75 mm Hg. This demonstrates the tremendous effect that CO_2 changes have in controlling respiration. By contrast, the change in respiration caused by changing the blood pH over a normal range from 7.3 to 7.5 is more than 10 times less effective.

TMP13 p. 542

65. D) The arterial O_2 tension has essentially no effect on V_A when it is higher than about 100 mm Hg, but ventilation approximately doubles when the arterial O_2 tension falls to 60 mm Hg and can increase as much as fivefold at very low O_2 tensions. This quantitative relationship between arterial O_2 tension and V_A was established in an experimental setting in which the arterial CO_2 tension and pH were held constant. The student can imagine that the ventilatory response to hypoxia would be blunted if the CO_2 tension were permitted to decrease.

TMP13 p. 543

66. B) In a normal person the alveolar gases are the same as the arterial blood. With rebreathing, the exhaled CO_2 is never removed and continues to accumulate in the bag. This increase in alveolar and thus arterial P_{CO_2} will be the stimulus for the increased breathing. The alveolar P_{O_2} will be decreased, not increased, with the decreased P_{O_2} stimulating breathing. A decreased P_{CO_2} will not stimulate ventilation. An increased pH, alkalosis, will not stimulate ventilation.

TMP13 pp. 541-543

67. A) Because strenuous exercise does not significantly change the mean arterial P_{O_2}, P_{CO_2}, or pH, it is unlikely that these play an important role in stimulating the immense increase in ventilation. Although the mean venous P_{O_2} decreases during exercise, the venous vasculature does not contain chemoreceptors that can sense P_{O_2}. The brain, upon transmitting motor impulses to the contracting muscles, is believed to transmit collateral impulses to the brain stem to excite the respiratory center. Also, the movement of body parts during exercise is believed to excite joint and muscle proprioceptors that then transmit excitatory impulses to the respiratory center.

TMP13 pp. 546-547

68. E) It is remarkable that the arterial P_{O_2}, P_{CO_2}, and pH remain almost exactly normal in a healthy athlete during strenuous exercise despite the 20-fold increase in O_2 consumption and CO_2 formation. This interesting phenomenon begs the question: What is it during exercise that causes the intense ventilation?

TMP13 pp. 546-547

69. D) A person with emphysema has an increase in airway resistance, a decrease in diffusing capacity (affecting gas exchange), an abnormal V/Q ratio (possible shunt), and a loss of large portions of the alveolar walls and capillaries. This loss of capillaries leads to an increase in pulmonary vascular resistance and the development of pulmonary hypertension.

TMP13 pp. 551-552

70. B) The basic mechanism of Cheyne-Stokes breathing can be attributed to a buildup of CO_2 that stimulates overventilation, followed by a depression of the respiratory center because of a low P_{CO_2} of the respiratory neurons. It should be clear that the greatest depth of breathing occurs when the neurons of the respiratory center are exposed to the highest levels of CO_2 (point W). This increase in breathing causes CO_2 to be blown off, and thus the P_{CO_2} of the lung blood is at its lowest value at about point Y in the figure. The P_{CO_2} of the pulmonary blood gradually increases from point Y to point Z, reaching its maximum value at point V. Thus, it is the phase lag between the P_{CO_2} at the respiratory center and the P_{CO_2} of the pulmonary blood that leads to this type of breathing. The phase-lag often occurs with left heart failure due to enlargement of the left ventricle, which increases the time required for blood to reach the respiratory center. Another cause of Cheyne-Stokes breathing is increased negative feedback gain in the respiratory control areas, which can be caused by head trauma, stroke, and other types of brain damage.

TMP13 pp. 546-548

71. D) The FVC is equal to the difference between the TLC and the RV. The TLC and RV are the points of intersection between the abscissa and flow-volume curve; that is, TLC = 5.5 liters and RV = 1.0 liter. Therefore, FVC = 5.5 − 1.0 = 4.5 liters.

TMP13 p. 550

72. D) The MEFV curve is created when a person inhales as much air as possible (point A, total lung capacity = 5.5 liters) and then expires the air with a maximum effort until no more air can be expired (point E, residual volume = 1.0 liter). The descending portion of the curve indicated by the downward pointing arrow represents the MEF at each lung volume. This descending portion of the curve is sometimes referred to as the "effort-independent" portion of the curve because the patient cannot increase expiratory flow rate to a higher level even when a greater expiratory effort is expended.

TMP13 p. 550

73. B) In obstructive diseases such as emphysema and asthma, the MEFV curve begins and ends at abnormally high lung volumes, and the flow rates are lower than normal at any given lung volume. The curve may also have a scooped out appearance, as shown in the figure. The other diseases listed as answer choices are constricted lung diseases (often called restrictive lung diseases). Lung volumes are lower than normal in constricted lung diseases.

TMP13 p. 550

74. A) Asbestosis is a constricted lung disease characterized by diffuse interstitial fibrosis. In constricted lung disease (more commonly called restrictive lung disease), the MEFV curve begins and ends at abnormally low lung volumes, and the flow rates are often higher than normal at any given lung volume, as shown in the figure. Lung volumes are expected to be higher than normal in asthma, bronchospasm, emphysema, old age, and in other instances in which the airways are narrowed or radial traction of the airways is reduced, allowing them to close more easily.

TMP13 p. 550

75. B) The figure shows that a maximum respiratory effort is needed during resting conditions because the MEF rate is achieved during resting conditions. It should be clear that his ability to exercise is greatly diminished. The man has smoked for 60 years and is likely to have emphysema. Therefore, the student can surmise that the TLC, FRC, and RV are greater than normal. The VC is only about 3.4 liters, as shown in the figure.

TMP13 pp. 550-551

76. A) The FVC is the VC measured with a forced expiration. The FEV_1 is the amount of air that can be expelled from the lungs during the first second of a forced expiration. The FEV_1/FVC for the normal individual (curve X) is 4 L/5 L = 80% and 2 L/4 L = 50% for the patient (curve Z). The FEV_1/FVC ratio has diagnostic value for differentiating between normal, obstructive, and constricted patterns of a forced expiration.

TMP13 p. 551

77. E) The FVC is the VC measured with a forced expiration. The FEV_1 is the amount of air that can be expelled from the lungs during the first second of a forced expiration. The FEV_1/FVC ratio for the healthy individual (X) is 4 L/5 L = 80%; FEV_1/FVC for patient Z is 3.0/3.5 = 86%. FEV_1/FVC is often increased in silicosis and other diseases characterized by interstitial fibrosis because of increased radial traction of the airways; that is, the airways are held open to a greater extent at any given lung volume, reducing their resistance to air flow. Airway resistance is increased (and therefore FEV_1/FVC is decreased) in asthma, bronchospasm, emphysema, and old age.

TMP13 p. 551

78. D) With consolidated pneumonia, the lung is filled with fluid and cellular debris, which results in a decreased area for diffusion. In addition, the V/Q ratio is decreased, which will lead to hypoxia (decreased Po_2 and content) and hypercapnia (increased Pco_2).

TMP13 pp. 552-553

79. D) With atelectasis of one lung, a collapse of the lung tissue occurs, which increases the resistance to blood flow. In addition, the hypoxia in the collapsed lung causes an additional vasoconstriction. The net effect is to shift blood to the opposite, ventilated lung, resulting in the majority of flow in the ventilated lung. A slight compromise in V/Q ratio will occur. With minimal changes in the V/Q ratio, there will be minimal changes in Po_2 and Pco_2. Thus there should be a slight decrease in arterial Po_2 and a slight decrease in saturation and content.

TMP13 p. 553

80. B) The loss of alveolar walls with destruction of associated capillary beds in the emphysematous lung reduces the elastic recoil and increases the compliance. The student should recall that compliance is equal to the change in lung volume for a given change in transpulmonary pressure; that is, compliance is equal to the slopes of the volume-pressure relationships shown in the figure. Asbestosis, silicosis, and tuberculosis are associated with deposition of fibrous tissue in the lungs, which decreases the compliance. Mitral obstruction and rheumatic heart disease can cause pulmonary edema, which also decreases the pulmonary compliance.

TMP13 p. 499

81. C) Curve X represents heavy exercise with a VT of about 3 liters. Note that the expiratory flow rate has reached a maximum value of nearly 4.5 L/sec during the heavy exercise. This effect occurred because a maximum expiratory air flow is required to move the air through the airways with the high ventilatory frequency associated with heavy exercise. Normal breathing at rest is represented by curve Z; note that the VT is less than 1 liter during resting conditions. Curve Y was recorded during mild exercise. An asthma attack or aspiration of meat would increase the resistance to air flow from the lungs, making it unlikely that expiratory air flow rate could approach its maximum value at a given lung volume. The VT should not increase greatly with pneumonia or tuberculosis, and it should not be possible to achieve a maximum expiratory air flow at a given lung volume with these diseases.

TMP13 pp. 550-551

82. **C)** A premature infant with respiratory distress syndrome has absent or reduced levels of surfactant. Loss of surfactant creates a greater surface tension. Because surface tension accounts for a large portion of lung elasticity, increasing surface tension will increase lung elasticity, making the lung stiffer and less compliant.

TMP13 p. 553

83. **C)** Asbestosis is associated with deposition of fibrous material in the lungs, which causes the pulmonary compliance (i.e., distensibility) to decrease and the elastic recoil to increase. Pulmonary compliance and elastic recoil change in opposite directions because compliance is proportional to 1/elastic recoil. It is somewhat surprising to learn that the elastic recoil of a rock is greater than the elastic recoil of a rubber band; that is, the more difficult it is to deform an object, the greater the elastic recoil of the object. The TLC, FRC, RV, and VC are decreased in all types of fibrotic lung disease.

TMP13 p. 499

84. **E)** Loss of lung tissue in emphysema leads to an increase in the compliance of the lungs and a decrease in the elastic recoil of the lungs. Pulmonary compliance and elastic recoil always change in opposite directions; that is, compliance is proportional to 1/elastic recoil. The TLC, RV, and FRC are increased in emphysema, but the VC is decreased.

TMP13 p. 499

85. **C)** There was an increase in P_{O_2}, but not to normal levels. The increase in P_{CO_2} means that the V_A decreased. In this patient the V_A was driven by the decreased O_2 levels. If P_{CO_2} increased, there is no increased pulmonary excretion of CO_2.

TMP13 pp. 541-542, 551-552

86. **D)** Diffusing capacity is directly related to alveolar surface area. It increases during exercise due to opening of capillaries and better V/Q match. The diffusing capacity of CO_2 is 20 times that of O_2. When one goes to a high altitude, an opening of blood vessels and alveoli occurs to increase the diffusion of O_2, resulting in an increased diffusing capacity.

TMP13 pp. 523-525

87. **B)** Total lung capacity and MEF are reduced in restrictive lung disease.

TMP13 p. 550

Aviation, Space, and Deep-Sea Diving Physiology

1. A diver is breathing 21% oxygen (O_2) at a depth of 132 feet. The diver's body temperature is 37°C, and partial pressure of carbon dioxide (P_{CO_2}) = 40 mm Hg. What is the alveolar partial pressure of oxygen (P_{O_2})?

   A) 149 mm Hg
   B) 380 mm Hg
   C) 578 mm Hg
   D) 738 mm Hg
   E) 3703 mm Hg

2. Upon returning to earth after 2 weeks in space, an astronaut will exhibit which of the following?

   A) An increased blood pressure
   B) An increased urinary output
   C) A decreased muscle tone
   D) An elevated cardiac output
   E) A normal blood volume

3. A man is planning to leave Miami (at sea level) and travel to Colorado to climb Mount Wilson (14,500 feet, barometric pressure = 450 mm Hg). Before his trip he takes acetazolamide, a carbonic anhydrase inhibitor that forces the kidneys to excrete bicarbonate. What response would be expected before he makes the trip?

   A) Alkalotic blood
   B) Normal ventilation
   C) Elevated ventilation
   D) Normal arterial blood gases

4. A diver carries a 1000-liter metal talk-box with an open bottom to a depth of 66 feet so that two divers can insert their heads and talk beneath the water. A person on the surface of the water pumps air into the box until the 1000-liter box is completely filled with air. How much air from the surface is required to fill the box (in liters)?

   A) 1000
   B) 2000
   C) 3000
   D) 4000
   E) 5000

5. Which set of changes best describes a Himalayan native living in the Himalayas, compared with a sea-level native living at sea level?

	Hematocrit	Arterial P_{O_2}	Arterial O_2 Content
A)	Decreased	Decreased	Decreased
B)	Decreased	Decreased	No difference
C)	Decreased	Increased	Decreased
D)	Decreased	Increased	No difference
E)	Increased	Decreased	Decreased
F)	Increased	Increased	Decreased
G)	Increased	Increased	No difference
H)	Increased	Decreased	No difference

6. Which of the following is true regarding a healthy recreational scuba diver at a depth of 66 feet in the Caribbean Sea?

   A) Her lungs are smaller than normal
   B) She has an elevated arterial P_{O_2} and a normal P_{CO_2}
   C) All gas partial pressures in her blood (O_2, nitrogen [N_2], CO_2, and water vapor) are elevated
   D) There are increases in both fraction of inspired oxygen (F_{IO_2}) and inspired nitrogen (F_{IN_2})

7. A pilot is flying a commercial, pressurized (730 mm Hg) airplane at 30,000 feet; the barometric pressure is 226 mm Hg. If the pilot's body temperature is normal and the alveolar P_{O_2} is 90 mm Hg, which of the following is true?

   A) Arterial P_{CO_2} is 40 mm Hg
   B) Alveolar ventilation will be increased
   C) Arterial pH will be 7.6
   D) Alveolar P_{CO_2} will be 45 mm Hg
   E) The pilot will be polycythemic

1. **D)** 132 feet is equivalent to 5 atmospheres of pressure (4 of water and 1 of air). The total barometric pressure is $760 \times 5 = 3800$. Alveolar P_{CO_2} would be normal at 40. Alveolar $P_{O_2} = (3800 - 47) \times 0.21 - (40/0.8) = 738$ mm Hg.
   TMP13 p. 569

2. **C)** During time in space, an astronaut will experience a decrease in muscle mass due to the lack of gravity. He or she will have a decreased blood volume but no increase in blood pressure. After coming back to earth, the astronaut will not have an elevated cardiac output due to the decreased blood volume. Therefore, when the astronaut returns to earth he or she will retain fluid to return the blood volume to normal and thus will have a decrease in urine output.
   TMP13 pp. 567-568

3. **C)** Acetazolamide is a medication that that forces the kidneys to excrete bicarbonate, the base form of CO_2. This excretion reacidifies the blood, balancing the effects of the hyperventilation that occurs at altitude in an attempt to get O_2. Such reacidification acts as a respiratory stimulant, particularly at night, reducing or eliminating the periodic breathing pattern common at altitude. This would increase ventilation, resulting in a decreased P_{CO_2}.
   TMP13 p. 563

4. **C)** Boyle's law states that $P_1V_1 = P_2V_2$, where P_1 and V_1 are the original pressure and volume and P_2 and V_2 are the new volume and pressure. The atmospheric pressure at a depth of 66 feet is three times greater than the atmospheric pressure at the surface of the water; that is, there is 1 atmosphere at the surface plus an additional atmosphere for each 33 feet below the surface. Therefore, it takes three times as much sea level air to fill the box when the box is submerged to a depth of 66 feet because the air is subjected to 3 atmospheres.
   TMP13 p. 569

5. **H)** Acclimatization to hypoxia includes an increase in pulmonary ventilation, an increase in red blood cells, an increase in diffusion capacity of the lungs, an increase in vascularity of the tissues, and an increase in the ability of the cells to use available O_2. The increase in hematocrit of high-altitude natives allows normal amounts of O_2 (or even greater than normal amounts of O_2) to be carried in the blood despite lower than normal arterial O_2 tension. For example, those native to elevations of 15,000 feet have an arterial O_2 tension of only 40 mm Hg, but because of greater amounts of hemoglobin in the blood, the quantity of O_2 carried in the blood is often greater than that in the blood of sea-level natives.
   TMP13 pp. 562-563

6. **B)** Water vapor pressure and CO_2 remain normal. All other partial pressures are increased. Tidal volume is normal because of the scuba gear. The compressed air is normal air: 79% N_2 and 21% O_2.
   TMP13 pp. 569-571

7. **A)** With a P_{O_2} of 90 mm Hg, there will be no drive to increase respiration. Therefore, the pilot will have normal ventilation with an arterial P_{CO_2} of 40, which will result in a normal pH of 7.4. Alveolar P_{CO_2} should be exactly the same as arterial P_{CO_2} and would not be 45 mm Hg. The pilot has no reason to be polycythemic because there is no evidence that he has been exposed to a chronic hypoxia.
   TMP13 pp. 562-563

The Nervous System: A. General Principles and Sensory Physiology

1. Which ion has the greatest electrochemical driving force in a typical neuron with a resting membrane potential of −65 millivolts?

   A) Chloride
   B) Potassium
   C) Sodium

2. A 2-year-old girl with fever is hyperventilating. Which of the following is most likely to occur in this girl?

   A) Decreased brain oxygenation only
   B) Decreased brain oxygenation and increased neuronal activity
   C) Decreased neuronal activity only
   D) Increased brain oxygenation only
   E) Increased brain oxygenation and decreased neuronal activity
   F) Increased neuronal activity only

3. Pain receptors in the skin are typically classified as which of the following?

   A) Encapsulated nerve endings
   B) A single class of morphologically specialized receptors
   C) The same type of receptor that detects position sense
   D) Free nerve endings

4. Which of the following best describes an expanded tip tactile receptor found in the dermis of hairy skin that is specialized to detect continuously applied touch sensation?

   A) Free nerve endings
   B) Merkel disc
   C) Pacinian corpuscle
   D) Ruffini endings

5. The release of neurotransmitter at a chemical synapse in the central nervous system is dependent upon which of the following?

   A) Synthesis of acetylcholinesterase
   B) Hyperpolarization of the synaptic terminal
   C) Opening of ligand-gated ion calcium channels
   D) Influx of calcium into the presynaptic terminal

6. Which of the following is best described as an elongated, encapsulated receptor found in the dermal pegs of glabrous skin that is especially abundant on lips and fingertips?

   A) Merkel disc
   B) Free nerve endings
   C) Meissner corpuscle
   D) Ruffini endings

7. A transmitter substance released from a presynaptic neuron activates a second messenger G-protein system in the postsynaptic neuron. Which one of the following postsynaptic responses to the transmitter substance is NOT a possible outcome?

   A) Activation of cyclic adenosine monophosphate (cAMP)
   B) Activation of cyclic guanosine monophosphate (cGMP)
   C) Activation of gene transcription
   D) Closing an ion channel
   E) Opening an ion channel

8. A 43-year-old man sustained a lower back injury that causes severe chronic pain. His physician prescribes benzodiazepine sedation medications to help him sleep. Which response best describes why this man has difficulty sleeping without medication?

   A) Depression of the amygdala
   B) Depression of reticular formation
   C) Excitation of the amygdala
   D) Excitation of reticular formation
   E) Loss of somatic sensations
   F) Loss of visceral sensations

9. A 15-year-old girl with epilepsy visits a physician for testing. The physician uses electroencephalography to study her brain waves during various activities. Which of the following is most likely to stimulate the greatest increase in brain activity in this girl?

   A) Hyperventilation
   B) Hypoventilation
   C) Hyperventilation plus flashing lights
   D) Hypoventilation plus flashing lights

10. Which of the following best describes the concept of specificity in sensory nerve fibers that transmit only one modality of sensation?

    A) Frequency coding principle
    B) Concept of specific nerve energy
    C) Singularity principle
    D) Labeled line principle

11. Which of the following is an encapsulated receptor found deep in the skin throughout the body, as well as in fascial layers, where it detects indentation of the skin (pressure) and movement across the surface (vibration)?

    A) Pacinian corpuscle
    B) Meissner's corpuscle
    C) Free nerve endings
    D) Ruffini endings

12. Which substance enhances the sensitivity of pain receptors but does not directly excite them?

    A) Bradykinin
    B) Serotonin
    C) Potassium ions
    D) Prostaglandins

13. Which of the following is an important functional parameter of pain receptors?

    A) Exhibit little or no adaptation
    B) Not affected by muscle tension
    C) Signal only flexion at joint capsules
    D) Can voluntarily be inhibited

14. The excitatory or inhibitory action of a neurotransmitter is determined by which of the following?

    A) The function of its postsynaptic receptor
    B) Its molecular composition
    C) The shape of the synaptic vesicle in which it is contained
    D) The distance between the pre- and postsynaptic membranes

15. A 39-year-old neurosurgeon picks up a scalpel, which activates numerous sensory receptors in her hand. An increase in which of the following best describes the basis for transduction of the sensory stimuli into nerve impulses?

    A) Activation of G protein
    B) Decreased ion permeability
    C) Decreased transmitter release
    D) Increased ion permeability
    E) Increased transmitter release
    F) Inhibition of G protein

16. Which ion has the lowest electrochemical driving force in a typical neuron with a resting membrane potential of −65 millivolts?

    A) Chloride
    B) Potassium
    C) Sodium

17. A physiology experiment is conducted in which a glass microelectrode in inserted into a Pacinian corpuscle to record receptor potentials during different levels of stimulation (from 0 percent to 100 percent). Increasing stimulus strength from 10 percent of maximum to 30 percent of maximum causes a 40 percent increase in the amplitude of the receptor potential. Increasing the stimulus potential from 70 percent of maximum to 90 percent of maximum is most likely to cause which increase in the amplitude of the receptor potential (in percent)?

    A) 10
    B) 40
    C) 60
    D) 80

18. Interneurons that utilize the neurotransmitter enkephalin to inhibit afferent pain signals are most likely to be found in which region of the central nervous system?

    A) Dorsal horn of spinal cord
    B) Postcentral gyrus
    C) Precentral gyrus
    D) δ-type A
    E) Type C fiber
    F) Ventral horn of spinal cord

19. Which system transmits somatosensory information with the highest degree of temporal and spatial fidelity?

    A) Anterolateral system
    B) Dorsal column–medial lemniscal system
    C) Corticospinal system
    D) Spinocerebellar system

20. The pathway of which system crosses in the ventral white commissure of the spinal cord within a few segments of entry and then courses to the thalamus contralateral to the side of the body from which the signal originated?

    A) Anterolateral system
    B) Dorsal column–medial lemniscal system
    C) Corticospinal system
    D) Spinocerebellar system

21. Neurons located in which area release serotonin as their neurotransmitter?

    A) Periaqueductal gray area
    B) Interneurons of the spinal cord
    C) Periventricular area
    D) Nucleus raphe magnus

22. Which system conveys information concerning highly localized touch sensation and body position (proprioceptive) sensation?

    A) Anterolateral
    B) Dorsal column–medial lemniscal
    C) Corticospinal
    D) Spinocerebellar

23. The first-order (primary afferent) cell bodies of the dorsal column–medial lemniscal system are found in which structure?

    A) Spinal cord dorsal horn
    B) Spinal cord ventral horn
    C) Dorsal root ganglia
    D) Nucleus cuneatus

24. Which structure carries axons from the nucleus gracilis to the thalamus?

    A) Fasciculus gracilis
    B) Fasciculus lemniscus
    C) Lateral spinothalamic tract
    D) Medial lemniscus

25. A 10-year-old boy cuts his finger with a pocketknife and immediately applies pressure to the damaged area with his other hand to partially alleviate the pain. Inhibition of pain signals by tactile stimulation of the skin is mediated by which type of afferent neurons from mechanoreceptors?

    A) α-type A
    B) β-type A
    C) δ-type A
    D) Type C

26. A pool of presynaptic neurons innervate the dendrites of a postsynaptic neuron. Electrical signals are transferred from the dendrites to the soma of the postsynaptic neuron by which process?

    A) Action potential
    B) Active transport
    C) Capacitive discharge
    D) Diffusion
    E) Electrotonic conduction

27. Which structure carries axons from neurons in the ventral posterolateral nucleus of the thalamus to the primary somatosensory cortex?

    A) Medial lemniscus
    B) External capsule
    C) Internal capsule
    D) Extreme capsule

28. Which of the following is characteristic of the events occurring at an excitatory synapse?

    A) There is a massive efflux of calcium from the presynaptic terminal
    B) Synaptic vesicles bind to the postsynaptic membrane
    C) Voltage-gated potassium channels are closed
    D) Ligand-gated channels are opened to allow sodium entry into the postsynaptic neuron

29. Stimulation of which brain area can modulate the sensation of pain?

    A) Superior olivary complex
    B) Locus ceruleus
    C) Periaqueductal gray area
    D) Amygdala

30. Which body part is represented superiorly and medially within the postcentral gyrus?

    A) Upper limb
    B) Lower limb
    C) Abdomen
    D) Genitalia

31. Which of the following is a group of neurons in the pain suppression pathway that uses enkephalin as a neurotransmitter?

    A) Postcentral gyrus
    B) Nucleus raphe magnus
    C) Periaqueductal gray area
    D) Type AB sensory fibers

Questions 32 and 33
A 19-year-old man has an automobile accident that completely eliminates all nerve traffic in the right half of the spinal cord at C2. Use this information to answer Questions 32 and 33.

32. Loss of which function is most likely in the right hand of this man?

    A) Crude touch and pain sensation
    B) Crude touch and temperature sensation
    C) Motor function and temperature sensation
    D) Motor function and vibration sense
    E) Vibration sense and crude touch
    F) Vibration sense and pain sensation

33. Loss of which function is most likely in the left hand of this man?

    A) Crude touch and pain sensation
    B) Crude touch and vibration sense
    C) Motor function and temperature sensation
    D) Motor function and vibration sense
    E) Vibration sense and pain sensation
    F) Vibration sense and crude touch

34. The highest degree of pain localization comes from which of the following?

    A) Simultaneous stimulation of free nerve endings and tactile fibers
    B) Stimulation of free nerve endings by bradykinin
    C) Nerve fibers traveling to the thalamus by way of the paleospinothalamic tract
    D) Stimulation of δ-type A fibers

35. Which of the following is the basis for referred pain?

    A) Visceral pain signals and pain signals from the skin synapse with separate populations of neurons in the dorsal horn
    B) Visceral pain transmission and pain transmission from the skin are received by a common set of neurons in the thalamus
    C) Visceral pain signals are rarely of sufficient magnitude to exceed the threshold of activation of dorsal horn neurons
    D) Some visceral pain signals and pain signals from the skin provide convergent input to a common set of neurons in the dorsal horn

36. Post-tetanic facilitation is thought to be the result of which of the following?

    A) Opening of voltage-gated sodium channels
    B) Opening of transmitter-gated potassium channels
    C) A buildup of calcium in the presynaptic terminal
    D) Electrotonic conduction

37. Within the primary somatosensory cortex, the various parts of the contralateral body surface are represented in areas of varying size that reflect which of the following?

    A) The relative size of the body parts
    B) The density of the specialized peripheral receptors
    C) The size of the muscles in that body part
    D) The conduction velocity of the primary afferent fibers

38. The gray matter of the primary somatosensory cortex contains six layers of cells. Which layer(s) receive the bulk of incoming signals from the somatosensory nuclei of the thalamus?

    A) I
    B) II and III
    C) III only
    D) IV

39. Which statement concerning visceral pain signals is correct?

    A) They are transmitted along sensory fibers that course mainly with sympathetic nerves in the abdomen and thorax
    B) They are not stimulated by ischemia in visceral organs
    C) They are transmitted only by the lightly myelinated δ-type A sensory fibers
    D) They are typically well localized

40. Pain from the stomach is referred to which area of the body?

    A) Upper right shoulder area
    B) Abdominal area above the umbilicus
    C) Proximal area of the anterior and inner thigh
    D) Abdominal area below the umbilicus

Questions 41–43

Each of the disorders in Questions 41–43 is characterized either by the production of excessive pain (hyperalgesia) or the loss of pain sensation.

41. Which disorder is characterized by excessive pain in a skin dermatomal distribution resulting from a viral infection of a dorsal root ganglion?

    A) Tic douloureux
    B) Thalamic pain syndrome
    C) Brown-Séquard syndrome
    D) Herpes zoster

42. Which disorder involves a loss of pain sensation on one side of the body coupled with the loss of proprioception, precise tactile localization, and vibratory sensations on the contralateral side of the body?

    A) Herpes zoster
    B) Thalamic pain syndrome
    C) Lateral medullary syndrome
    D) Brown-Séquard syndrome

43. Which disorder is characterized by the loss of pain sensation throughout one entire side of the body and the opposite side of the face?

    A) Brown-Séquard syndrome
    B) Thalamic pain syndrome
    C) Herpes zoster
    D) Lateral medullary syndrome ,PICA

44. Stimulation by touching or pulling on which structure is least likely to cause a painful sensation?

    A) The postcentral gyrus
    B) The dura overlying the postcentral gyrus
    C) Branches of the middle meningeal artery that lie superficial to the dura over the postcentral gyrus
    D) Branches of the middle cerebral artery that supply the postcentral gyrus

45. Vibratory sensation depends on the detection of rapidly changing, repetitive sensations. The high-frequency end of the repetitive stimulation scale is detected by which structure?

    A) Merkel discs
    B) Meissner corpuscles
    C) Pacinian corpuscles
    D) Free nerve endings

46. The ability to detect two points simultaneously applied to the skin is based on which physiologic mechanism?

    A) Presynaptic inhibition
    B) Lateral inhibition
    C) Medial inhibition
    D) Feed-forward inhibition

47. Which electrical event is characteristic of inhibitory synaptic interactions?

    A) A neurotransmitter agent that selectively opens ligand-gated chloride channels is the basis for an inhibitory postsynaptic potential
    B) Because the Nernst potential for chloride is about −70 mV, chloride ions tend to move out of the cell along its electrochemical gradient
    C) A neurotransmitter that selectively opens potassium channels will allow potassium to move into the cell
    D) An increase in the extracellular sodium concentration usually leads directly to an inhibitory postsynaptic potential

48. Which somatosensory deficit is NOT typically seen after the development of lesions that involve the postcentral gyrus?

    A) Inability to discretely localize touch sensation over the contralateral face and upper limb
    B) Inability to judge the weight of easily recognizable objects
    C) Inability to accurately assess the texture of common objects by touching them with the fingers
    D) Inability to move the contralateral arm and leg

49. Which statement concerning sensory neurons or their functional properties is true?

    A) All sensory fibers are unmyelinated
    B) In spatial summation, increasing signal strength is transmitted by using progressively greater numbers of sensory fibers
    C) Increased stimulus intensity is signaled by a progressive decrease in the receptor potential
    D) Continuous subthreshold stimulation of a pool of sensory neurons results in disfacilitation of those neurons
    E) Temporal summation involves signaling of increased stimulus strength by decreasing the frequency of action potentials in the sensory fibers

50. A 23-year-old gymnast lifts her right leg above her head while in the standing position. Activation of a single pyramidal cell in the motor cortex leads to stimulation of 2000 muscle fibers in her right quadriceps muscle. Which of the following best describes the type of neuronal circuitry activated in this woman when she lifts her leg?

    A) Converging
    B) Diverging
    C) Inhibitory
    D) Reverberatory

51. An input neuron to a diverging circuit causes the membrane potential of a target neuron to change from −65 millivolts to −55 millivolts. Which of the following best describes this change in membrane potential (in millivolts)?

    A) Excitatory postsynaptic potential = +10
    B) Excitatory postsynaptic potential = −10
    C) Inhibitory postsynaptic potential = +10
    D) Inhibitory postsynaptic potential = −10

52. Prolonged changes in neuronal activity are usually achieved through the activation of which of the following?

    A) Voltage-gated chloride channels
    B) Transmitter-gated sodium channels
    C) G-protein–coupled channels
    D) Voltage-gated potassium channels

53. Position sense, or more commonly proprioceptive sensation, involves muscle spindles and which of the following?

    A) Skin tactile receptors
    B) Deep receptors in joint capsules
    C) Both tactile and joint capsule receptors
    D) Pacinian corpuscles

54. Migraine headaches often begin with a prodromal symptom such as nausea, loss of vision, visual aura, or other sensory hallucinations. Which of the following is believed to be the cause of such prodromes?

    A) Increased blood flow to brain tissue in the visual or other sensory cortex
    B) A selective loss of gamma-aminobutyric acid neurons in the various sensory areas of cortex
    C) Constipation
    D) Vasospasm leading to ischemia and a disruption of neuronal activity in the relevant sensory areas of cortex

55. Which statement accurately describes a feature of temperature sensation by the nervous system?

    A) Cold receptors continue to be activated even if skin temperature is lowered well below its freezing point
    B) Both cold and warm receptors each have very specific, nonoverlapping ranges of temperature sensitivity
    C) Warm and cold receptors respond to both steady state temperatures and to changes in temperature
    D) Temperature receptor function is the result of ion conduction changes and not changes in their metabolic rate

56. For a sensory nerve fiber that is connected to a Pacinian corpuscle located on palmar surface of the right hand, the synaptic connection with the subsequent neuron in the corresponding sensory pathway is located in

    A) The right dorsal column nucleus
    B) The left dorsal column nucleus
    C) The dorsal horn of the right side of the spinal cord
    D) The dorsal horn of the left side of the spinal cord

57. The sensation of temperature is signaled mainly by warm and cold receptors whose sensory fibers travel in association with the sensory fibers carrying pain signals. Which statement best characterizes the transmission of signals from warm receptors?

    A) Warm receptors are well characterized histologically

    B) Signals from warm receptors are mainly transmitted along slow-conducting type C sensory fibers

    C) Warm receptors are located well below the surface of the skin in the subcutaneous connective tissue

    D) There are 3 to 10 times more warm receptors than cold receptors in most areas of the body

58. Like other sensory systems, the somatosensory system has a descending component that functions to regulate the overall sensitivity of the system. Which of the following selections best describes the function of the corticofugal signals transmitted from the somatosensory cortex downward to the thalamus and dorsal column nuclei?

    A) Increase or decrease the perception of signal intensity

    B) Decrease the ability to detect body position sense

    C) Remove the thalamus from the processing of somatosensory signals

    D) Allow ascending information to bypass the nucleus cuneatus and gracilis

59. Which statement concerning the generation of an action potential is correct?

    A) When the membrane potential in the soma/axon hillock dips below "threshold," an action potential is initiated

    B) The action potential is initiated in synaptic boutons

    C) The least number of voltage-gated sodium channels in an axon is found near the node of Ranvier

    D) Once an action potential is initiated, it will always run its course to completion

60. Which statement concerning synaptic transmission is correct?

    A) When a specific population of synaptic terminals is spread over the considerable surface of a neuron, their collective effects cannot spatially summate and lead to initiation of an action potential

    B) Even if the successive discharges of an excitatory synapse occur sufficiently close in time, they cannot temporally summate and initiate an action potential

    C) A neuron is "facilitated" when its membrane potential is moved in the less negative or depolarizing direction

    D) Even when rapidly stimulated by excitatory synaptic input for a prolonged period, neurons typically do not exhibit synaptic fatigue

1. **C)** The electrochemical driving force (V_{DF}) for an ion can be calculated as follows: $V_{DF} = V_m - V_{eq}$, where V_m is the membrane potential and V_{eq} is the equilibrium potential of the ion. A calculator is available at http://physiology-web.com/calculators/electrochemical_driving_force_calculator.html. A positive value indicates outward flux of the ion, and a negative value indicates inward flux of the ion. A typical equilibrium potential for sodium (calculated using the Nernst equation) is +62 millivolts, so the electrochemical driving force for sodium is $-65 - 62 = -127$ millivolts. This means that a 127-millivolt force attempts to drive sodium into the cell. The equilibrium potential is about -86 millivolts for potassium and about -70 millivolts for chloride; hence, the electrochemical driving force for these two ions is +21 and +5 millivolts, respectively (and both ions tend to be driven out of the cell).
   TMP13 pp. 587-588

2. **B)** Hyperventilation lowers the carbon dioxide tension of the blood, which leads to increases in the pH of the body tissues, including the brain. Alkalinity increases neuronal activity in the brain. Carbon dioxide also has the potent effect of increasing cerebral blood flow; thus, hyperventilation can lead to decreased cerebral blood flow with a subsequent decrease in oxygenation of the brain.
   TMP13 pp. 592, 787

3. **D)** Pain receptors in the skin are free nerve endings.
   TMP13 p. 621

4. **B)** Merkel discs are found in the dermis of hairy skin and signal continuous touch.
   TMP13 p. 608

5. **D)** The release of neurotransmitter depends on the influx of calcium through voltage-gated channels. When this influx occurs, synaptic vesicles fuse with the presynaptic membrane and release the transmitter agent into the synaptic cleft.
   TMP13 p. 582

6. **C)** Meissner corpuscles are found in the dermal pegs.
   TMP13 pp. 596, 607-608

7. **D)** A so-called second messenger system can be activated by a transmitter substance released from an initial neuron by first causing the release of a G protein into the second neuron's cytoplasm. Neurotransmitter activation of G proteins is not known to cause closure of an ion channel. G proteins can activate G-protein–gated ion channels for both sodium and potassium, as well as gene transcription, and cAMP and cGMP. G proteins also can activate intracellular enzymes that have a variety of different functions.
   TMP13 pp. 583-584

8. **D)** Individuals experiencing severe chronic pain have difficulty sleeping because the ascending pain pathways provide excitatory input to reticular formation elements that constitute the reticular activating system; this system maintains the alert, waking state. The overall function of the amygdala is thought to make the person's behavioral response appropriate for each occasion; it does not play a major role in establishing the awake state. Loss of visceral sensations or somatic sensations would likely help the man sleep.
   TMP13 pp. 623-624

9. **C)** Hyperventilation plus flashing lights can sometimes initiate an epileptic seizure in a susceptible person who is poorly medicated. Flashing lights alone activate neurons in the occipital cortex that can sometimes lead to increases in electrical activity throughout the brain. Hyperventilation (taking long, deep breaths) lowers carbon dioxide levels in the blood, causing the brain to become alkalotic; this activation method is commonly used to increase brain activity during electroencephalography.
   TMP13 p. 592

10. **D)** The association of one sensory modality with one type of nerve fiber is the basis for the labeled line theory.
    TMP13 p. 595

11. **A)** Pacinian corpuscles detect pressure and movement across the skin surface and are encapsulated receptors found deep in the skin throughout the body.
    TMP13 pp. 597, 608

12. **D)** Prostaglandins are believed to enhance the sensitivity of pain receptors but do not actually excite them.
    TMP13 p. 621

13. **A)** Pain receptors exhibit little or no functional adaptation.
    TMP13 pp. 621-622

14. **A)** The function of a transmitter agent is solely dependent on the postsynaptic receptor to which it binds.
    TMP13 p. 582

15. **D)** Virtually all mechanical stimuli cause an increase in ion permeability (usually to sodium) in mechanoreceptors. If the membrane potential of the mechanoreceptor reaches a critical threshold value, an action potential is initiated. The G-protein "second messenger" system is typically involved with prolonged postsynaptic neuronal excitation or inhibition; transduction in mechanoreceptors is rapid and transient. Transmitter release does

not occur at the level of the mechanoreceptor, but if a mechanoreceptor is activated, afferent nerve impulses do stimulate transmitter release at the nerve terminal in the central nervous system.

TMP13 pp. 582-583

16. **A)** The equilibrium potential for chloride averages about –70 millivolts in a typical neuron, so with a resting membrane potential of –65 millivolts, the electrochemical driving force for chloride is 5 millivolts. The electrochemical driving force for sodium is about 127 millivolts; potassium has a value of about 21 millivolts during basal conditions.

TMP13 pp. 587-588

17. **A)** The amplitude of the receptor potential from a Pacinian corpuscle increases greatly with a step increase in stimulus intensity at lower levels of stimulus strength, and to a lesser extent with a similar step increase at higher levels of stimulus strength, as shown in the figure below. This relationship between stimulus strength and amplitude of receptor potential allows the Pacinian corpuscle to discern small changes in stimulus strength at low levels of stimulation and yet still respond to changes in stimulus strength when the intensity of stimulation is high.

TMP13 pp. 597-598

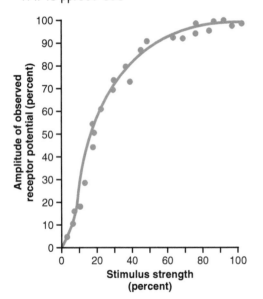

Data from Loëwenstein WR: Excitation and inactivation in a receptor membrane. Ann N Y Acad Sci 94:510, 1961.

18. **A)** Interneurons in the dorsal horn of the spinal cord use enkephalin as a transmitter substance that effectively inhibits pain transmission from tissues of the body. The somatosensory cortex is located in the postcentral gyrus, and the primary motor cortex is located in the precentral gyrus; neither are thought to use enkephalin to inhibit pain transmission. Myelinated δ-type A fibers and unmyelinated type C fibers are not interneurons. Interneurons are physically short neurons that form a connection between other neurons that are usually close together. There are distinguished from "projection" neurons that project to more distant regions of the brain or spinal cord.

TMP13 pp. 625-626

19. **B)** Temporal and spatial fidelity is enhanced in the dorsal column–medial lemniscal system compared with the anterolateral system.

TMP13 p. 610

20. **A)** Fibers in the anterolateral system cross in the anterior white commissure within a few segments of their entry before ascending on the contralateral side. Signals ascending in the dorsal column–medial lemniscal system do not cross until they reach the dorsal column nuclei in the medulla.

TMP13 pp. 616-617

21. **D)** Neurons of the nucleus raphe magnus release serotonin at their nerve endings. In the endogenous pain suppression system, the termination of these neurons is in the spinal cord on interneurons that in turn release enkephalin and block the incoming signals from the pain fibers.

TMP13 p. 625

22. **B)** The sensations of highly localized touch and body position are carried in the dorsal column–medial lemniscal system.

TMP13 p. 610

23. **C)** Primary afferent neuronal cell bodies are found in the dorsal root ganglia.

TMP13 pp. 609-610

24. D) The medial lemniscus conveys axons from the nucleus gracilis and cuneatus to the thalamus (see the figure below).
   TMP13 p. 610

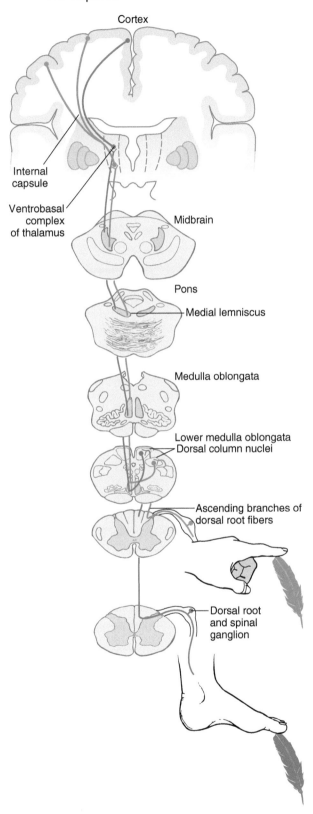

Cortex

Internal capsule

Ventrobasal complex of thalamus

Midbrain

Pons

Medial lemniscus

Medulla oblongata

Lower medulla oblongata
Dorsal column nuclei

Ascending branches of dorsal root fibers

Dorsal root and spinal ganglion

25. B) Stimulation of β-type A fibers from peripheral tactile receptors can decrease transmission of pain signals by a type of lateral inhibition; this process is mediated by inhibitory interneurons in the dorsal column of the spinal cord. α-Type A neurons project to skeletal muscles, causing them to contract. δ-Type A fibers and type C fibers conduct pain signals to the dorsal column of the spinal cord.
   TMP13 pp. 599-600

26. E) Transmission of electrical signals in dendrites occurs by electrotonic conduction. Dendrites have few voltage-gated sodium channels, which makes it virtually impossible for action potentials to be initiated in this portion of a typical neuron. A neuron can be considered as a type of capacitor that discharges during an action potential, but this occurs in the axon, not the dendrites. Electrotonic conduction does not occur by diffusion or active transport.
   TMP13 pp. 590-591

27. C) The internal capsule conveys axons from the ventral posterolateral thalamic nucleus to the primary somatosensory cortex.
   TMP13 p. 610

28. D) Ligand-gated channels open and allow entry of sodium. This entry is accompanied by the influx of calcium, binding of synaptic vesicles to the presynaptic membrane, and electrical changes in the postsynaptic membrane.
   TMP13 pp. 582-583

29. C) The periaqueductal gray area in the midbrain contains neurons that contribute to the descending pain suppression system.
   TMP13 p. 625

30. B) The lower limb representation is found in the superior and medial portion of the postcentral gyrus (see the figure below).
TMP13 p. 612

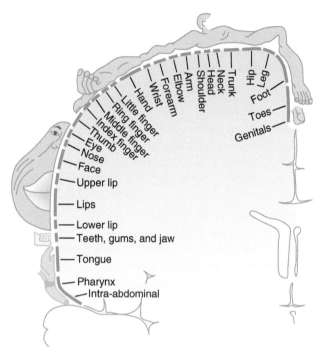

31. C) Neurons in the periaqueductal gray area use enkephalin as a transmitter agent.
TMP13 p. 625

32. D) Most motor neurons cross to the contralateral side in the pyramidal decussation of the medulla oblongata, which is proximal to the damaged area. Fine sensory sensations (vibration sense, fine touch, proprioception, and two-point discrimination) transmitted in the dorsal-column medial lemniscal pathway cross to the contralateral side in the medulla. Therefore, both motor function and vibration sense are lost on the same side (ipsilateral) as the cord lesion.
TMP13 pp. 610, 709

33. A) Crude touch, pain sensations, and temperature sensations travel in the anterolateral pathway of the spinal cord; the afferent neurons from the receptor organs decussate in the spinal cord close to the point of entry. Hence, these sensations are lost on the side opposite of the lesion.
TMP13 pp. 609-610

34. A) In general, the sensation of pain is poorly localized. However, when a tactile receptor and a pain receptor are stimulated simultaneously, the pain sensation is localized with greater accuracy.
TMP13 p. 624

35. D) Visceral pain fibers can provide input to anterolateral tract cells that also receive somatic pain from the skin surface. The convergence of these two types of pain signals onto single spinal cord neurons is thought to be the basis for referred pain.
TMP13 p. 626

36. C) Post-tetanic facilitation is the neuronal phenomenon in which a neuron is more easily excited after a brief period of activity. This phenomenon is thought to be due to the buildup of calcium in the presynaptic membrane caused by the prior neuronal activity. Subsequent neuronal impulses release neurotransmitter more readily as a result of this preplaced calcium from the prior stimulus.
TMP13 pp. 589-590

37. B) The size of the representation of various body parts in the primary somatosensory cortex is correlated with the density of cutaneous receptors in that body part.
TMP13 p. 612

38. D) Layer IV of the somatosensory cortex receives the bulk of the input from the somatosensory nuclei of the thalamus.
TMP13 p. 612

39. A) Visceral pain signals from structures in the abdomen and thorax travel toward the spinal cord in association with fibers of the sympathetic system.
TMP13 pp. 627-628

40. B) Pain from the stomach is referred to the upper abdominal area. In general, it will be above the level of the umbilicus.
TMP13 p. 627

41. D) Herpes zoster is a disorder characterized by excessive pain in a dermatomal distribution that results from a viral infection of a dorsal root ganglion.
TMP13 p. 628

42. D) The Brown-Séquard syndrome is characterized by the loss of pain sensation on one side of the body coupled with a loss of discriminative sensations, such as proprioception and vibratory sensation, on the opposite side of the body.
TMP13 p. 628

43. D) The lateral medullary syndrome exhibits one of the most characteristic patterns of sensory loss in clinical neurology; pain sensation is lost over one side of the body from feet to neck and on the opposite side of the face. Moreover, the side of facial pain loss indicates the side of the lesion.
TMP13 p. 628

44. A) Touching or pulling on the postcentral gyrus is least likely to evoke a painful sensation because brain tissue lacks pain receptors.
TMP13 p. 629

45. C) High-frequency repetitive stimulation (indentation/pressure) of the skin is sensed by Pacinian corpuscles.
TMP13 p. 608

46. B) The process of lateral inhibition, illustrated in the figure below, underlies the ability to discriminate two points simultaneously applied.
TMP13 p. 603

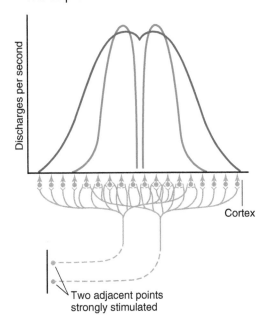

Cortex

Two adjacent points strongly stimulated

47. A) The opening of ligand-gated chloride channels and movement of chloride ions into the cell leads to hyperpolarization of the membrane. Neither increasing the extracellular sodium concentration nor the movement of potassium into the cell leads to hyperpolarization of the membrane.
TMP13 p. 589

48. D) Paralysis of the contralateral arm and leg is a motor deficit, and such a deficit would not typically be observed after damage to the primary somatosensory cortex.
TMP13 p. 613

49. B) In spatial summation, increasing signal strength is transmitted by using greater numbers of sensory fibers.
TMP13 p. 600

50. B) A diverging neuronal pathway amplifies nerve signals; activation of a single pyramidal cell in motor cortex can stimulate as many as 10,000 muscle fibers. In a converging circuit, multiple input fibers converge upon a single postsynaptic neuron, which allows summation of information from multiple sources. An inhibitory circuit often has inhibitory interneurons that stop the spread of a nerve signal. Reverberatory circuits have

positive feedback elements that allow a nerve impulse to continue on for a prolonged time.
TMP13 p. 602

51. A) The positive increase in membrane potential to a less negative value is called the excitatory postsynaptic potential (EPSP). Because the resting membrane potential is −65 millivolts and the final membrane potential is −55 millivolts, the EPSP is +10 millivolts. EPSPs are always positive. Inhibitory postsynaptic potentials are always negative because the membrane potential is lowered to a more negative value.
TMP13 p. 588

52. C) Activation of G proteins usually changes the long-term response characteristics of the neuron.
TMP13 p. 583

53. C) Proprioceptive sensation depends on tactile and joint capsule receptors.
TMP13 p. 628

54. D) Vasospasm and eventually ischemia in a sensory area of cortex is thought to be the basis for the prodromal symptoms experienced by patients with migraines.
TMP13 p. 629

55. C) Both warm and cold receptors are able to respond to steady-state temperatures, as well as changes in temperature.
TMP13 p. 631

56. A) The Pacinian corpuscle transmits a modality of sensation (vibration) that is transmitted in the dorsal column–medial lemniscal system. The first synaptic connection in this sensory pathway is in the dorsal column nuclei on the ipsilateral side of the body.
TMP13 p. 610

57. B) Warm receptors mainly transmit signals along relatively slow-conducting type C fibers.
TMP13 p. 630

58. A) Descending cortical modulation of somatosensation involves an increase or decrease in the perception of signal intensity.
TMP13 pp. 610-611

59. D) The action potential is described as an "all or none" process. Once initiated, the action potential runs its course to completion.
TMP13 p. 589

60. C) A facilitated neuron is one whose resting membrane potential is closer to the threshold for activation; that is, less negative or in the depolarizing direction.
TMP13 p. 590

The Nervous System: B. The Special Senses

1. A 10-year-old boy looks at ants through a magnifying glass. He finds that the ants must be 10 centimeters from the convex lens to be in focus. Which value best describes the refractive power of the lens (in diopters)?

   A) 0.1
   B) 1.0
   C) 10
   D) 100
   E) 1000

2. Which of the following best describes the "blind spot" of the eye?

   A) Located 5 degrees lateral to the central point of vision
   B) The exit point of the optic nerve
   C) Contains only rods and thus has monochromatic vision
   D) Contains no blood vessels
   E) The area where chromatic aberration of the lens is the greatest

3. A 6-year-old boy with albinism is taken to the ophthalmologist because of difficulty seeing. Testing shows that his visual acuity is reduced. Which of the following is the most likely cause of the decrease in visual acuity in this boy?

   A) Cataracts
   B) Hyperopia
   C) Myopia
   D) Photophobia
   E) Presbyopia

4. A 53-year-old woman with celiac disease visits the physician because of difficulty seeing at night. The woman has frequent, foul-smelling stools. Stool analysis reveals a high content of partially digested fat. A decrease in blood levels of which of the following is the most likely cause of her night blindness?

   A) 2-Monoglycerides
   B) Amino acids
   C) Free fatty acids
   D) Glucose
   E) Vitamin A
   F) Vitamin B_{12}

5. Which substance will elicit the sensation of bitter taste?

   A) Aldehydes
   B) Alkaloids
   C) Amino acids
   D) Hydrogen ions
   E) Ketones

6. Damage to the sixth cranial nerve will produce which deficit in eye movement? *Abducens*

   A) Inability to move the eyes in a vertical up-and-down motion
   B) Inability to rotate the eyes within the eye socket
   C) Inability to move the eyes laterally toward the midline
   D) Inability to move the eyes laterally away from the midline
   E) Vertical strabismus

7. The condition of cataracts is usually the result of which process or condition?

   A) Denaturation of the proteins in the lens of the eye
   B) Elongated eye globe
   C) Unresponsive and dilated pupil
   D) Coagulation of the proteins in the lens of the eye
   E) Increase in intraocular pressure

8. Which substance will elicit the sensation of sour taste?

   A) Aldehydes
   B) Alkaloids
   C) Amino acids
   D) Hydrogen ions
   E) Ketones

9. Which taste sensation is the most sensitive (i.e., has the lowest stimulation threshold)?

   A) Acid
   B) Bitter
   C) Salty
   D) Sour
   E) Sweet

10. An 85-year-old woman visits the ophthalmologist because of difficulty seeing. The patient is given an eye examination, and bifocal lenses are prescribed. The physician notes that the lenses of her eyes are clear. The woman sees well with her new prescription glasses. Which of the following best describes the most likely vision problem in this woman?

    A) Cataracts
    B) Glaucoma
    C) Hyperopia
    D) Myopia
    E) Presbyopia

11. Which of the following is the middle ear ossicle that is attached to the tympanic membrane?

    A) Columella
    B) Incus
    C) Malleus
    D) Modiolus
    E) Stapes –oval window.

12. Light entering the eye passes through which retinal layer first?

    A) Inner nuclear layer
    B) Outer nuclear layer
    C) Outer plexiform layer
    D) Photoreceptor layer
    E) Retinal ganglion layer

13. A 25-year-old student with 20/20 vision looks up from his book to view his girlfriend sitting on the other side of the room. Which of the following is most likely to occur when the student changes his view from his book to his girlfriend?

    A) Thicker lens, contraction of ciliary muscle
    B) Thicker lens, relaxation of ciliary muscle
    C) Thinner lens, contraction of ciliary muscle
    D) Thinner lens, relaxation of ciliary muscle

14. A 60-year-old woman visits the ophthalmologist because of eye pain. Tests show that her right eye has an intra-ocular pressure of 22 mm Hg and her left eye has an intra-ocular pressure of 25 mm Hg. Which of the following is the most likely cause of eye pain in this woman?

    A) Decreased hydraulic resistance of trabecular meshwork
    B) Decreased production of aqueous humor
    C) Increased hydraulic resistance of trabecular meshwork
    D) Increased production of aqueous humor

15. Ganglion cells attached to photoreceptors located on the temporal portion of the retina project to which structure?

    A) Contralateral lateral geniculate nucleus
    B) Ipsilateral lateral geniculate nucleus
    C) Ipsilateral medial geniculate nucleus
    D) Calcarine fissure
    E) Contralateral medial geniculate nucleus

16. When parallel light rays pass through a concave lens, which of the following will occur?

    A) The rays converge toward each other
    B) The rays diverge away from each other
    C) The rays maintain a parallel relationship
    D) The rays reflect back in the direction from where they came
    E) The rays refract to one focal point

17. A 40-year-old woman is admitted emergently to the hospital because of sudden, severe pain in her right eye. Tests show an intraocular pressure of 30 mm Hg in her right eye; the intraocular pressure of her left eye is 15 mm Hg. Which of the following is the most likely cause of eye pain in this woman?

    A) Acute angle-closure glaucoma
    B) Chronic glaucoma
    C) Conjunctivitis
    D) Corneal abrasion
    E) Open-angle glaucoma
    F) Optic neuritis

18. Which compartment of the cochlea contains the organ of Corti?

    A) Ampulla } vestibule
    B) Saccule
    C) Scala media
    D) Scala tympani
    E) Scala vestibuli

19. Which molecules combine to form rhodopsin?

    A) Bathorhodopsin and 11-cis-retinal
    B) Bathorhodopsin and all-trans-retinal
    C) Bathorhodopsin and scotopsin
    D) Scotopsin and 11-cis-retinal
    E) Scotopsin and all-trans-retinal

20. Analysis of visual detail occurs in which secondary visual area?

    A) Brodmann's area 18
    B) Inferior ventral and medial regions of the occipital and temporal cortex
    C) Frontal lobe
    D) Occipitoparietal cortex
    E) Posterior midtemporal area

Questions 21–23
A 23-year-old student is trapped in an elevator with no light. Twenty minutes later the student finds an emergency light and turns it on. Use this information to answer Questions 21–23.

21. Which substance is most likely to increase in the rods of the retina when the light is turned on?

    A) Cyclic adenosine monophosphate (cAMP)
    B) Cyclic guanosine monophosphate (cGMP)
    C) Metarhodopsin II
    D) Rhodopsin
    E) Vitamin A

22. Which of the following best describes the permeability to sodium and potassium in rod cells in response to the light?

A) Decreased sodium permeability, decreased potassium permeability
B) Decreased sodium permeability, increased potassium permeability
C) Decreased sodium permeability, no change in potassium permeability
D) Increased sodium permeability, decreased potassium permeability
E) Increased sodium permeability, increased potassium permeability
F) Increased sodium permeability, no change in potassium permeability

23. Which of the following best describes the electrical response of the rods to light?

A) Action potential
B) Capacitive discharge
C) Depolarization
D) Hyperpolarization

24. Which substance is responsible for the umami taste sensation?

A) Acetic acid
B) Potassium tartrate
C) Long-chained organic substances containing nitrogen
D) Fructose
E) Glutamate

25. Which cell type(s) have action potentials in the retina of the human eye?

A) Bipolar cells and ganglion cells
B) Bipolar cells only
C) Bipolar cells, horizontal cells, and ganglion cells
D) Ganglion cells and horizontal cells
E) Ganglion cells only
F) Horizontal cells only

26. Olfactory receptor cells belong to which group of cells?

A) Bipolar neurons
B) Fibroblasts
C) Modified epithelial cells
D) Multipolar neurons
E) Pseudounipolar neurons

27. Which of the following best describes when the transmission of sound waves in the cochlea occurs?

A) When the foot of the stapes moves inward against the oval window and the round window bulges outward
B) When the foot of the stapes moves inward against the round window and the oval window bulges outward
C) When the head of the malleus moves inward against the oval window and the round window bulges outward
D) When the incus moves inward against the oval window and the round window bulges outward
E) When the incus moves inward against the round window and the oval window bulges outward

28. Under low or reduced light conditions, which chemical compound is responsible for the inward-directed sodium current in the outer segments of the photoreceptors?

A) Metarhodopsin II
B) cGMP
C) 11-cis retinal
D) cAMP
E) 11-trans retinal

29. Which cells in layer IV of the primary visual cortex detect orientation of lines and borders?

A) Border cells
B) Complex cells
C) Ganglion cells
D) Hypercomplex cells
E) Simple cells

Questions 30 and 31
A 20-year-old soldier sustains a noise-induced hearing loss over a period of 6 months from multiple exposures to loud sounds. Use this information to answer Questions 30 and 31.

30. Loss of which structure is most likely to contribute to the hearing deficit?

A) Cochlea
B) Inner hair cells
C) Organ of Corti
D) Scala media
E) Scala vestibuli

31. An increase in which of the following is the most likely cause of this hearing loss?

A) Connexin 26
B) Endolymph
C) Perilymph
D) Reactive oxygen species

32. Which event occurs in photoreceptors during phototransduction in response to light?

A) Phosphodiesterase activity decreases
B) Transducin activity decreases
C) Hydrolysis of cGMP increases
D) Neurotransmitter release increases
E) The number of open voltage-gated calcium channels increases

33. During photoreception, all the following increase except

A) cGMP phosphodiesterase
B) Transducin
C) cAMP
D) Metarhodopsin II
E) Sodium influx into the outer segment of the rod

Questions 34 and 35

A 50-year-old woman visits an otolaryngologist for sudden bouts of dizziness that subside after about 20 minutes. She also has temporary hearing losses and a feeling of fullness in her right ear; low-pitched buzzing sounds occur intermittently in her right ear. Physical examination shows nystagmus during a dizzy spell. Use this information to answer Questions 34 and 35.

34. Which of the following is the most likely diagnosis?

    A) Acoustic neuroma
    B) Aural polyp
    C) Exostosis
    D) Incus erosion
    E) Meniere's disease   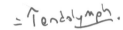 = Tendolymph.

35. An increase in which of the following is the most likely cause of this patient's condition?

    A) Endolymph pressure only
    B) Endolymph volume only
    C) Endolymph volume and pressure
    D) Perilymph pressure only
    E) Perilymph volume only
    F) Perilymph volume and pressure

36. The condition of myopia is usually corrected by which type of lens?

    A) Compound lens
    B) Convex lens
    C) Spherical lens
    D) Concave lens
    E) Cylindrical lens

37. Which lobe of the cerebral cortex contains the small bilateral cortical area that controls voluntary fixation movements?

    A) Frontal
    B) Limbic
    C) Occipital
    D) Parietal
    E) Temporal

38. Which sensory system has the smallest range of intensity discrimination?

    A) Auditory
    B) Gustatory
    C) Olfactory
    D) Somatosensory
    E) Visual

39. Which molecules move from the endolymph into the stereocilia and depolarize the hair cell?

    A) Calcium ions
    B) Chloride ions
    C) Hydrogen ions
    D) Potassium ions
    E) Sodium ions

40. The stereocilia of hair cells are embedded in which membrane?

    A) Basilar
    B) Reissner's
    C) Tectorial
    D) Tympanic
    E) Vestibular

41. Which cranial nerve is correctly paired with the extra-ocular muscle it innervates?

    A) Abducens nerve–medial rectus
    B) Oculomotor nerve–inferior oblique
    C) Oculomotor nerve–lateral rectus
    D) Oculomotor nerve–superior oblique
    E) Trochlear nerve–superior rectus

42. After olfactory receptor cells bind odor molecules, a sequence of intracellular events occurs that culminates in the entrance of specific ions that depolarize the olfactory receptor cell. Which ions are involved?

    A) Calcium
    B) Chloride
    C) Hydrogen
    D) Potassium
    E) Sodium

43. For the eye to adapt to intense light, which of the following may occur?

    A) Bipolar cells will continuously transmit signals at the maximum rate possible
    B) Photochemicals in both rods and cones will be reduced to retinal and opsins
    C) The levels of rhodopsin will be very high
    D) The size of the pupil will increase
    E) Vitamin A will convert into retinal

44. In the central auditory pathway, which option represents the correct sequence of structures in the pathway?

    A) Cochlear nuclei–superior olive–inferior colliculus via the lateral lemniscus–medial geniculate–auditory cortex
    B) Cochlear nuclei–inferior olive–inferior colliculus via the medial lemniscus–medial geniculate–auditory cortex
    C) Cochlear nuclei–superior olive–superior colliculus via the lateral lemniscus–lateral geniculate–auditory cortex
    D) Cochlear nuclei–inferior olive–inferior colliculus via the lateral lemniscus–lateral geniculate–auditory cortex
    E) Cochlear nuclei–trapezoid body–dorsal acoustic stria–inferior colliculus via the lateral lemniscus–medial geniculate–auditory cortex

45. Which statement regarding the transmission of auditory information from the ear to the cerebral cortex is correct?

    A) Inferior colliculus neurons synapse in the cochlear nuclei of the brain stem
    B) Neurons with cell bodies in the spiral ganglion of Corti synapse in the inferior colliculus
    C) The majority of neurons from the cochlear nuclei synapse in the contralateral superior olivary nucleus
    D) There is no crossing over of information between the right and left auditory pathways in the brain stem
    E) Trapezoid neurons synapse in the cochlear nuclei of the brain stem

46. Which statement regarding color vision is correct?

    A) Green is perceived when only green cones are stimulated
    B) The stimulation ratio of the three types of cones allows specific color perception
    C) The wavelength of light corresponding to white is shorter than that corresponding to blue
    D) When no stimulation of red, green, or blue cones occurs, there will be the sensation of seeing white
    E) Yellow is perceived when green and blue cones are stimulated equally

47. Which event prompts the auditory system to interpret a sound as loud?

    A) A decreased number of inner hair cells become stimulated
    B) A decreased number of outer hair cells become stimulated
    C) Hair cells excite nerve endings at a diminished rate
    D) The amplitude of vibration of the basilar membrane decreases
    E) The amplitude of vibration of the basilar membrane increases

48. Which statement is correct concerning the elements of the retina?

    A) The total number of cones in the retina is much greater than the total number of rods
    B) Each individual cone responds to all wavelengths of light
    C) Photoreceptor activation (rods and cones) results in hyperpolarization of the receptor
    D) The central fovea contains only rods
    E) The pigment layer of the retina contains the photo-receptors

49. The condition of hyperopia is usually caused by which anomaly of the eye?

    A) Decreased production of melanin
    B) Uneven curvature of the cornea
    C) An eyeball that is shorter than normal
    D) An eyeball that is longer than normal
    E) A lens system that is too powerful and focuses the object in front of the retina

50. Which statement regarding the two types of deafness is correct?

    A) An audiogram of a person with conduction deafness would show much greater loss for air conduction than for bone conduction of sound
    B) An audiogram of a person with nerve deafness would show much greater loss for bone conduction than for air conduction of sound
    C) Conduction deafness occurs when the cochlea or cochlear nerve is impaired
    D) Nerve deafness occurs when the physical structures that conduct the sound into the cochlea are impaired
    E) Prolonged exposure to very loud sounds is more likely to cause deafness for high-frequency sounds than for low-frequency sounds

51. When a person turns the head to the left about the axis of the neck, the motion begins when the chin is directly over the right shoulder and ends with the chin directly over the left shoulder. Which option best describes the eye movements associated with this type of head rotation in a normal person?

    A) While the head is turning, the eyes will be moving to the right and saccadic eye motion will be to the left
    B) While the head is turning, the eyes will be moving in the same direction as the head rotation and the saccadic eye motion will be to the left
    C) While the head is turning, the eyes will be moving to the right and the saccadic eye motion will be to the right
    D) While the head is turning, the eyes will remain stationary within the orbits and the saccadic eye motion will be to the right
    E) While the head is turning, the eyes will be moving to the left and the saccadic eye motion will be to the right

52. Olfactory information transmitted to the orbitofrontal cortex passes through which thalamic nucleus?

    A) Dorsomedial
    B) Lateral geniculate
    C) Medial geniculate
    D) Ventral posterolateral
    E) Ventral posteromedial

53. A 29-year-old student with 20/20 vision looks at a beautiful scene. The axons of ganglion cells transmitting visual signals in the form of action potentials to the primary visual cortex are most likely to synapse in which structure?

    A) Lateral geniculate nucleus
    B) Medial geniculate nucleus
    C) Optic chiasm
    D) Optic radiation
    E) Superior cervical ganglion
    F) Superior colliculus

54. The function of the round window can best be described by which statement?

    A) It provides the connection point for the stapes
    B) It serves to damp out low frequency sounds such as your own voice
    C) It transmits the frequency information into the cochlea from the tympanic membrane
    D) It serves as the pressure relief valve for the cochlea
    E) It transmits amplitude information into the cochlea from the tympanic membrane

55. Which muscle is contracted as part of the pupillary light reflex?

    A) Ciliary muscle
    B) Pupillary dilator muscle
    C) Pupillary sphincter muscle
    D) Radial fibers of the iris
    E) Superior oblique muscle

Questions 56 and 57
A 24-year-old woman sustains a laceration on the right side of the neck in a motor vehicle accident. Physical examination shows that her right pupil is constricted, her right eyelid droops, the skin is dry on the right side of her face, and the conjunctiva of her right eye is red. Use this information to answer Questions 56 and 57.

56. What is the most likely diagnosis?

    A) Cone-rod dystrophy
    B) Horner's syndrome
    C) Iris heterochromia
    D) Retinoblastoma
    E) Xerophthalmia

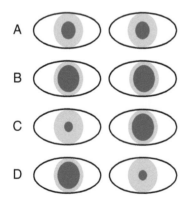

57. Which test result shown in the above figure is most likely after topical treatment with cocaine in both eyes?

    A) A
    B) B
    C) C
    D) D

58. Which neurotransmitter is released by both rods and cones at their synapses with bipolar cells?

    A) Acetylcholine
    B) Dopamine
    C) Glutamate
    D) Glycine
    E) Serotonin

59. Which of the following allows the visual apparatus to accurately determine the distance of an object from the eye (depth perception)?

    A) Monocular vision
    B) The location of the retinal image on the retina
    C) The phenomenon of stationary parallax
    D) The phenomenon of stereopsis
    E) The size of the retinal image if the object is of unknown size

60. Which of the following provides about two thirds of the 59 diopters of refractive power of the eye?

    A) Anterior surface of the cornea
    B) Anterior surface of the lens
    C) Iris
    D) Posterior surface of the cornea
    E) Posterior surface of the lens

61. Which photoreceptor responds to the broadest spectrum of wavelengths of light?

    A) Rod receptors
    B) Green cone receptors
    C) Blue cone receptors
    D) Red cone receptors
    E) Cells containing melanin in the pigment layer

62. Which structure secretes the intraocular fluid of the eye?

    A) Ciliary processes
    B) Cornea
    C) Iris
    D) Lens
    E) Trabeculae

63. Which type of papillae is located in the posterior part of the tongue?

    A) Circumvallate
    B) Foliate
    C) Fungiform
    D) Fungiform and circumvallate
    E) Papilla of Vater

64. Which statement regarding retinal ganglion cells is correct?

  A) One W ganglion cell from the periphery of the retina typically transmits information from one rod
  B) One X ganglion cell from the fovea typically transmits information from as many as 200 cones
  C) W ganglion cells respond best to directional movement or vision under very bright conditions
  D) X ganglion cells respond best to color images and are the most numerous of the three types of ganglion cells
  E) Y ganglion cells respond best to rapid changes in the visual image and are the most numerous of the three types of ganglion cells

65. Auditory information is relayed through which thalamic nucleus?

  A) Dorsomedial
  B) Lateral geniculate
  C) Medial geniculate
  D) Ventral posterolateral
  E) Ventral posteromedial

66. Which of the following describes the phenomenon of taste preference?

  A) A central nervous system process
  B) The result of neonatal stimulation of circumvallate papilla
  C) A learned behavior in animals
  D) A result of taste bud maturation
  E) A result of taste bud proliferation after exposure to glutamic acid

67. The primary auditory cortex lies primarily in which lobe of the cerebral cortex?

  A) Frontal
  B) Limbic
  C) Occipital
  D) Parietal
  E) Temporal

68. The first central synapse for neurons transmitting the sweet taste sensation is in which structure?

  A) Dorsal sensory nucleus of vagus nerve
  B) Nucleus of solitary tract
  C) Nucleus of olfactory nerve
  D) Nucleus of hypoglossal nerve
  E) Nucleus of facial nerve

69. Which statement best describes the underlying basis of the dark current in the outer segment of the photoreceptors?

  A) Dark current results from the influx of sodium ions via c-AMP–dependent sodium channels
  B) Dark current results from the influx of sodium ions via c-GMP–dependent sodium channels

  C) Dark current results from the efflux of potassium ions via c-GMP–dependent potassium channels
  D) Dark current results from the efflux of sodium ions via c-GMP–dependent sodium channels
  E) Dark current results from the efflux of sodium ions via c-AMP–dependent sodium channels

70. Which structure functions to ensure that each of the three sets of extraocular muscles is reciprocally innervated so that one muscle of the pair relaxes while the other contracts?

  A) Edinger-Westphal nucleus
  B) Medial longitudinal fasciculus
  C) Pretectal nucleus
  D) Superior colliculus
  E) Suprachiasmatic nucleus

71. The intraocular fluid of the eye flows from the canal of Schlemm into which location?

  A) Anterior chamber
  B) Aqueous veins
  C) Lens
  D) Posterior chamber
  E) Trabeculae

72. Which retinal cells have action potentials?

  A) Amacrine cells
  B) Bipolar cells
  C) Ganglion cells
  D) Horizontal cells
  E) Photoreceptors

73. Which brain stem structure plays a major role in determining the direction from which a sound originates?

  A) Cochlear nucleus
  B) Inferior colliculus
  C) Lateral lemniscus
  D) Superior olivary nucleus
  E) Trapezoid

74. A 25-year-old student studies for a test in medical physiology. The visual contrast of the subject matter is enhanced due to lateral inhibition of the visual input by which cell type in the retina?

  A) Amacrine cells
  B) Bipolar cells
  C) Ganglion cells
  D) Horizontal cells

75. Which type of papillae is located in the folds along the lateral surfaces of the tongue?

  A) Circumvallate
  B) Foliate
  C) Fungiform
  D) Fungiform and circumvallate
  E) Papilla of Vater

1. **C)** The refractive power of a lens (in diopters) = 1 meter/ focal length; if the subject matter is in focus when a convex lens is 1 meter from the subject matter, the lens has a refractive power of 1 meter/1 meter = 1 diopter. Thus, there is an inverse relationship between focal length and refractive power; a thicker convex lens has a shorter focal length and a greater refractive power. In this problem, the lens must be 10 centimeters from the subject matter to be in focus (focal length = 100 millimeters); therefore, 1000 millimeters/100 millimeter = 10 diopters. Because the retina of the eye is about 17 millimeters behind the lens, the refractive power of the lens of the eye is about 59 diopters.
TMP13 pp. 637-638

2. **B)** The blind spot is located 15 degrees lateral to the central point of vision. It is the location where fibers that make up the optic nerve exit the globe of the eye. There are no photoreceptors in this location.
TMP13 p. 665

3. **D)** Photophobia is discomfort or pain to the eyes due to light exposure; it is a medical condition, not a fear or phobia. The lack of melanin (black pigment) in the irises of the eyes makes them somewhat translucent, so they cannot block light effectively. The lack of melanin in the pigment layer of the retina causes light to scatter inside the globe of the eye, which decreases contrast and visual acuity.
TMP13 pp. 648-649

4. **E)** Vitamin A is a fat-soluble vitamin that can be excreted in the feces along with fat in persons with celiac disease and other diseases that cause malabsorption of intestinal contents. A lack of vitamin A can cause a decrease in production of retinal, which is necessary for synthesis of rhodopsin in the rods of the retina. Decreased levels of rhodopsin in the rods can lower the sensitivity of the retina to light, thus causing night blindness.
TMP13 pp. 648-649

5. **B)** The taste sensation of bitter is caused by many organic substances that contain nitrogen, as well as by alkaloids.
TMP13 p. 685

6. **D)** The sixth cranial nerve is also known as the *abducens nerve*. The abducens nerve innervates the lateral rectus muscle, which is attached to the lateral surface of the globe of the eye. Contraction of the lateral rectus muscle results in movement of the eyeball laterally away from the midline of the face in an abducting manner—thus the name *abducens nerve*.
TMP13 pp. 665-666

7. **D)** The condition of cataracts causes the lens of the eye to become opaque and resemble the look of water in a waterfall or rapids in a river, thus the name, cataract. A cataract results from the progressive coagulation of the proteins that make up the lens. One can think of this coagulation as similar to the white of an egg turning opaque as it is cooked. Heating the egg white results in coagulation of the proteins contained within it.
TMP13 p. 642

8. **D)** The taste sensation of sour is proportional to the logarithm of the hydrogen ion concentration caused by acids. The taste sensation of sweet is caused by a long list of chemicals, including sugars, alcohols, aldehydes, ketones, and amino acids.
TMP13 p. 685

9. **B)** The bitter taste sense is much more sensitive than the other sensations because it provides an important protective function against many dangerous toxins in food.
TMP13 p. 686

10. **E)** A person with presbyopia cannot accommodate for near and far vision, which means that the lenses of the eyes have lost their elasticity and thus cannot change their focal point. A child with good vision has 14 diopters of accommodation; this accommodation decreases throughout life until, at approximately 70 years, the lenses cannot change their shape and the power of accommodation is then zero. People with zero power of accommodation are said to be presbyopic.
TMP13 p. 640

11. **C)** The malleus is attached to the tympanic membrane, and the stapes is attached to the oval window. The incus has articulations with both of these bones.
TMP13 p. 673

12. **E)** Light passes through the eye to the retina in the posterior portion of the eye. The most anterior layer of the retina, through which light passes first, is the retinal ganglion layer. Light then passes through the other cell layers of the retina until it reaches the photoreceptors in the posterior region of the retina.
TMP13 p. 647

13. **D)** Light rays from distant objects do not require as much refraction (bending) as do light rays from objects close at hand. Therefore, a thinner lens with less curvature is required for viewing distant objects. The process of accommodation adjusts the thickness of the lens for near and far vision by contracting or relaxing the ciliary muscle that surrounds the lens of the eye; contraction

of the ciliary muscle thickens the lens, and relaxation causes the lens to become thinner.
TMP13 pp. 639-640

14. C) This woman has open-angle glaucoma, which is the most common type of glaucoma. Glaucoma is the second leading cause of blindness worldwide after cataracts. Blindness occurs because of damage to the optic nerve. The high intraocular pressure causes blood vessels and axons of the optic nerve to be compressed at the optic disc, which leads to poor nutrition with possible death of the neurons. The main cause of open-angle glaucoma is reduced flow of aqueous humor through the trabecular meshwork because of tissue debris, white blood cells, deposition of fibrous material, and other factors that increase the hydraulic resistance of the meshwork.
TMP13 p. 646

15. B) The axons of the ganglion cells make up the fibers of the optic nerve. The first synapse in the visual system takes place in the lateral geniculate nucleus. Ganglion cells attached to photoreceptors on the temporal side of the retina project to the same-sided or ipsilateral lateral geniculate nucleus. Fibers from the nasal side of the retina cross over to the opposite or contralateral lateral geniculate nucleus in the optic chiasm. The medial geniculate nucleus is a sensory relay for the auditory system.
TMP13 p. 661

16. B) A concave lens diverges light rays; in contrast, a convex lens will converge light rays toward each other. If a convex lens has the appropriate curvature, parallel light rays will be bent so that all pass through a single point, called the *focal point.*
TMP13 p. 636

17. A) This woman has acute angle-closure glaucoma, which is a medical emergency. Sudden closure of the iridocorneal angle prevents aqueous humor from reaching its outflow pathway in the canal of Schlemm. Intraocular pressure can increase rapidly and cause blindness without immediate treatment. Chronic glaucoma and open-angle glaucoma are the same disease. Conjunctivitis (pinkeye) is an inflammation of the conjunctiva. A corneal abrasion is a scratch on the cornea; it can be very painful. Optic neuritis is inflammation of the optic nerve.
TMP13 p. 646

18. C) The ampulla and saccule are part of the vestibular apparatus, not the cochlear apparatus. The cochlea has three main compartments, with fluid movement occurring in the scala vestibuli and scala media in response to sound vibrations. The organ of Corti is contained within the scala media.
TMP13 pp. 674-675

19. D) Rhodopsin is the light-sensitive chemical in rods. Scotopsin and all-trans retinal are the breakdown products of rhodopsin, which has absorbed light energy. The all-trans retinal is converted into 11-cis retinal, which can recombine with scotopsin to form rhodopsin.
TMP13 pp. 649-650

20. B) Visual information from the primary visual cortex (Brodmann's area 17) is relayed to Brodmann's area 18 and then into other areas of the cerebral cortex for further processing. Analysis of three-dimensional position, gross form, and motion of objects occurs in the posterior midtemporal area and occipitoparietal cortex. Analysis of visual detail and color occurs in the inferior ventral and medial regions of the occipital and temporal cortex.
TMP13 pp. 662-664

21. C) Photons activate rhodopsin to become metarhodopsin II in the rods of the retina, which means that exposure to light decreases the concentration of rhodopsin and increases the concentration of metarhodopsin II, also called *activated rhodopsin.* Metarhodopsin II leads to a decrease in cGMP through a series of biochemical reactions; cAMP levels are unchanged. Vitamin A levels are not likely to change with exposure to light.
TMP13 pp. 647, 649-651

22. C) Activated rhodopsin (metarhodopsin II) closes cGMP-gated sodium channels by lowering levels of cGMP; this action decreases sodium permeability. Potassium permeability is not affected.
TMP13 pp. 650-651

23. D) Exposure of rods to light causes cGMP-gated sodium channels in the cell membrane to close; this action causes rods to hyperpolarize from a resting value of about −40 millivolts to as low as −70 millivolts. Action potentials do not occur in rods or cones. A capacitive discharge occurs during the course of an action potential.
TMP13 p. 651

24. E) The term *umami* is derived from the Japanese word for savory or delicious and is often described as similar to the taste of meat. Glutamate is the chemical believed to elicit the umami taste sensation.
TMP13 p. 686

25. E) Ganglion cells are the only cell type in the retina that have action potentials. The axons of ganglion cells comprise the optic nerve. Bipolar cells, cones, rods, horizontal cells, and other cell types in the retina signal information by electrotonic conduction, which allows a graded response proportional to light intensity.
TMP13 pp. 655, 656, 658

26. A) The receptor cells for the smell sensation are bipolar nerve cells derived originally from the central nervous system itself.
TMP13 p. 689

27. **A)** The malleus is connected to the tympanic membrane, the incus articulates with the malleus and stapes, and the stapes is connected to the oval window.
TMP13 p. 673

28. **B)** In low light conditions, the level of cGMP is high. cGMP-dependent sodium channels in the outer portions of the rods and cones allow sodium ions to pass from the extracellular space to the intracellular space of the photoreceptor. This passage results in a membrane potential that is somewhat lower than the resting membrane potential of a typical neuron. The movement of the sodium ions and resulting electrical potential change as a result of this enhanced permeability is known as the *dark current.*
TMP13 pp. 650-651

29. **E)** The simple cells of the primary visual cortex detect orientation of lines and borders, whereas the complex cells detect lines oriented in the same direction but are not position specific. That is, the line can be displaced moderate distances laterally or vertically, and the same few neurons will be stimulated as long as the line is the same direction.
TMP13 p. 664

30. **B)** Noise-induced hearing loss (NIHL) is the most common acquired cause of hearing loss worldwide. NIHL is usually caused by damage and eventual death of the inner hair cells located in the organ of Corti of the cochlea; these cells do not grow back. The inner hair cells are the actual sensory receptors of the organ of Corti. The scala media and scala vestibuli are fluid-filled coiled tubes that comprise the cochlea.
TMP13 pp. 682, 683

31. **D)** Prolonged exposure to excessive sound levels or loud sounds overstimulates hair cells, causing them to produce large amounts of reactive oxygen species, which can cause oxidative cell death. Animal studies have shown that antioxidant vitamins administrated the day after noise exposure can reduce the hearing loss, but pretreatment is more effective. Low levels of connexin 26 due to gene mutation are thought to constitute a congenital hearing loss. Perilymph is the fluid contained in the scala vestibuli and scala tympani of the cochlea; endolymph is the fluid contained in the scala media and membranous labyrinth.
TMP13 pp. 682-683

32. **C)** In the dark state, cGMP helps maintain the open state of the sodium channels in the outer membrane of the rod. Hydrolysis of cGMP by light causes these sodium channels to close. Less sodium is able to enter the rod outer segment, thus hyperpolarizing the rod.
TMP13 pp. 651-652

33. **E)** During photoreception, the active compound metarhodopsin is formed, which in turn activates a G protein called *transducin.* The transducin activates a cGMP phosphodiesterase that destroys cGMP. cGMP-dependent sodium channels close, and the influx of sodium ions into the outer segment of the photoreceptors decreases.
TMP13 pp. 650-652

34. **E)** This woman has Meniere's disease, which is a disorder of the inner ear that affects hearing and balance. The disease results from excess endolymph in the scala media and membranous labyrinth. The cause is not known, but it appears to have a genetic component. Symptoms include vertigo, nystagmus, low-pitched tinnitus, and sudden but temporary hearing loss; hearing loss can become permanent. Acoustic neuroma is a slow-growing benign tumor that develops on the auditory nerve. An aural polyp is a growth in the auditory canal that may be attached to the tympanic membrane, or it may grow from the middle ear. An exostosis is the formation of new bone on the surface of an existing bone; it sometimes occurs in the auditory canal of swimmers after prolonged exposure to cold water and is sometimes called "surfer's ear." The incus bone is anvil-shaped and is one of the three ossicles in the middle ear.
TMP13 pp. 677, 678

35. **C)** Increases in both volume and pressure of endolymph in the membranous labyrinth produce the symptoms of Meniere's disease; the reason for this buildup of endolymph is unknown. The membranous labyrinth is composed mainly of the cochlea and balance organs (semicircular canals, utricle, and saccule). Repeated rupturing and healing of the endolymphatic sac of the membranous labyrinth can account for the intermittent symptoms of Meniere's disease. The endolymphatic sac is thought to regulate hydrostatic pressure of endolymph by simple expansion or collapse; it may also have secretory and absorption functions.
TMP13 pp. 677, 678

36. **D)** In myopia the focal point of the lens system of the eye is in front of the retina. A concave lens will diverge light rays. By placing the proper concave lens in front of the eye, the divergence of light rays will move the focal point from in front of the retina to a position on the retina.
TMP13 p. 641

37. **A)** A bilateral premotor cortical region of the frontal lobes controls voluntary fixation movements. A lesion of this region makes it difficult for a person to "unlock" their eyes from one point of fixation and then move them to another point.
TMP13 pp. 666-667

38. C) Concentrations that are only 10 to 50 times above threshold values will evoke maximum intensity of smell, which is in contrast to most other sensory systems of the body, where the range of intensity discrimination may reach 1 trillion to 1. This phenomenon can perhaps be explained by the fact that smell is concerned more with detecting the presence or absence of odors than with quantitative detection of their intensities.
TMP13 p. 690

39. D) Although most cells in the nervous system depolarize in response to sodium entry, hair cells are one group of cells that depolarize in response to potassium entry.
TMP13 p. 677

40. C) The scala media is bordered by the basilar membrane and Reissner's membrane and contains a tectorial membrane. The apical border of hair cells has stereocilia that are embedded in the tectorial membrane.
TMP13 p. 677

41. B) The abducens nerve innervates the lateral rectus muscle. The trochlear nerve innervates the superior oblique muscle. The oculomotor nerve innervates the medial rectus, inferior oblique, superior rectus, and inferior rectus muscles.
TMP13 p. 666

42. E) Even the minutest concentration of a specific odorant initiates a cascading effect that opens extremely large numbers of sodium channels. This phenomenon accounts for the exquisite sensitivity of the olfactory neurons to even the slightest amount of odorant.
TMP13 p. 690

43. B) The reduction of rhodopsin and cone pigments by light reduces the concentrations of photosensitive chemicals in rods and cones. Thus, the sensitivity of the eye to light is correspondingly reduced. This phenomenon is called *light adaptation*.
TMP13 pp. 652-653

44. A) Auditory fibers enter the cochlear nucleus. Fibers from the cochlear nucleus pass to the inferior colliculus via the lateral lemniscus. Fibers from the inferior colliculus travel to the medial geniculate nucleus and from there to the primary auditory cortex.
TMP13 p. 679

45. C) Neurons with cell bodies in the spiral ganglion of Corti synapse in the cochlear nuclei. The majority of the cochlear nuclei neurons synapse in the contralateral superior olivary nucleus. Crossing over occurs in at least three places in the pathway, and a preponderance of auditory transmission is in the contralateral pathway. From the superior olivary nucleus, the auditory pathway then passes upward through the lateral lemniscus, with most auditory fibers terminating at the inferior colliculus. From there, the pathway continues on to the medial geniculate nucleus and then to the primary auditory cortex.
TMP13 p. 679

46. B) Research has shown that the nervous system perceives the sensation of a specific color by interpreting the set of ratios of stimulation of the three types of cones. Investigators used only red, green, and blue monochromatic lights mixed in different combinations. All gradations of colors the human eye can detect were detected with only these three colors.
TMP13 pp. 653-654

47. E) The auditory system determines loudness in at least three ways. First, the amplitude of vibration of the basilar membrane increases so that hair cells excite nerve endings at more rapid rates. Second, more and more hair cells on the fringes of the resonating portion of the basilar membrane become stimulated. Third, outer hair cells become recruited at a significant rate.
TMP13 pp. 676, 678

48. C) Unlike most other sensory receptors that depolarize when activated, the photoreceptors produce the opposite response, which is hyperpolarization. The total number of rods is much greater than the number of cones. Cones respond to a very specific range of wavelengths of light. The pigment layer is posterior to the retinal layer that contains the photoreceptors.
TMP13 p. 650

49. C) In hyperopia the focal point of the eye's lens system is behind the retina. This is usually the result of an eyeball that is too short in the anterior to posterior direction.
TMP13 p. 640

50. A) With nerve deafness, there is damage to the cochlea, auditory nerve, or neural pathway. The ability to hear sound as tested by both air conduction and bone conduction is greatly reduced or lost with nerve deafness. However, with conduction deafness, the person retains the ability to hear sound by bone conduction, but not by air conduction.
TMP13 p. 682

51. A) In the situation described, the eyes will fix on an object in the visual field and remain on that object while the head is turning to the left, resulting in eye movement to the right as the head is turned to the left. When the object is no longer in the central field of vision, the eyes will exhibit a quick jumping movement to the left (i.e., in the direction of the head rotation) and fix on a new object in the visual field. This jump is called a *saccade*. This process will repeat until the head has turned all the way to the left. During saccadic eye movement, vision is suppressed.
TMP13 pp. 667-668

52. A) A newer olfactory pathway has been found that projects to the dorsomedial thalamic nucleus and then to the orbitofrontal cortex. However, the older olfactory pathways bypass the thalamus to reach the cortex, in contrast to other sensory systems, which have thalamic relays.
TMP13 p. 691

53. A) Ganglion cells of the retina have synaptic connections within the lateral geniculate nucleus (LGN); from there the visual signals (action potentials) are transmitted to the primary visual cortex. Ganglion cells in the nasal half of the retina synapse in the contralateral LGN, whereas ganglion cells from the temporal half of the retina synapse in the ipsilateral LGN. Decussation occurs in the optic chiasm. Postsynaptic neurons in the LGN travel in the optic radiations and synapse in a fan-shaped manner in the primary visual cortex.

TMP13 pp. 661-662

54. D) The cochlea is a structure of tubes and chambers that is filled with fluid. The fluid is not compressible. As the stapes moves back and forth against the oval window, the increase and decrease in pressure caused by that in-and-out movement of the oval window is relieved by the opposite back-and-forth movement of the round window.

TMP13 p. 675

55. C) In a normal individual, shining a light in either eye will result in both pupils constricting due to contraction of the pupillary sphincter muscles. In contrast, the pupillary dilator muscle dilates the pupil. The ciliary muscle is involved in focusing the eye (accommodation).

TMP13 p. 672

56. B) This woman has Horner's syndrome, which is not a disease but rather a symptom of a disease or other problem. In this problem, lacerations to the right side of the neck have damaged the sympathetic nerves to the right eye and right side of the face. Other causes of Horner's syndrome include aortic dissection that compresses adjacent tissues, carotid dissection, Pancoast lung tumor, and tuberculosis, and it can also be congenital. Disruption of sympathetic nerves to the eye causes ipsilateral miosis, ptosis, and dilated blood vessels in the conjunctiva. Cone-rod dystrophy is a chronic disease in which the rods and cones deteriorate over time. Iris heterochromia is a difference in the color of the irises of the two eyes, which often occurs in persons with Horner's syndrome before the age of 2 years but not in adults, in whom eye color has been established. Retinoblastoma is a cancer of the eye in children. Xerophthalmia (also called *dry eye syndrome*) is a disease caused by dryness of the eye.

TMP13 p. 670

57. D) Cocaine blocks the reuptake of norepinephrine, increasing its concentration at the nerve terminal. Norepinephrine relaxes the pupillary dilator muscle (also called the *pupillary sphincter*), causing the pupil to become larger. Failure of cocaine to cause pupillary dilation indicates disruption of the sympathetic nerves to the pupillary dilator muscle because norepinephrine is not being released at the nerve-muscle junction.

A more recent approach is to apply an α-adrenergic agonist (such as apraclonidine) to both eyes. The pupillary dilator muscle responds to denervation by increasing the number of its α-1 receptors. The weak α-1 adrenergic properties of apraclonidine have no effect on the normal pupillary dilator muscle but cause extensive dilation of the hypersensitive, denervated pupillary dilator muscle. Thus, with application of apraclonidine, the correct answer would be C because the right eye is denervated and thus hypersensitive to α-1 adrenergic stimulation.

TMP13 p. 670

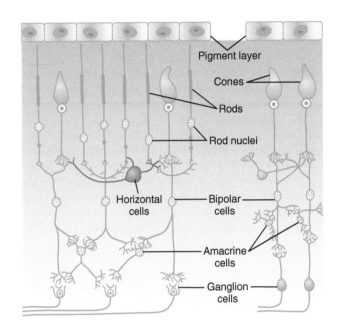

58. C) At least eight types of neurotransmitter substances have been identified for amacrine cells. The neurotransmitters used for bipolar and horizontal cells are unclear, but it is well established that rods and cones release glutamate at their synapses with bipolar cells (see figure above).

TMP13 p. 655

59. D) Because one eye is a little more than 2 inches to the side of the other eye, the images on the two retinas differ from one another. This binocular parallax (stereopsis) allows a person with two eyes far greater ability than a person with only one eye to judge relative distances when objects are nearby.

TMP13 p. 644

60. A) The principal reason why the anterior surface of the cornea provides most of the refractive power of the eye is that the refractive index of the cornea is markedly different from that of air.

TMP13 p. 638

61. D) Intuitively, one would guess that the rod photo-receptor would have the greatest range of spectral sensitivity. However, it is the red cone that has the broadest spectral sensitivity, followed by the rods, the green cones, and finally the blue cones, which have the narrowest range of spectral sensitivity.
TMP13 p. 652

62. A) Ciliary processes secrete all the aqueous humor of the intraocular fluid at an average rate of 2 to 3 μl/min. These processes are linear folds that project from the ciliary muscle into the space behind the iris. The intraocular fluid flows from behind the iris through the pupil into the anterior chamber of the eye.
TMP13 p. 645

63. A) Circumvallate papillae are located in the posterior part of the tongue, fungiform papillae in the anterior part of the tongue, and foliate papillae on the lateral part of the tongue. The papilla of Vater empties pancreatic secretions and bile into the duodenum.
TMP13 p. 687

64. D) There are three distinct groups of retinal ganglion cells, designated as W, X, and Y cells. W cells transmit rod visual signals. Y cells are the least numerous and transmit information about rapid changes in the visual image. X cells are the most numerous and receive input from cones regarding the visual image and color vision.
TMP13 pp. 657-658

65. C) The medial geniculate nucleus is the thalamic nucleus that conveys auditory information from the brain stem to the primary auditory cortex.
TMP13 p. 679

66. A) Taste preference, although not completely understood, is believed to involve a central process.
TMP13 p. 688

67. E) Most of the primary auditory cortex is in the temporal lobe, but the association auditory cortices extend over much of the insular lobe and even onto the lateral portion of the parietal lobe.
TMP13 p. 680

68. B) The termination of taste fibers for all taste sensations is in the nucleus of the solitary tract in the medulla.
TMP13 pp. 687-688

69. B) cGMP-dependent sodium channels in the outer portions of the rods and cones allow sodium ions to pass from the extracellular space to the intracellular space of the photoreceptor. This process results in a membrane potential that is somewhat lower than the resting membrane potential of a typical neuron. The movement of the sodium ions and resulting electrical potential change as a result of this enhanced permeability is known as the *dark current.*
TMP13 p. 650

70. B) The medial longitudinal fasciculus is a pathway for nerve fibers entering and leaving the oculomotor, trochlear, and abducens nuclei of the brain stem, thus allowing communication to coordinate the contraction of the various extraocular eye muscles.
TMP13 p. 666

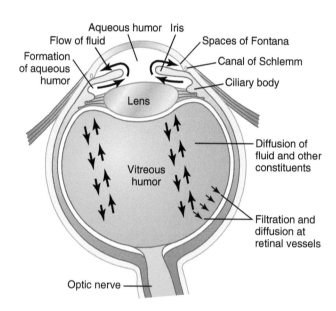

71. B) Intraocular fluid flows from the anterior chamber of the eye, between the cornea and the iris through a meshwork of trabeculae into the canal of Schlemm, which empties into extraocular aqueous veins (see the figure above).
TMP13 p. 645

72. C) Only ganglion cells have action potentials. Photoreceptors, bipolar cells, amacrine cells, and horizontal cells all appear to operate through graded potentials.
TMP13 p. 655

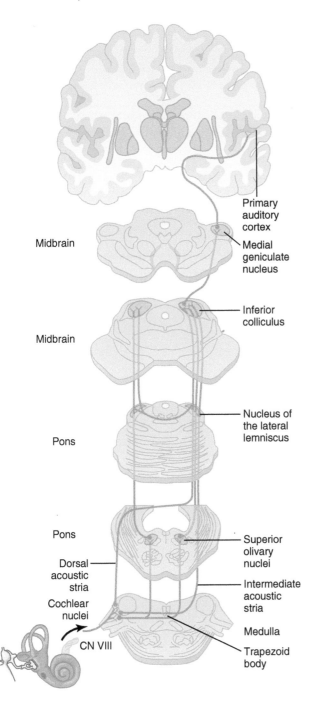

Primary auditory cortex

Midbrain

Medial geniculate nucleus

Inferior colliculus

Midbrain

Nucleus of the lateral lemniscus

Pons

Pons

Superior olivary nuclei

Dorsal acoustic stria

Intermediate acoustic stria

Cochlear nuclei

Medulla

CN VIII

Trapezoid body

73. D) The superior olivary nuclei (see the figure at left) receive auditory information from both ears and begin the process of detecting the direction from which a sound comes. The lateral part of the superior olivary nucleus does so by comparing the difference in intensities of sound reaching the two ears, whereas the medial part of the superior olivary nucleus detects time lag between signals entering both ears.
TMP13 pp. 681-682

74. D) The outputs of horizontal cells are always inhibitory; their lateral connections with synaptic bodies of photoreceptors (rods and cones) and dendrites of bipolar cells provide lateral inhibition to ensure transmission of visual patterns with proper visual contrast. Lateral inhibition is critical in all sensory systems to sharpen the sensory signals. There are many types of amacrine cells with at least six types of functions; they transmit signals both horizontally and vertically, forming connections with many different cell types. Bipolar cells transmit signals vertically from photoreceptors and horizontal cells to ganglion cells and amacrine cells in the inner plexiform layer of the retina. Ganglion cells transmit output signals from the retina through the optic nerve to the brain.
TMP13 pp. 656-657

75. A) Foliate papillae are located in the folds along the lateral surfaces of the tongue, fungiform papillae are located in the anterior part of the tongue, and circumvallate papillae are located in the posterior part of the tongue. The papilla of Vater empties pancreatic secretions and bile into the duodenum.
TMP13 p. 687

The Nervous System: C. Motor and Integrative Neurophysiology

1. A 76-year-old man has a stroke that severely impairs his speech. Which area of his brain is most likely damaged?

   A) Primary motor cortex
   B) Premotor area
   C) Broca's area
   D) Cerebellum

2. A 17-year-old boy sustains serious head and neck trauma during a football game. Physical examination shows a positive Babinski sign. What part of the brain has most likely been damaged in this boy?

   A) Anterior motor neurons
   B) Cerebellum
   C) Corticospinal tract
   D) Premotor cortex

3. Which statement best describes a functional role for the lateral hemispheres of the cerebellum?

   A) Control and coordinate movements of the axial muscles, as well as the shoulder and hip
   B) Control movements that involve distal limb musculature
   C) Function with the cerebral cortex to plan movements
   D) Stimulate motor neurons through their connections to the spinal cord

4. In which type of neuron does the axon form synaptic junctions with the skeletal muscle cells (extrafusal fibers) that comprise the major part of a muscle?

   A) Alpha motor neuron
   B) Pyramidal neuron
   C) Gamma motor neuron
   D) Granule cell
   E) Purkinje cell

5. Which of the following would produce an increase in cerebral blood flow?

   A) Increase in carbon dioxide concentration
   B) Increase in oxygen concentration
   C) Decrease in the activity of cerebral cortex neurons
   D) Decrease in carbon dioxide concentration
   E) Decrease in arterial blood pressure from 120 mm Hg to 90 mm Hg

6. As the axons of motor neurons leave the spinal cord and course peripherally to skeletal muscle, they must pass through which structure?

   A) Posterior column
   B) Posterior root
   C) Ventral white commissure
   D) Posterior horn
   E) Anterior root

7. Which spinal cord level contains the entire population of preganglionic sympathetic neurons?

   A) C5-T1
   B) C3-C5
   C) S2-S4
   D) T1-L2
   E) T6-L1

Questions 8 and 9

A left-side subdural hematoma develops in a 23-year-old man after an automobile accident. Physical examination shows papilledema 3 days after the accident. Use this information to answer Questions 8 and 9.

8. Which of the following is most likely to be increased in this patient?

   A) Cerebral blood flow
   B) Cerebrospinal fluid production
   C) Cerebrospinal fluid volume
   D) Intracranial pressure
   E) Intracranial venous volume

9. Collapse of which of the following structures is most likely to lead to a decrease in brain oxygenation in this patient?

   A) Arteries
   B) Capillaries
   C) Lateral ventricles
   D) Subarachnoid space
   E) Veins

10. Preganglionic sympathetic axons pass through which of the following structures?

    A) Dorsal root
    B) Dorsal primary rami
    C) White rami
    D) Gray rami
    E) Ventral primary rami

11. Which statement best describes a functional role for the intermediate zone of the cerebellum?

  A) Controls and coordinates movements of the axial muscles, as well as the shoulder and hip
  B) Controls movements that involve distal limb musculature
  C) Functions with the cerebral cortex to plan movements
  D) Stimulates motor neurons through its connections to the spinal cord

12. Which body part is represented most laterally and inferiorly within the primary motor cortex?

  A) Face
  B) Hand
  C) Neck
  D) Abdomen
  E) Lower limb

13. The gigantocellular neurons of the reticular formation release which neurotransmitter?

  A) Norepinephrine
  B) Serotonin
  C) Dopamine
  D) Acetylcholine
  E) Glutamate

14. Astrocytes participating in the metabolic control of cerebral blood flow have the following three events associated with the process: (1) prostaglandin release, (2) a calcium wave, and (3) glutamate spillover. Which sequence best describes the correct temporal order of these three events?

  A) 2, 1, 3
  B) 1, 2, 3
  C) 3, 1, 2
  D) 1, 3, 2
  E) 3, 2, 1
  F) 2, 3, 1

15. A 15-year-old girl is taken to see a physician because of a sore throat. An antibiotic is prescribed that can enter most tissues of the body but cannot penetrate the blood-brain barrier. The blood-brain barrier can be attributed primarily to which cell type?

  A) Astrocyte
  B) Endothelial cell
  C) Glial cell
  D) Macrophage
  E) Pericyte
  F) Smooth muscle cell

16. In which type of neuron does the axon form synaptic junctions with skeletal muscle cells (intrafusal fibers) within the muscle spindles?

  A) Alpha motor neuron
  B) Pyramidal neuron
  C) Gamma motor neuron
  D) Granule cell
  E) Purkinje cell

17. Which statement best describes a functional role for the cerebellar vermis?

  A) Controls and coordinates movements of the axial muscles, as well as the shoulder and hip
  B) Controls movements that involve distal limb musculature
  C) Functions with the cerebral cortex to plan movements
  D) Stimulates motor neurons through its connections to the spinal cord

18. Which projection system is contained in the superior cerebellar peduncle?

  A) Pontocerebellar
  B) Cerebellothalamic
  C) Posterior spinocerebellar
  D) Corticospinal

Questions 19 and 20
A 29-year-old man steps on a broken bottle with his bare right foot. His right leg immediately lifts while his left leg extends before he can consciously react to the pain. Use this information to answer Questions 19 and 20.

19. This action is attributable to which reflex?

  A) Walking reflex
  B) Stretch reflex
  C) Patellar tendon reflex
  D) Golgi tendon reflex
  E) Flexor withdrawal reflex

20. Which of the following best describes the type of reflex arc and sensory receptor for this reflex?

	Reflex Arc	Sensory Receptor
A)	Disynaptic	Pacinian corpuscle
B)	Disynaptic	Nociceptor
C)	Monosynaptic	Pacinian corpuscle
D)	Monosynaptic	Golgi tendon organ
E)	Polysynaptic	Nociceptor
F)	Polysynaptic	Muscle spindle

21. Which brain structure serves as the major controller of the limbic system?

  A) Hypothalamus
  B) Hippocampus
  C) Amygdala
  D) Mammillary body
  E) Fornix

22. A large portion of the cerebral cortex does not fit into the conventional definition of motor or sensory cortex. Which term refers to the type of cortex that receives input primarily from several other regions of the cerebral cortex?

  A) Cortex that is agranular
  B) Secondary somatosensory cortex
  C) Association cortex
  D) Supplementary motor cortex
  E) Secondary visual cortex

23. The two hemispheres of the brain are connected by which nerve fibers or pathways?

    A) Lateral lemniscus
    B) Corticofugal fibers
    C) Corpus callosum
    D) Arcuate fasciculus
    E) Medial longitudinal fasciculus

24. The fibers of the corticospinal tract pass through which structure?

    A) Medial lemniscus
    B) Medullary pyramid
    C) Posterior funiculus
    D) Medial longitudinal fasciculus
    E) Anterior roots

25. The condition of prosopagnosia usually results from dysfunction or damage to which area of the cerebral cortex?

    A) Prefrontal area
    B) Junction of the parietal and temporal lobe on the nondominant side of the brain
    C) Frontal eye fields
    D) Underside of the medial occipital and temporal lobes
    E) Limbic association areas of frontal and anterior temporal lobes

26. Lesions of which area of the brain would have the most devastating effect on verbal and symbolic intelligence?

    A) Hippocampus
    B) Amygdala
    C) Wernicke's area on the nondominant side of the brain
    D) Broca's area
    E) Wernicke's area on the dominant side of the brain

27. Which term applies to the combination of a motor neuron and all the skeletal muscle fibers contacted by that motor neuron?

    A) Golgi tendon organ
    B) Motor unit
    C) Propriospinal neurons
    D) Skeletal muscle fibers

28. Which maneuver will attenuate the stretch reflex in skeletal muscle?

    A) Sectioning the dorsal root of a spinal nerve
    B) Disruption of the spinocerebellar tract
    C) Disruption of the corticospinal tract
    D) Sectioning the medial lemniscus on the contralateral side of the skeletal muscle in question
    E) Creating a lesion in the contralateral globus pallidus

29. A stroke involving the middle cerebral artery on the left side is likely to cause which symptom? →? right side .

    A) Paralysis of the left side of the face and left upper extremity   right
    B) Paralysis of left lower extremity
    C) Complete loss of vision in both eyes
    D) Loss of ability to comprehend speech
    E) Loss of vision in the left half of both eyes

30. The creation of memory can be interrupted by which activity?

    A) Phosphorylation of a potassium channel to block activity
    B) Activation of adenylate cyclase
    C) Unnatural loss of consciousness
    D) Increase in protein synthesis
    E) Activation of cyclic guanosine monophosphate (cGMP) phosphodiesterase

31. Which structure serves to connect Wernicke's area to Broca's area in the cerebral cortex?

    A) Arcuate fasciculus
    B) Lateral lemniscus
    C) Medial longitudinal fasciculus
    D) Anterior commissure
    E) Internal capsule

32. Broca's area is a specialized portion of motor cortex. Which condition best describes the deficit resulting from damage to Broca's area?

    A) Spastic paralysis of the contralateral hand
    B) Paralysis of the muscles of the larynx and pharynx
    C) Inability to use two hands to grasp an object
    D) Inability to direct the two eyes to the contralateral side
    E) Inability to speak whole words correctly ✓

33. Which projection system is contained in the inferior cerebellar peduncle?

    A) Pontocerebellar
    B) Cerebellothalamic
    C) Posterior spinocerebellar
    D) Corticospinal
    E) Dorsospinocerebellar

34. Signals from motor areas of the cortex reach the contralateral cerebellum after first passing through which structure?

    A) Thalamus
    B) Caudate nucleus
    C) Red nucleus
    D) Basilar pontine nuclei
    E) Dorsal column nuclei

35. Cerebrospinal fluid (CSF) provides a cushioning effect both inside and outside the brain. Which space that lies outside the brain or spinal cord contains CSF?

    A) Lateral ventricle
    B) Third ventricle
    C) Cisterna magna
    D) Epidural space
    E) Aqueduct of Sylvius

Questions 36 and 37

A 40-year-old woman visits the physician because of uncontrolled movements of her arms, legs, head, face, and upper body. These symptoms have increased progressively during the past 12 months. She is also depressed and irritable, and she repeats the same question six times during the 30-minute office visit. Gene analyses show expansion of a CAG triplet repeat on chromosome 4. Use this information to answer Questions 36 and 37.

36. Which diagnosis is most likely?

    A) Alzheimer's disease
    B) Bipolar disorder
    C) Brain tumor
    D) Huntington's disease
    E) Parkinson's disease

37. Which of the following is most likely to be decreased in this woman?

    A) Acetylcholine neurons in the magnocellular forebrain nucleus
    B) Dopamine neurons in the substantia nigra
    C) γ-Aminobutyric acid (GABA) neurons in the caudate nucleus and putamen - ~overa~
    D) Serotonin neurons in the raphe nuclei

38. Which projection system is contained in the middle cerebellar peduncle?

    A) Pontocerebellar
    B) Cerebellothalamic
    C) Posterior spinocerebellar
    D) Corticospinal
    E) Ventrospinocerebellar

39. The peripheral sensory input that activates the ascending excitatory elements of the reticular formation comes mainly from which of the following?

    A) Pain signals
    B) Proprioceptive sensory information
    C) Corticospinal system
    D) Medial lemniscus
    E) Input from Pacinian corpuscles

40. Cells of the adrenal medulla receive synaptic input from which type of neuron?

    A) Preganglionic sympathetic
    B) Postganglionic sympathetic
    C) Preganglionic parasympathetic
    D) Postsynaptic parasympathetic
    E) Presynaptic parasympathetic

41. Which activity will increase the sensitivity of the stretch reflex?

    A) Cutting the dorsal root fibers associated with the muscle in which the stretch reflex is being examined
    B) Increasing the activity of the medullary reticular nuclei
    C) Bending the head forward
    D) Enhanced activity in the fusimotor (gamma motor neuron) system
    E) Stimulating the lateral hemispheres of the cerebellum

42. Neurological disease associated with the cerebellum produces which type of symptoms?

    A) Resting tremor
    B) Athetosis
    C) Rigidity
    D) Ataxia
    E) Akinesia

43. Preganglionic parasympathetic neurons that contribute to the innervation of the descending colon and rectum are found in which structure?

    A) Superior cervical ganglion
    B) Dorsal motor nucleus of the vagus
    C) Superior mesenteric ganglion
    D) Ciliary ganglion
    E) Spinal cord levels S2 and S3

44. A complex spike pattern in the Purkinje cells of the cerebellum can be initiated by stimulation of which brain area?

    A) Inferior olivary complex
    B) Brain stem reticular nuclei
    C) Neurons in red nucleus
    D) Superior olivary complex
    E) Dorsal vestibular nucleus

45. In a muscle spindle receptor, which type of muscle fiber is responsible for the dynamic response?

    A) Extrafusal muscle fiber
    B) Static nuclear bag fiber
    C) Nuclear chain fiber
    D) Dynamic nuclear bag fiber
    E) Smooth muscle fiber

46. Which structure serves as an "alternative pathway" for signals from the motor cortex to the spinal cord?

    A) Red nucleus
    B) Basilar pontine nuclei
    C) Caudate nucleus
    D) Thalamus
    E) Dorsal column nuclei

47. The phenomenon of decerebrate rigidity can be explained, at least in part, by which of the following?

    A) Stimulation of type 1b sensory neurons
    B) Loss of cerebellar inputs to the red nucleus
    C) Overactivity of the medullary reticular nuclei involved in motor control
    D) Unopposed activity of the pontine reticular nuclei
    E) Degeneration of the nigrostriatal pathway

48. Like the primary visual cortex, the primary motor cortex is organized into vertical columns composed of cells linked together throughout the six layers of the cortex. The cells that contribute axons to the corticospinal tract are concentrated in which cortical layer?

    A) Layer I
    B) Layer II
    C) Layer III
    D) Layer IV
    E) Layer V — CST/ CBT.

Questions 49 and 50

A 60-year-old man is taken to the physician because of a tremor in his hands, trouble sleeping, constipation, and dizziness. Physical examination shows a resting tremor, rigidity, and bradykinesia. The man is alert, engaging, and optimistic. He speaks in a low, soft voice. Use this information to answer Questions 49 and 50.

49. Which diagnosis is most likely?

    A) Alzheimer's disease
    B) Bipolar disorder
    C) Brain tumor
    D) Huntington's disease
    E) Parkinson's disease

50. Which of the following is most likely to be decreased in this man?

    A) Serotonin neurons in the raphe nuclei
    B) GABA neurons in the caudate nucleus and putamen
    C) Dopamine neurons in the substantia nigra
    D) Acetylcholine neurons in the magnocellular forebrain nucleus

51. Motor cortex neurons receive feedback from muscles activated by the corticospinal system. This feedback arises from which of the following structures?

    A) Red nucleus
    B) Spinocerebellar tracts
    C) Skin surface of fingers used to grasp an object
    D) Muscle spindles in muscles antagonistic to those used to make the movement
    E) Vestibular nuclei

52. The sweat glands and piloerector muscles of hairy skin are innervated by which type of fibers?

    A) Cholinergic postganglionic parasympathetic
    B) Cholinergic postganglionic sympathetic
    C) Adrenergic preganglionic parasympathetic
    D) Adrenergic postganglionic sympathetic
    E) Adrenergic preganglionic sympathetic

53. In a neurophysiology experiment conducted with monkeys, the amygdalae are surgically ablated bilaterally. Which of the following is most likely to be increased 6 months after ablation of the amygdala?

    A) Despondence
    B) Memory
    C) Paranoia
    D) Sex drive
    E) Tremors

54. In controlling the fine muscles of the hands and fingers, corticospinal axons can synapse primarily with which of the following?

    A) Posterior horn neurons
    B) Spinal cord interneurons
    C) Spinal cord motor neurons
    D) Purkinje cells
    E) Renshaw cells

55. Which of the following foramina allows cerebrospinal fluid to pass directly from the ventricular system into the subarachnoid space?

    A) Foramen of Magendie
    B) Aqueduct of Sylvius
    C) Third ventricle
    D) Lateral ventricle
    E) Arachnoid villi

56. Which epileptic condition involves a postictal depression period lasting from several minutes to perhaps as long as several hours?

    A) Generalized tonic-clonic seizure
    B) Absence seizure
    C) Jacksonian seizure
    D) Phase-out clonic seizure
    E) Temporal lobe seizure

57. An area in the dominant hemisphere, when damaged, may leave the sense of hearing intact but not allow words to be arranged into a comprehensive thought. Which term is used to identify this portion of the cortex?

    A) Primary auditory cortex
    B) Wernicke's area
    C) Broca's area
    D) Angular gyrus
    E) Limbic association cortex

58. Afferent signals from the periphery of the body travel to the cerebellum in which nerve tract?

    A) Ventral spinocerebellar
    B) Fastigioreticular
    C) Vestibulocerebellar
    D) Reticulocerebellar
    E) Dorsal spinocerebellar

59. Which cells receive direct synaptic input from Golgi tendon organs?

    A) Type Ia inhibitory interneurons
    B) Dynamic gamma motor neurons
    C) Alpha motor neurons
    D) Type Ib inhibitory interneurons
    E) Type II excitatory interneurons

60. Which neurotransmitter is used by the axons of locus coeruleus neurons that distribute throughout much of the brain?

    A) Norepinephrine
    B) Dopamine
    C) Serotonin
    D) Acetylcholine

Questions 61 and 62
A 45-year-old man visits the physician because of difficulties performing simple tasks that involve repetitive movements. The physician asks the patient to turn one hand upward and downward at a rapid pace. The man quickly loses all perception of the instantaneous position of the hand, which results in a series of stalled attempts and jumbled movements. Use this information to answer Questions 61 and 62.

61. Which term best describes this patient's movements?

    A) Agraphesthesia
    B) Astereognosis
    C) Dysarthria
    D) Dysdiadochokinesia
    E) Hemineglect

62. Which area of his brain is most likely to have a lesion?

    A) Cerebellum
    B) Limbic system
    C) Medulla oblongata
    D) Premotor cortex
    E) Primary motor cortex

63. The excitatory or inhibitory effect of a postganglionic sympathetic fiber is determined by which feature or structure?

    A) Function of the postsynaptic receptor to which it binds
    B) Specific organ innervated
    C) Ganglion where the postganglionic fiber originates
    D) Ganglion containing the preganglionic fiber
    E) Emotional state of the individual

64. Which of the following correctly describes the relationship of CSF pressure to the venous pressure in the superior sagittal sinus?

    A) A few millimeters higher
    B) A few millimeters lower
    C) Equal to
    D) Twice the value
    E) One-half the value

65. A vascular lesion that causes degeneration of corticospinal axons in the basilar pons will most likely lead to which condition?

    A) Paralysis primarily involving muscles around the contralateral shoulder and hip joints
    B) Paralysis of the muscles of mastication
    C) Loss of voluntary control of discrete movements of the contralateral hand and fingers
    D) Inability to speak clearly
    E) Inability to convert short-term memory to long-term memory

66. Fine motor movement of the index finger can be elicited by stimulation of which brain area?

    A) Primary motor cortex
    B) Lateral cerebellar hemisphere
    C) Premotor cortex
    D) Supplemental motor area
    E) Red nucleus

67. Which type of cholinergic receptor is found at synapses between preganglionic and postganglionic neurons of the sympathetic system?

    A) Muscarinic
    B) Nicotinic
    C) Alpha
    D) Beta-1
    E) Beta-2

68. A 23-year-old basketball player mentally rehearses free throw shots while lying in bed. Which option best describes the area of the brain that is involved in generating a motor image of this action in the absence of actual movement?

    A) Basal ganglia
    B) Cerebellum
    C) Limbic system
    D) Premotor cortex
    E) Primary motor cortex

69. The perivascular space (Virchow-Robin space) in the brain is formed between the wall of small penetrating vessels and which structure?

    A) Dura mater
    B) Arachnoid membrane
    C) Pia mater
    D) Choroid plexus
    E) Ependymal cells

70. Which type of seizure is associated with a spike and dome electroencephalogram pattern during the seizure activity?

    A) Generalized tonic-clonic
    B) Temporal lobe
    C) Jacksonian
    D) Absence
    E) Apoplectic

71. Which substance has the lowest concentration in the cerebrospinal fluid compared with the cerebral blood plasma?

    A) Chloride
    B) Glucose
    C) Potassium
    D) Protein
    E) Sodium

72. The formation of cerebrospinal fluid by the choroid plexus includes (1) osmosis of water, (2) active transport of sodium, and (3) passive diffusion of chloride. Which sequence best describes the correct temporal order of these processes?

    A) 2, 3, 1
    B) 3, 2, 1
    C) 1, 3, 2
    D) 3, 1, 2
    E) 1, 2, 3
    F) 2, 1, 3

Questions 73 and 74
A 10-year-old girl is taken to the physician because of difficulty walking. Physical examination shows loss of tendon reflexes in the knees and ankles and reduced two-point discrimination in the hands and feet. Repeat visits to the physician show a progressive worsening of these symptoms during the next 2 years. However, the girl is always alert and seems to have normal reasoning abilities. Her uncle had similar problems at age 12 years and later developed scoliosis followed by loss of hearing and vision. Use this information to answer Questions 73 and 74.

73. What is the most likely diagnosis?

    A) Friedreich's ataxia
    B) Huntington's disease
    C) Multiple sclerosis
    D) Parkinson's disease
    E) Poliomyelitis

74. What is the most likely cause of these symptoms in this girl?

    A) A lesion in the premotor cortex
    B) A lesion in the primary motor cortex
    C) Malformation of the cerebellum
    D) Malformation of the frontal lobe
    E) Nerve degeneration
    F) Nerve proliferation

75. Which neurotransmitter is used by the axons of substantia nigra neurons that project to the caudate and putamen?

    A) Norepinephrine
    B) Dopamine
    C) Serotonin
    D) Acetylcholine
    E) GABA

76. Damage limited to the primary motor cortex (area 4) is thought to cause hypotonia in the affected muscles. However, most cortical lesions, particularly those caused by vascular infarcts, generally involve the primary motor cortex in addition to surrounding areas of cortex or cortical efferent axons. The latter type of cortical lesion will cause which of the following?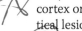

    A) Spastic muscle paralysis
    B) Flaccid muscle paralysis
    C) No paralysis—only jerky, fast movements
    D) Complete blindness in the contralateral eye
    E) Loss of sensation in the contralateral foot

77. The term *limbic cortex* includes the orbitofrontal cortex, subcallosal gyrus, cingulate gyrus, and which area?

    A) Supplementary motor cortex
    B) Postcentral gyrus
    C) Lingual gyrus
    D) Parahippocampal gyrus
    E) Paracentral lobule

78. Which substance activates adrenergic alpha and beta receptors equally well?

    A) Acetylcholine
    B) Norepinephrine
    C) Epinephrine
    D) Serotonin
    E) Dopamine

79. The posterior and lateral hypothalamus, in combination with the preoptic area, are involved in the control of which of the following functions?

    A) Cardiovascular functions involving blood pressure and heart rate
    B) Regulation of thirst and water intake
    C) Stimulation of uterine contractility and milk ejection from the breast
    D) Signaling that food intake is sufficient (satiety)
    E) Secretion of hormones from the anterior lobe of the pituitary gland

80. In the patellar tendon reflex, which of the following items will synapse directly on alpha motor neurons that innervate the muscle being stretched?

    A) Ia sensory fiber
    B) Ib sensory fiber
    C) Excitatory interneurons
    D) Gamma motor neurons
    E) Inhibitory interneurons

81. Occlusion of which structure would lead to communicating hydrocephalus?

    A) Aqueduct of Sylvius
    B) Lateral ventricle
    C) Foramen of Luschka
    D) Foramen of Magendie
    E) Arachnoid villi

82. Evaluation of a patient reveals the following deficits: (1) decreased aggressiveness and ambition and inappropriate social responses; (2) inability to process sequential thoughts in order to solve a problem; and (3) inability to process multiple bits of information that could then be recalled instantaneously to complete a thought or solve a problem. Damage to which brain region could be responsible for such deficits?

   A) Premotor cortex
   B) Parieto-occipital cortex in the nondominant hemisphere
   C) Broca's area
   D) Limbic association cortex
   E) Prefrontal association cortex

83. A lesion in Wernicke's cortical area in the dominant hemisphere is most likely to produce which symptoms?

   A) Impaired language skills
   B) Impaired motor skills
   C) Inability to form new memories
   D) Inability to plan future movements
   E) Reduced cerebellar activity
   F) Reduced cerebral cortex activity

84. Which of the following represents the structural basis of the blood-CSF barrier?

   A) Tight junctions between the ependymal cells forming the ventricular walls
   B) Arachnoid villi
   C) Tight junctions between adjacent choroid plexus cells
   D) Astrocyte foot processes
   E) Tight junctions between adjacent endothelial cells of brain capillaries

85. The withdrawal reflex is initiated by stimulation delivered to which receptor?

   A) Muscle spindle
   B) Joint capsule receptor
   C) Cutaneous free nerve ending
   D) Golgi tendon organ
   E) Pacinian corpuscle

86. A 21-year-old woman is a right-handed musician of considerable talent. Which brain structure is most likely to have been physically larger in the dominant hemisphere compared with the nondominant hemisphere at birth?

   A) Anterior temporal lobe
   B) Posterior temporal lobe
   C) Premotor cortex
   D) Primary motor cortex
   E) Primary somatosensory area
   F) Sensory association area

87. Nasal, lacrimal, salivary, and gastrointestinal glands are stimulated by which substance?

   A) Acetylcholine
   B) Norepinephrine
   C) Epinephrine
   D) Serotonin
   E) Dopamine

88. The neurons located in the locus coeruleus release which neurotransmitter at their synaptic terminals?

   A) Norepinephrine
   B) Dopamine
   C) GABA
   D) Acetylcholine
   E) Serotonin

89. Which of the following reflexes best describes incoming pain signals that elicit movements performed by antagonistic muscle groups on either side of the body?

   A) Crossed extensor reflex
   B) Withdrawal reflex
   C) Reciprocal inhibition
   D) Autogenic inhibition

90. Which portion of the cerebellum functions in the planning of sequential movement?

   A) Vermis and fastigial nucleus
   B) Intermediate zone and fastigial nucleus
   C) Lateral hemisphere and interposed nucleus
   D) Cerebrocerebellum and dentate nucleus
   E) Spinocerebellum and interposed nucleus

91. Which reflex is correctly paired with the sensory structure that mediates the reflex?

   A) Autogenic inhibition—muscle spindle
   B) Reciprocal inhibition—Golgi tendon organ
   C) Reciprocal inhibition—Pacinian corpuscle
   D) Stretch reflex—muscle spindle
   E) Golgi tendon reflex—Meissner corpuscle

92. Damage to which brain area leads to the inability to comprehend the written or the spoken word?

   A) Insular cortex on the dominant side of the brain
   B) Anterior occipital lobe
   C) Junction of the parietal, temporal, and occipital lobes
   D) Medial portion of the precentral gyrus
   E) Most anterior portion of the temporal lobe

93. A computed tomography scan of a newborn boy shows agenesis of the corpus callosum. Which of the following is most likely to occur in this child during the next 5 years as he matures?

   A) Inability to form new memories
   B) Inability to understand spoken words
   C) Inability to verbally express words
   D) Reduction in communication between the two hemispheres
   E) Tameness and inability to recognize expressions of fear

94. A 67-year-old man has a stroke. One week later, he experiences sudden and uncontrolled flailing, ballistic movements of his limbs. Which part of the man's brain is most likely to have been damaged by the stroke?

    A) Globus pallidus
    B) Lateral hypothalamus
    C) Red nucleus
    D) Subthalamic nucleus
    E) Ventrobasal complex of thalamus

95. A physiology experiment is conducted in which a test dose of norepinephrine is administered intravenously to the front limbs of rats, causing a 25 percent reduction in blood flow to the front limbs compared with basal values. Next, the stellate ganglion is removed. Three days later the same dose of norepinephrine is administered intravenously. Which option best describes the most likely change in front limb blood flow (compared with basal values) within 30 minutes after norepinephrine is administered to the ganglionectomized rats?

    A) 25 percent increase
    B) 25 percent reduction
    C) 5 percent increase
    D) 5 percent reduction
    E) 75 percent increase
    F) 75 percent reduction

96. In an otherwise normal person, dysfunction of which brain area will lead to behavior that is not appropriate for the given social occasion?

    A) Ventromedial nuclei of hypothalamus
    B) Amygdala
    C) Corpus callosum
    D) Fornix
    E) Uncus

97. The function of which organ or system is dominated by the sympathetic nervous system?

    A) Systemic blood vessels
    B) Heart
    C) Gastrointestinal gland secretion
    D) Salivary glands
    E) Gastrointestinal motility

98 Schizophrenia is thought to be caused in part by excessive production and release of which neurotransmitter agent?

    A) Norepinephrine
    B) Serotonin
    C) Acetylcholine
    D) Substance P
    E) Dopamine

99. Stimulation of which subcortical area can lead to contraction of a single muscle or small groups of muscles?

    A) Dentate nucleus of the cerebellum
    B) Ventrobasal complex of the thalamus
    C) Red nucleus
    D) Subthalamic nucleus
    E) Nucleus accumbens

100. Bilateral lesions involving the ventromedial hypothalamus will lead to which of the following deficits?

    A) Decreased eating and drinking
    B) Loss of sexual drive
    C) Excessive eating, rage and aggression, hyperactivity
    D) Uterine contractility, mammary gland enlargement
    E) Obsessive compulsive disorder

101. Under awake, resting conditions, brain metabolism accounts for about 15 percent of the total metabolism of the body; this rate is among the highest metabolic rates of all tissues in the body. Which cellular population of the nervous system contributes most substantially to this high rate of metabolism?

    A) Astrocytes
    B) Neurons
    C) Ependymal cells
    D) Choroid plexus cells
    E) Brain endothelial cells

102. Which structure(s) in the cerebellum has/have a topographical representation of the body?

    A) Dentate nucleus
    B) Lateral hemispheres
    C) Flocculonodular lobe
    D) Vermis and intermediate hemisphere
    E) Cerebellar peduncle

103. Which structure is an important pathway for communication between the limbic system and the brain stem?

    A) Mamillothalamic tract
    B) Fornix
    C) Anterior commissure
    D) Indusium griseum
    E) Medial forebrain bundle

104. A 75-year-old woman is taken to the physician because of worsening forgetfulness. She has trouble playing cards with her friends because she cannot remember what game is being played. She recently got lost during a walk in the neighborhood she has lived in for 35 years. Which substance is most likely to be increased in the brain of this woman?

    A) alpha-1 antitrypsin
    B) alpha-amylase
    C) beta-amyloid peptide
    D) beta-endorphin
    E) gamma-glutamyl hydrolase
    F) gamma-glutamyl transferase

105. Which of the following best describes the cerebellar deficit in which there is a failure to perform rapid alternating movements indicating a failure of "progression" from one part of the movement to the next?

    A) Past-pointing
    B) Intention tremor
    C) Dysarthria
    D) Cerebellar nystagmus
    E) Dysdiadochokinesia

106. Which structure in the vestibular apparatus is responsible for the detection of angular acceleration?

    A) Statoconia
    B) Macula
    C) Semicircular canals
    D) Saccule
    E) Ampullae

107. The concept of "autonomic tone" is quite advantageous because it allows the nervous system to have much finer control over the function of an organ or organ system than would otherwise be possible. This ability is exemplified in the control of systemic arterioles. Which action would lead to vasodilation of systemic arterioles?

    A) Increased activity of preganglionic parasympathetic neurons
    B) Decreased activity of postganglionic parasympathetic neurons
    C) Increased activity of postganglionic sympathetic neurons
    D) Decreased activity of postganglionic sympathetic neurons
    E) Increased activity of preganglionic sympathetic neurons

108. A person who has had a traumatic brain injury seems to be able to understand the written and spoken word but cannot create the correct sounds to be able to speak a word that is recognizable. This person most likely has damage to which area of the brain?

    A) Wernicke's area
    B) Broca's area
    C) Angular gyrus
    D) Dentate nucleus
    E) Prefrontal lobe

Questions 109 and 110
A 45-year-old man is taken to the psychiatrist because of delusional behavior in the workplace. The man accused a co-worker of scheming with his neighbor to transplant poison ivy in his backyard. This plot was revealed to the man by a voice in his head. Other examples of delusional thinking and voices in the man's head are abundant. Use this information to answer Questions 109 and 110.

109. What is the most likely diagnosis?

    A) Bipolar disorder
    B) Dissociative identity disorder
    C) Multiple personality disorder
    D) Schizophrenia

110. A decrease in size of which brain structure is most likely in this man?

    A) Globus pallidus
    B) Hippocampus
    C) Lateral hypothalamus
    D) Red nucleus
    E) Subthalamic nucleus

111. Which structure is maximally sensitive to linear head movement in the vertical plane?

    A) Macula of the utricle
    B) Macula of the saccule
    C) Crista ampullaris of the anterior semicircular duct
    D) Crista ampullaris of the horizontal semicircular duct

112. Retrograde amnesia is the inability to recall long-term memories. Damage to which brain region leads to retrograde amnesia?

    A) Hippocampus
    B) Dentate gyrus
    C) Amygdaloid complex
    D) Thalamus
    E) Mammillary nuclei of hypothalamus

113. Which component of the basal ganglia plays the major role in the control of cognitive (memory-guided) motor activity?

    A) Globus pallidus
    B) Substantia nigra
    C) Caudate nucleus
    D) Putamen
    E) Subthalamic nucleus

114. A 9-month-old boy is brought to the emergency department by his grandmother because of irritability and vomiting. The parents dropped the baby off at the grandmother's house 1 hour ago; their current whereabouts are not known. Magnetic resonance imaging shows retinal hemorrhages in both eyes, a subdural hematoma, and cerebral edema. Which of the following is most likely to be increased in this infant?

    A) Brain oxygenation
    B) Cerebral venous volume
    C) Intracranial pressure
    D) Visual acuity

115. Stimulation of the punishment center can inhibit the reward center, demonstrating that fear and punishment can take precedence over pleasure and reward. Which of the following cell groups is considered the punishment center?

    A) Lateral and ventromedial hypothalamic nuclei
    B) Periventricular hypothalamus and midbrain central gray area
    C) Supraoptic nuclei of hypothalamus
    D) Anterior hypothalamic nucleus

116. Drugs that stimulate specific adrenergic receptors are called *sympathomimetic drugs*. Which drug is a sympathomimetic drug?

    A) Reserpine
    B) Phentolamine
    C) Propranolol
    D) L-dopa
    E) Phenylephrine

117. Although the sympathetic nervous system is often activated in such a way that it leads to mass activation of sympathetic responses throughout the body, it can also be activated to produce relatively discrete responses. Which option is an example of a local or discrete sympathetic action?

    A) Heating of a patch of skin causes a relatively restricted vasodilation in the heated region
    B) Food in the mouth causes salivation
    C) Emptying of the bladder may cause reflexive emptying of the bowel
    D) Dust particles in the eye cause increased tear fluid release
    E) Bright light introduced into one eye

118. An experimental drug is administered intravenously to six healthy volunteers. A unanimous finding in all six volunteers is decreased induction of sleep. A decrease in production of which substance is most likely in these volunteers after treatment with the experimental drug?

    A) Acetylcholine
    B) Dopamine
    C) Glutamate
    D) Norepinephrine
    E) Serotonin

119. A 10-year-old boy jumps off the porch and lands on the balls of his feet. The increase in muscle tension causes a sudden, complete relaxation of the affected muscles. Which sensory receptor is most likely to mediate this relaxation of muscles when tension is increased?

    A) Free nerve ending
    B) Golgi tendon organ
    C) Krause corpuscle
    D) Muscle spindle
    E) Pacinian corpuscle

120. Which structure connects the hippocampus to the limbic system?

    A) Mamillothalamic tract
    B) Fornix
    C) Anterior commissure
    D) Medial forebrain bundle
    E) Arcuate fasciculus

121. A wide variety of neurotransmitters have been identified in the cell bodies and afferent synaptic terminals in the basal ganglia. A deficiency of which transmitter is typically associated with Parkinson's disease?

    A) Norepinephrine
    B) Dopamine
    C) Serotonin
    D) GABA
    E) Substance P

122. The condition of athetosis results when which area of the brain is dysfunctional?

    A) Globus pallidus
    B) Substantia nigra
    C) Ventral anterior complex of the thalamus
    D) Putamen
    E) Purkinje cell layer of the cerebellum

1. **C)** Broca's area is a region of the premotor area of one hemisphere (usually the left). Damage to Broca's area does not prevent a person from vocalizing but makes it impossible to speak whole words other than occasional simple words such as "yes" or "no." The primary motor cortex works with other areas of the brain to plan and execute movements. The cerebellum plays a critical role in motor control; it does not initiate movement but contributes to coordination, precision, and accurate timing of movements.
    TMP13 pp. 708, 709

2. **C)** A positive Babinski sign (also called the *Babinski reflex*) occurs normally in children up to 2 years of age. The reflex occurs after the sole of the foot has been stroked with a blunt instrument; the big toe moves upward and the other toes fan out. A positive Babinski sign in adults can indicate damage to the corticospinal tract.
    TMP13 pp. 705-706

3. **C)** The lateral cerebellar hemispheres function with the cerebral cortex in the planning of complex movements.
    TMP13 p. 722

4. **A)** Alpha motor neurons form direct synaptic contact with skeletal extrafusal muscle fibers, whereas gamma motor neurons form synaptic junctions with intrafusal muscle fibers. Pyramidal, granule, and Purkinje neurons are located in the central nervous system and have no direct contact with skeletal muscle.
    TMP13 p. 696

5. **A)** The most potent stimulator of cerebral blood flow is a local increase in carbon dioxide concentration, followed in order by a decrease in oxygen concentration and an increase in local neuronal activity.
    TMP13 p. 788

6. **E)** Axons of motor neurons in the anterior horn exit the spinal cord through the anterior root. The posterior root serves as the entry point for sensory fibers coming into the posterior horn region of the spinal cord. The posterior column and ventral white commissure are fiber tracts located solely within the spinal cord.
    TMP13 pp. 695-696

7. **D)** All preganglionic sympathetic neurons are located in the intermediolateral cell column (lateral horn); this cell group extends from T1 to L2.
    TMP13 p. 774

8. **D)** A subdural hematoma can lead to increased intracranial pressure because it takes up space in the cranium; papilledema (optic disc swelling) suggests an increase in intracranial pressure. The increase in intracranial pressure does not affect production of CSF, but it may cause decreased CSF volume because the high pressure pushes CSF into venous blood through the arachnoidal villi and also compresses the volume of brain structures that contain CSF. Cerebral blood flow should remain normal with small increases in intracranial pressure, but larger increases can decrease cerebral blood flow.
    TMP13 pp. 792-793

9. **E)** The veins have lower pressures compared with arteries and capillaries, making them easier to compress. When the veins are compressed, the capillary pressure increases, which increases the ultrafiltration of fluid from the capillaries into the interstitial spaces, thereby increasing the intracranial pressure even more. The increase in intracranial pressure can cause compression of lateral ventricles and the subarachnoid space, but this mechanism is compensatory rather than a cause for deterioration of blood flow and brain oxygenation.
    TMP13 p. 793

10. **C)** Preganglionic sympathetic axons pass through the white communicating rami to enter the sympathetic trunk. Postganglionic sympathetic axons course through gray rami and might be found in dorsal and ventral primary rami.
    TMP13 p. 773

11. **B)** The intermediate zone of the cerebellum influences the function of distal limb muscles.
    TMP13 p. 722

12. **A)** The face region of the motor cortex is most inferior and lateral in the territory of the middle cerebral artery, whereas the lower limb is in the paracentral lobule in the territory of the anterior cerebral artery.
    TMP13 p. 708

13. **D)** The gigantocellular neurons of the reticular formation reside in the pons and mesencephalon. These neurons release acetylcholine, which functions as an excitatory neurotransmitter in most brain areas.
    TMP13 p. 753

14. **E)** Increased neuronal activity in the brain causes the neurotransmitter glutamate to diffuse from the site of release at the synapses into the adjacent tissues. The

glutamate triggers a calcium wave in astrocytes, which leads to astrocytic release of vasodilatory prostaglandins that cause arterioles to dilate. In this way, the local blood flow to the tissues can be matched with the metabolic activity of the neurons.
TMP13 p. 788

15. **B)** The endothelial cells lining all blood vessels in the brain constitute the blood-brain barrier. The purpose of the blood-brain barrier is to protect the chemical environment of the brain from rapid changes in composition that occur normally in the rest of the body fluids. Brain capillary endothelial cells have special structural and biochemical attributes that impede diffusion of ions, nutrients, and fat-soluble substances; these substances can diffuse through the endothelial barrier and thereby enter into all other tissues of the body.
TMP13 p. 793

16. **C)** Gamma motor neurons form direct synaptic contact with the skeletal muscle fibers known as *intrafusal fibers.* Extrafusal muscle fibers are innervated by alpha motor neurons, whereas Purkinje, granule, and pyramidal neurons have no synaptic contact with muscles in the periphery.
TMP13 p. 696

17. **A)** The cerebellar vermis is involved with the control of axial muscles and proximal limb muscles in the shoulder and hip.
TMP13 p. 722

18. **B)** Cerebellothalamic projections are contained in the superior cerebellar peduncle.
TMP13 p. 724

19. **E)** In this example, the flexor withdrawal reflex is activated by a painful stimulus to the right foot. Flexor muscles in the right leg and extensor muscles in the left leg are simultaneously stimulated to contract, causing reflex removal of the foot from the painful stimulus while shifting body weight to the other leg. The patellar tendon reflex (also called *knee jerk*), which is activated by tapping the patellar tendon, is a type of stretch reflex. The Golgi tendon reflex provides a negative feedback mechanism that prevents the development of too much tension in a muscle.
TMP13 pp. 702-704

20. **E)** The flexor withdrawal reflex is a polysynaptic reflex arc activated by stimulation of nociceptors in the skin. Multiple excitatory and inhibitory interneurons in the spinal cord are involved. The stretch reflex is a monosynaptic reflex arc involving two neurons. The Golgi tendon reflex is a disynaptic reflex arc because the reflex involves two synapses—an afferent and efferent neuron synapse with an inhibitory interneuron in the spinal cord.
TMP13 pp. 702-704

21. **A)** The hypothalamus, despite its small size, is the most important control center for the limbic system. It controls most of the vegetative and endocrine functions of the body and many aspects of behavior.
TMP13 p. 755

22. **C)** The association cortex is defined by the fact that it receives multiple inputs from a wide variety of sensory areas of cortex. It is the true multimodal cortex.
TMP13 pp. 739-740

23. **C)** The corpus callosum is the main fiber pathway for communication between the two hemispheres of the brain.
TMP13 pp. 741-742

24. **B)** Corticospinal fibers pass through the medullary pyramid.
TMP13 pp. 709-710

25. **D)** Prosopagnosia is the inability to recognize faces. This inability occurs in people who have extensive damage on the medial undersides of both occipital lobes and along the medioventral surfaces of the temporal lobes.
TMP13 p. 740

26. **E)** The somatic, visual, and auditory association areas all meet one another at the junction of the parietal, temporal, and occipital lobes. This area is known as *Wernicke's area.* This area on the dominant side of the brain plays the single greatest role for the highest comprehension levels we call intelligence.
TMP13 pp. 740-741

27. **B)** The combination of a motor neuron and all the muscle fibers innervated by that motor neuron is called a *motor unit.*
TMP13 p. 696

28. **E)** Broca's aphasia typically involves an inability to speak words correctly in the absence of any true paralysis of the laryngeal or pharyngeal musculature.
TMP13 pp. 708-709

29. **D)** A stroke involving the left middle cerebral artery is likely to cause an aphasic syndrome that may involve the loss of speech comprehension and/or the loss of the ability to produce speech sounds. Any paralysis resulting from the lesion would affect the right side of the body; similarly, any visual field deficits would affect the right visual field of each eye.
TMP13 p. 741

30. **E)** For an event or sensory experience to be remembered, it must first be consolidated. The consolidation of memory takes time. A disruption of consciousness during the process of consolidation will prevent the development of memory for the event or sensory experience.
TMP13 pp. 748-749

31. A) The connection between Wernicke's area and Broca's area in made by the arcuate fasciculus.
TMP13 pp. 743-744

32. A) Type 1a sensory fibers that innervate the stretch receptors of the muscle spindle travel in the appropriate spinal nerve that provides both the sensory and motor innervation of the muscle. The spinal nerves carry both afferent and efferent fibers. The afferent fibers (which contain the sensory fibers innervating the muscle spindle) pass through the dorsal root. Cutting the dorsal root will remove the afferent limb of the stretch reflex arc.
TMP13 pp. 696, 698-699

33. C) Posterior spinocerebellar fibers pass through the inferior cerebellar peduncle.
TMP13 p. 723

34. D) The main pathway linking the cerebral cortex and the cerebellum involves cortical projections to the ipsilateral basilar pontine nuclei, the cells of which then project to the contralateral cerebellum.
TMP13 pp. 722-723

35. C) The cerebrospinal fluid outside the brain and spinal cord is located within the subarachnoid space. Dilated regions of the subarachnoid space are identified as cisterns. The cisterna magna is one of the largest cisterns and is positioned at the caudal end of the fourth ventricle between the cerebellum and posterior surface of the medulla.
TMP13 p. 790

36. D) This woman has Huntington's disease. This hereditary disorder results from expansion of a CAG triplet repeat in the Huntingtin gene on chromosome 4. Typical symptoms are listed in the question stem. Huntington's disease is a neurodegenerative disorder that at first causes flicking movements in individual muscles and then progresses to distortional movements of the entire body; severe dementia develops along with the motor dysfunctions.
TMP13 pp. 734-735

37. C) The abnormal movements of Huntington's disease are thought to be caused by loss of GABA-secreting neurons in the caudate nucleus and putamen; acetylcholine-secreting neurons in many parts of the brain are also thought to be affected. The axon terminals of GABA-secreting neurons normally inhibit portions of the globus pallidus and substantia nigra. This loss of inhibition is thought to allow spontaneous outbursts of globus pallidus and substantia nigra activity that cause the distortional movements.
TMP13 pp. 734-735

38. A) Pontocerebellar axons are contained in the middle cerebellar peduncle.
TMP13 pp. 722-723

39. A) Pain signals traveling through the anterolateral system, but not any of the discriminative sensations coursing through the medial lemniscal system, provide input to the cells in the reticular formation that give rise to ascending projections to the intralaminar nuclei of the thalamus.
TMP13 pp. 751-752

40. A) Preganglionic sympathetic axons synapse on cells in the adrenal medulla that function as postganglionic sympathetic neurons.
TMP13 p. 774

41. D) Gamma motor neurons innervate the contractile ends of the muscle spindle receptor. Stimulation of gamma motor neurons will cause the ends of the spindle to contract, which in turn will stretch the center of the spindle receptor in the muscle in which the spindle receptor is embedded. The activity of the gamma motor neurons is influenced by the fusimotor system. Enhanced activity of this system will lead to an increase in gamma motor tone and increase the sensitivity of the muscle spindle as a stretch receptor.
TMP13 pp. 699-670

42. D) The cerebellum is responsible for coordinating and timing motor activity. Disorders of the cerebellum are associated with lack of coordination of motor activity. An example of this lack of coordination is ataxia, which is an unsteady gait.
TMP13 p. 729

43. E) Preganglionic parasympathetic neurons that contribute to the innervation of the descending colon and rectum are found at S2 and S3 levels of the spinal cord.
TMP13 p. 775

44. A) Complex spike output from the Purkinje cells of the cerebellum is a response to activation of climbing fibers in cerebellar neural circuitry. All climbing fibers originate in the inferior olivary nucleus.
TMP13 p. 724

45. D) The dynamic nuclear bag fiber responds to the rate of change of length of the muscle spindle receptor. This fiber is responsible for the dynamic response of the muscle spindle.
TMP13 p. 698

46. A) Cortical projections to the red nucleus provide an alternative pathway for the cerebral cortex to control flexor muscles through the rubrospinal tract.
TMP13 pp. 710-711

47. D) The pontine reticular nuclei are tonically active. These nuclei have a stimulatory effect on the antigravity muscles of the body. The pontine nuclei are normally opposed by the medullary reticular nuclei. The medullary nuclei are not tonically active and require stimulation from higher brain centers to counterbalance the signal from the pontine nuclei. Decerebrate rigidity

results when the stimulatory signal from higher brain areas to the medullary nuclei is absent. This absence allows an unopposed and vigorous activation of the antigravity muscles, resulting in extension of the arms and legs and contraction of the axial muscles of the spinal column.
TMP13 p. 714

48. **E)** Corticospinal axons originate from cell bodies (pyramidal neurons) in layer V of the motor areas of the cortex.
TMP13 pp. 709-710

49. **E)** This man has Parkinson's disease. No laboratory biomarkers exist for Parkinson's disease, and imaging results are unremarkable. Diagnosis requires two of three cardinal signs that include (1) resting tremor, (2) rigidity, and (3) bradykinesia (or slow movement); this man has all three signs. Parkinson's disease affects about 1 percent of persons older than 60 years. Progressive disability can be slowed but not halted by treatment.
TMP13 p. 734

50. **C)** This man with Parkinson's disease has a loss of pigmented dopaminergic neurons of the substantia nigra pars compacta that send dopamine-secreting nerve fibers to the caudate nucleus and putamen. The causes of the abnormal motor movements are poorly understood; however, dopamine is an inhibitory transmitter in the caudate nucleus and putamen. It is therefore possible that overactivity of the caudate nucleus and putamen could result from decreased dopamine levels in this patient with Parkinson's disease; these brain structures are largely responsible for voluntary movement.
TMP13 p. 734

51. **C)** The palmar (volar) surfaces of the skin contain receptors that project through the medial lemniscal system to the primary somatosensory cortex. When these fingers are flexed and grasp an object, the cutaneous receptors send signals to the primary somatosensory cortex. These cortical neurons then project to the adjacent motor cortex and the pyramidal neurons that sent the original message down the corticospinal tract to cause contraction of the finger flexors. The motor cortex neurons are then said to be "informed of the muscle contractions" that they originally specified.
TMP13 pp. 711-712

52. **B)** Sweat glands and the piloerector smooth muscle of hairy skin are innervated by the population of cholinergic postganglionic sympathetic neurons.
TMP13 p. 775

53. **D)** Bilateral ablation of the amygdala causes behavioral changes known as *Klüver-Bucy syndrome.* These changes include lack of fear, extreme curiosity, forgetfulness, oral fixation, and a strong sex drive. The sex drive can be so strong that monkeys will attempt to copulate with immature animals, animals of the wrong sex, and even animals of the wrong species. Although similar brain legions in humans are rare, afflicted people have similar symptoms. The amygdala is thought to make the person's behavioral response appropriate for each occasion.
TMP13 p. 760

54. **C)** Although the majority of corticospinal axons synapse with the pool of spinal cord interneurons, some will synapse directly with the motor neurons that innervate muscles controlling the wrist and finger flexors.
TMP13 p. 712

55. **A)** The foramen of Magendie and the two lateral foramina of Luschka form the communication channels between the ventricular system within the brain and the subarachnoid space that lies outside the brain and spinal cord.
TMP13 pp. 790-791

56. **A)** A generalized tonic-clonic epileptic seizure is associated with the sudden onset of unconsciousness and an overall steady but uncoordinated contracture of many muscles of the body followed by alternating contractions of flexor and extensor muscles—that is, tonic-clonic activity. This effect is the result of widespread and uncontrolled activity in many parts of the brain. It takes the brain from a few minutes to a few hours to recover from this vigorous activity.
TMP13 pp. 769-770

57. **B)** Wernicke's area in the dominant hemisphere is responsible for interpreting spoken language. Damage to Wernicke's area will eliminate comprehension of spoken language.
TMP13 pp. 740-741

58. **E)** Afferent signals to the cerebellum travel primarily in the dorsal and ventral spinocerebellar tracts. The dorsal spinocerebellar tract carries signals from the muscle spindle receptors and Golgi tendon receptors, as well as large tactile receptors of the skin and joint proprioceptors. The ventral spinocerebellar tract carries information from the anterior portion of the spinal cord. This tract relays information regarding which motor signals from the motor areas of the brain have arrived at the level of the spinal cord.
TMP13 p. 723

59. **D)** Golgi tendon organs provide direct synaptic input to type Ib inhibitory interneurons. Type Ia interneurons and alpha motor neurons receive input from muscle spindle afferents, whereas dynamic gamma motor neurons and excitatory interneurons receive their input from supraspinal systems.
TMP13 p. 701

60. **A)** Neurons in the locus coeruleus utilize the neurotransmitter norepinephrine in their widespread projections throughout the brain.
TMP13 pp. 752-753

61. **D)** Dysdiadochokinesia is the inability to perform rapid alternating movements. Patients with hemineglect are unaware of items to one side of space. Astereognosis is the inability to recognize objects by touch. Agraphesthesia is a disorientation of the skins sensation across its space (e.g., it is difficult to identify a number or letter traced on the hand). Dysarthria is a failure of progression in talking.
TMP13 pp. 729-730

62. **A)** The cerebellum plays major roles in the timing of motor activities and in rapid, smooth progression from one muscle movement to the next. Lesions of the cerebellum can also cause dysmetria, ataxia, past pointing, nystagmus, dysarthria, intention tremor, and hypotonia. The premotor cortex and primary motor cortex plan and execute movements. The limbic system is involved with behavior, motivation, emotion, long-term memory, and olfaction.
TMP13 pp. 721-724

63. **A)** The excitatory or inhibitory effect of a postganglionic sympathetic fiber is determined solely by the type of receptor to which it binds.
TMP13 p. 777

64. **A)** CSF will flow across the valve-like arachnoid villi when the CSF pressure is only a few millimeters higher than the pressure within the superior sagittal sinus.
TMP13 p. 792

65. **C)** The most characteristic deficit after damage to corticospinal tract neurons involves discrete voluntary movement of the contralateral hand and fingers.
TMP13 p. 713

66. **A)** A large area of the primary motor cortex is dedicated to activating the muscles that control the movement of the fingers. Stimulation of the primary motor cortex usually results in very discrete contractions of small groups of muscles. Stimulation of the premotor cortex results in the contraction of large groups of muscles, and stimulation of the supplemental motor area results in bilateral movements.
TMP13 pp. 707-708

67. **B)** Nicotinic cholinergic receptors are found at synapses between preganglionic and postganglionic sympathetic neurons.
TMP13 p. 777

68. **D)** The premotor cortex generates nerve signals for complex patterns of movement rather than discrete patterns generated in the primary motor cortex. The most anterior part of the premotor area first develops a motor image of the total muscle movement that is to be performed. Next, the successive pattern of muscle activity required to achieve the image excites neurons in the posterior premotor cortex; from here, signals are sent directly to the primary motor cortex to excite specific muscles or by way of the basal ganglia and thalamus and then to the primary motor cortex.
TMP13 p. 701

69. **C)** The perivascular space (also known as the *Virchow-Robin space*) is formed between the outer wall of small vessels penetrating into the brain and the pia mater, which lines the outer surface of the brain and is only loosely attached to the brain.
TMP13 p. 792

70. **D)** The spike and dome pattern is characteristic of an absence seizure.
TMP13 p. 770

71. **D)** The concentration of protein in the CSF is only 1 percent to 2 percent of that of plasma; interstitial fluid in the tissues of the brain has an equally low protein concentration. This low protein concentration of CSF can be attributed to the blood-brain barrier, which is impermeable to protein. The concentration of sodium in CSF is slightly less than that of plasma, the chloride concentration is about 15 percent greater than that of plasma, the potassium concentration is 40 percent of that of plasma, and the glucose concentration of CSF is about 30 percent of that of plasma.
TMP13 p. 791

72. **A)** Active transport of sodium ions through the epithelial cells lining the choroid plexus is followed by passive diffusion of chloride ions to maintain electroneutrality. The osmotic gradient created by the sodium and chloride ions causes the immediate osmosis of water into the CSF. The osmolarity of CSF is identical to that of blood plasma.
TMP13 pp. 790-791

73. **A)** This patient has Friedreich's ataxia, which is an autosomal-recessive ataxia resulting from a mutation on chromosome 9. It accounts for about 50 percent of all hereditary ataxias. Huntington's disease is a neurodegenerative disease that affects muscle coordination and causes a decline in cognitive function and psychiatric problems. Multiple sclerosis is an inflammatory disease in which the myelin covering of nerve cells in the brain and spinal cord is damaged, resulting in a wide range of symptoms that include physical, mental, and psychiatric problems.
TMP13 pp. 729-730

74. **E)** The major pathological finding in Friedreich's ataxia is degeneration and loss of axons, especially in the spinal cord and spinal roots; this effect increases with age and duration of disease. Most major nerve tracts in the spinal cord show demyelination, and the spinal cord itself

becomes thin. There are no lesions in the premotor cortex or primary motor cortex, and the frontal lobe remains normal. The disorder does not affect cognitive functions, and unmyelinated sensory fibers are spared.
TMP13 pp. 729-730

75. **B)** Cells in the pars compacta portion of the substantia nigra use the neurotransmitter dopamine in their projections to the caudate and putamen.
TMP13 p. 733

76. **A)** Lesions that damage primary motor cortex and other surrounding motor cortical areas lead to spastic paralysis in the affected muscles.
TMP13 p. 713

77. **D)** The parahippocampal gyrus is an important component of the limbic cortex, or limbic lobe.
TMP13 pp. 754-755

78. **C)** Epinephrine activates alpha- and beta-adrenergic receptors equally well. Norepinephrine excites both types of receptors but has a markedly greater effect on alpha receptors.
TMP13 p. 777

79. **A)** The posterior and lateral hypothalamus, in combination with the preoptic hypothalamus, form an important group of cells controlling cardiovascular functions such as heart rate and blood pressure.
TMP13 pp. 755-756

80. **A)** Ia sensory fibers synapse directly with alpha motor neurons, whereas Ib sensory fibers synapse with inhibitory interneurons. Excitatory interneurons play an important role in the withdrawal reflex. Gamma motor neurons receive input primarily from supraspinal systems.
TMP13 pp. 698-700

81. **E)** Noncommunicating hydrocephalus results when a blockage of CSF flow occurs within the ventricular system or at the sites of communication between the ventricular system and the subarachnoid space. Communicating hydrocephalus occurs when a blockage occurs either within the subarachnoid space or at the arachnoid villi, thus preventing communication between the subarachnoid space and the superior sagittal sinus.
TMP13 p. 793

82. **E)** Behavioral deficits, changes in personality, and diminished problem-solving ability are all signs of damage to the prefrontal association cortex.
TMP13 pp. 741-742

83. **A)** Wernicke's cortical area is the major brain area for language comprehension. A person with a lesion in Wernicke's area may be able to understand either the spoken word or the written word but would not be able to interpret the thought that is expressed.
TMP13 pp. 739-740

84. **C)** The tight junctions formed between adjacent choroid epithelial cells represent the structural basis of the blood-CSF barrier. The blood-brain barrier is formed by the tight junctions between adjacent endothelial cells of brain capillaries.
TMP13 pp. 793-794

85. **C)** The withdrawal reflex is activated by stimuli from free nerve endings. Muscle spindles provide the afferent signals for the stretch reflex, and Golgi tendon organs are the source of stimuli for the inverse myotatic reflex.
TMP13 pp. 701-702

86. **B)** The posterior temporal lobe is larger at birth in the dominant hemisphere of the brain, which is the left hemisphere in 95 percent of people. Because of the tendency to direct one's attention to the better developed region, the rate of learning in the cerebral hemisphere that gains the first start increases rapidly, whereas learning remains slight in the opposite, less-used side. Hence, the left hemisphere normally becomes dominant over the right.
TMP13 pp. 741-742

87. **A)** The nasal, lacrimal, salivary, and gastrointestinal glands are stimulated by cholinergic postganglionic parasympathetic neurons.
TMP13 pp. 778, 780

88. **A)** The neurons located in the locus coeruleus release norepinephrine at their nerve terminals.
TMP13 pp. 752-753

89. **A)** The crossed extensor reflex depends on incoming pain signals distributed to both sides of the spinal cord via excitatory interneurons.
TMP13 p. 703

90. **D)** The cerebrocerebellum and the dentate nucleus are involved with the thalamus and cortex in the planning of complex movements.
TMP13 p. 722

91. **D)** The stretch reflex is mediated by muscle spindles. Autogenic inhibition involves Golgi tendon organs. Reciprocal inhibition is also related to muscle spindles.
TMP13 pp. 698-699

92. **C)** The junction of the parietal, temporal, and occipital lobe is commonly referred to as *Wernicke's area*. This area of the brain is responsible for the ability to comprehend both the written and spoken word.
TMP13 p. 739

93. **D)** The corpus callosum connects the left and right cerebral hemispheres and hence facilitates communication between them. Agenesis of the corpus callosum is a rare defect in which there is a complete or partial absence of the corpus callosum.
TMP13 pp. 709-710, 742

94. **D)** Damage to the subthalamic nucleus of the basal ganglia often leads to flailing movements of an entire limb; this condition is called *hemiballismus*. Stroke is the most common cause of hemiballismus in adults, but this condition is rare. The globus pallidus is part of the basal ganglia and is involved with movement; however, damage to the globus pallidus does not cause hemiballismus. The lateral hypothalamus is mostly concerned with hunger. The red nucleus serves as an alternative pathway for transmitting cortical signals to the spinal cord; it controls the crawling of babies and may be responsible for swinging the arms while walking. The ventrobasal complex of thalamus is a sensory relay area of the brain.
    TMP13 p. 732

95. **F)** The greater reduction in blood flow to the front limbs is caused by denervation supersensitivity of norepinephrine receptors. The mechanism of denervation supersensitivity is poorly understood, but it is most likely caused by an actual increase in the number of norepinephrine receptors on the muscle vasculature. These additional receptors greatly enhance the vasoconstrictor effects of norepinephrine.
    TMP13 p. 777

96. **B)** The amygdala seems to function in behavioral awareness at a semiconscious level. The amygdala also is thought to project into the limbic system the individual's current status with respect to his or her surroundings. Therefore, the amygdala is believed to help pattern behavior appropriate for each occasion.
    TMP13 p. 760

97. **A)** The innervation and function of systemic blood vessels is influenced primarily, if not exclusively, by the sympathetic nervous system.
    TMP13 p. 780

98. **E)** Schizophrenia is thought to be caused in part by excessive release of dopamine. Occasionally, patients with Parkinson's disease exhibit schizophrenic symptoms because of uncontrolled L-dopa therapy and the subsequent production of dopamine.
    TMP13 p. 771

99. **C)** The magnocellular portion of the red nucleus has a somatographic representation of all the muscles of the body, similar to the motor cortex. Stimulation of this area in the red nucleus results in contraction of a single muscle or small groups of muscles.
    TMP13 p. 711

100. **C)** Lesions involving the ventromedial hypothalamus lead to excessive eating (hyperphagia), excessive drinking, rage and aggression, and hyperactivity.
    TMP13 p. 757

101. **B)** The high metabolic rate in the nervous system is primarily due to the high metabolic activity in neurons, even in the resting state.
    TMP13 p. 794

102. **D)** The vermis and the intermediate zone of the cerebellar hemisphere have a distinct topographic representation of the body. These areas are responsible for coordinating the contraction of the muscles of the body for intended motion.
    TMP13 p. 722

103. **E)** The medial forebrain bundle extends from the septal and orbitofrontal regions of the cerebral cortex downward through the center of the hypothalamus to the brain stem reticular area. This structure serves as an important communication system between the limbic system and the brain stem.
    TMP13 p. 755

104. **C)** This woman has Alzheimer's disease. Increased amounts of beta-amyloid peptide is found in the brains of patients with Alzheimer's disease. The peptide accumulates in amyloid plaques with diameters up to several hundred millimeters in widespread areas of the brain, including the cerebral cortex, hippocampus, basal ganglia, thalamus, and cerebellum. A key role for excess accumulation of beta-amyloid peptide in the pathogenesis of Alzheimer's disease is suggested by multiple observations.
    TMP13 pp. 771-772

105. **E)** Dysdiadochokinesia is a cerebellar deficit that involves a failure of progression from one part of a movement to the next. Consequently, movements that include rapid alternation between flexion and extension are most severely affected.
    TMP13 p. 729

106. **C)** Linear acceleration is in a straight line; angular acceleration is that which occurs by turning about a point. The semicircular canals respond to the turning motions of the head and body.
    TMP13 p. 717

107. **D)** Decreased activity of postganglionic sympathetic neurons leads to vasodilation of systemic arterioles. In contrast, increased activity in postganglionic sympathetics results in vasoconstriction.
    TMP13 p. 782

108. **B)** Damage to Broca's area leads to motor aphasia, or the inability to form words correctly.
    TMP13 p. 744

109. **D)** This man has schizophrenia, which is characterized by a breakdown of cognitive and emotional responses. Dissociative identity disorder was formerly called *multiple personality disorder*. Bipolar disorder

is characterized by episodes of elevated mood (mania) alternating with episodes of depression.
TMP13 p. 771

110. B) A consistent finding in most schizophrenics is that the hippocampus is reduced in size. The hippocampus is part of the limbic system. Incoming sensory information activates various parts of the hippocampus that, in turn, initiate behavioral reactions for different purposes. Removal of the hippocampus makes it impossible to learn new information based on verbal symbolism; however, past memories are preserved.
TMP13 p. 771

111. B) Hair cells in the macula of the saccule are maximally sensitive to linear head movement in the vertical plane.
TMP13 p. 716

112. D) Lesions involving the thalamus lead to retrograde amnesia, because they are believed to interfere with the process of retrieving long-term memory stored in other portions of the brain.
TMP13 p. 749

113. C) The caudate nucleus is involved in the basal ganglia circuits that control memory-guided motor activity.
TMP13 pp. 732-733

114. C) This infant has shaken baby syndrome. The subdural hematoma has increased intracranial pressure, which in turn has caused cerebral edema. The venous vasculature in the brain is compressed due to the high intracranial pressure. Continued compression of brain structures can lead to worsening cerebral edema with decreased oxygenation of the brain.
TMP13 p. 793

115. B) The punishment center is primarily localized to the periventricular hypothalamus and the midbrain central gray area.
TMP13 p. 758

116. A) Athetosis is a slow and continuous writhing movement of the arm, neck, or the face. It results from damage or dysfunction of the globus pallidus.
TMP13 p. 731

117. A) An example of a relatively restricted or local sympathetic action is the vasodilation or vasoconstriction of blood vessels that occurs upon warming or cooling of a patch of skin. When a bright light is introduced to one eye, the pupils of both eyes constrict. The pupillary light reflex is a multiple-neuron event that involves the Edinger-Westphal nucleus of the brainstem; it is not a local event.
TMP13 p. 782

118. E) The most conspicuous stimulation area for causing sleep is the raphe nuclei in the lower half of the pons and in the medulla. Many nerve endings of fibers from raphe neurons secrete serotonin. When the formation of serotonin is blocked by drugs, sleep is often disrupted for hours to days. Therefore, it has been assumed that serotonin is a transmitter associated with the production of sleep.
TMP13 pp. 764-765

119. D) The Golgi tendon organ senses tension in the tendons. When tension becomes exceedingly high, an inhibitory reflex is activated that causes relaxation of the entire muscle, which serves to protect the muscle from tearing. However, the Golgi tendon organ is also thought to play a key role in maintaining equal tension in the muscle fibers of a skeletal muscle so that imbalances in tension among the different muscle fibers can be equalized.
TMP13 p. 701

120. B) The fornix connects the hippocampus to the anterior thalamus, hypothalamus, and the limbic system.
TMP13 p. 756

121. B) Degeneration of the dopaminergic cells in the pars compacta of the substantia nigra is thought to be the primary defect in Parkinson's disease.
TMP13 pp. 733-734

122. E) Phenylephrine is a sympathomimetic drug that stimulates adrenergic receptors. Reserpine, phentolamine, and propranolol are sympathetic antagonists.
TMP13 p. 758

Gastrointestinal Physiology

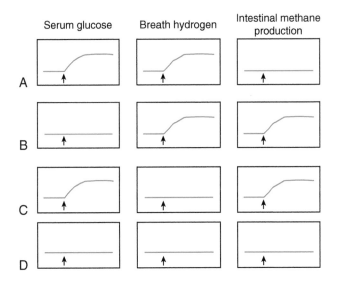

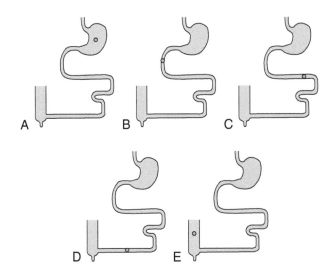

1. A 21-year-old woman visits her physician because of nausea, diarrhea, light-headedness, and flatulence. After an overnight fast, the physician administers 50 grams of oral lactose at time zero (indicated by the arrows in the above figure). Which combination is most likely in this patient during the next 3 hours?

   A) A
   B) B
   C) C
   D) D

2. A 43-year-old man eats a meal consisting of 40 percent protein, 10 percent fat, and 50 percent carbohydrate. Thirty minutes later the man feels the urge to defecate. Which reflex results in the urge to defecate when the duodenum is stretched?

   A) Duodenocolic
   B) Enterogastric
   C) Intestino-intestinal
   D) Rectosphincteric

3. A 23-year-old man consumes a meal containing 30 percent protein, 15 percent fat, and 55 percent carbohydrate. At which of the locations depicted in the above figure are bile salts most likely to be absorbed by an active transport process?

   A) A
   B) B
   C) C
   D) D
   E) E

4. The ileum and distal jejunum of a 34-year-old man are ruptured in an automobile accident. The entire ileum and a portion of the jejunum are resected. What is most likely to occur in this man?

   A) Atrophic gastritis
   B) Constipation
   C) Gastric ulcer
   D) Gastroesophageal reflux disease (GERD)
   E) Vitamin B_{12} deficiency

5. Which ion has the highest concentration in saliva under basal conditions?

   A) Bicarbonate
   B) Chloride
   C) Potassium
   D) Sodium

6. A 10-year-old boy consumes a cheeseburger, fries, and chocolate shake. The meal stimulates the release of several gastrointestinal hormones. The presence of fat, carbohydrate, or protein in the duodenum stimulates the release of which hormone from the duodenal mucosa?

   A) Cholecystokinin (CCK)
   B) Glucose-dependent insulinotropic peptide (GLIP)
   C) Gastrin
   D) Motilin
   E) Secretin

7. A clinical experiment is conducted in which one group of subjects is given 50 grams of glucose intravenously and another group is given 50 grams of glucose orally. Which factor can explain why the oral glucose load is cleared from the blood at a faster rate compared with the intravenous glucose load?

   A) CCK-induced insulin release
   B) CCK-induced vasoactive intestinal peptide (VIP) release
   C) GLIP-induced glucagon release
   D) GLIP-induced insulin release
   E) VIP-induced GLIP release

8. Digestion of which of the following is impaired to the greatest extent in patients with achlorhydria?

   A) Carbohydrate
   B) Fat
   C) Protein

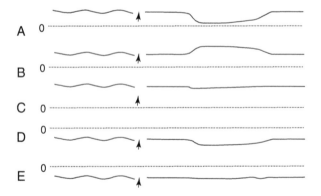

9. A 33-year-old man visits his physician because his chest hurts when he eats, especially when he eats meat. He also belches excessively and has heartburn. His wife says he has bad breath. A radiograph shows a dilated esophagus. Which pressure tracing shown in the above figure was most likely taken at the lower esophageal sphincter (LES) of this patient before and after swallowing (indicated by the arrow)? The dotted line represents a pressure of 0 mm Hg.

   A) A
   B) B
   C) C
   D) D
   E) E

10. The proenzyme pepsinogen is secreted mainly from which of the following structures?

    A) Acinar cells of the pancreas
    B) Ductal cells of the pancreas
    C) Epithelial cells of the duodenum
    D) Gastric glands of the stomach

11. Which hormone is released by the presence of fat and protein in the small intestine and has a major effect in decreasing gastric emptying?

    A) CCK
    B) GLIP
    C) Gastrin
    D) Motilin
    E) Secretin

12. Compared with plasma, saliva has the highest relative concentration of which ion under basal conditions?

    A) Bicarbonate
    B) Chloride
    C) Potassium
    D) Sodium

13. Which of the following can inhibit gastric acid secretion?

	Somatostatin	Secretin	GLIP	Enterogastrones	Nervous Reflexes
A)	No	No	Yes	No	Yes
B)	No	Yes	No	No	No
C)	No	Yes	No	Yes	No
D)	Yes	No	No	Yes	Yes
E)	Yes	No	Yes	No	No
F)	Yes	Yes	Yes	Yes	Yes

14. The gastrointestinal hormones have physiological effects that can be elicited at normal concentrations, as well as pharmacological effects that require higher than normal concentrations. What is the direct physiological effect of the various hormones on gastric acid secretion?

	Gastrin	Secretin	Cholecystokinin	GLIP	Motilin
A)	No effect	Stimulate	Stimulate	No effect	No effect
B)	Stimulate	Inhibit	No effect	Inhibit	No effect
C)	Stimulate	Inhibit	No effect	No effect	No effect
D)	Stimulate	Inhibit	Inhibit	Stimulate	Stimulate
E)	Stimulate	Stimulate	Inhibit	Inhibit	No effect

15. The cephalic phase of gastric secretion accounts for about 30 percent of the acid response to a meal. Which of the following can completely eliminate the cephalic phase of gastric secretion?

    A) Antacids (e.g., Rolaids)
    B) Antigastrin antibody
    C) Atropine
    D) Histamine H_2 blocker
    E) Vagotomy
    F) Sympathectomy

16. Migrating motility complexes (MMCs) occur about every 90 minutes between meals and are thought to be stimulated by the gastrointestinal hormone motilin. An absence of MMCs causes an increase in which of the following?

    A) Duodenal motility
    B) Gastric emptying
    C) Intestinal bacteria
    D) Mass movements
    E) Swallowing

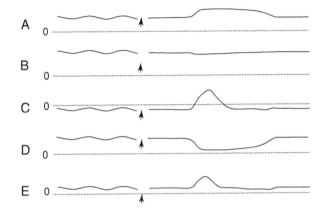

17. Which manometric recording in the above figure illustrates normal function of the esophagus at midthoracic level before and after swallowing (indicated by the arrow)? The dotted lines represent a pressure of 0 mm Hg.

    A) A
    B) B
    C) C
    D) D
    E) E

18. Gastric emptying is tightly regulated to ensure that chyme enters the duodenum at an appropriate rate. Which event promotes gastric emptying under normal physiological conditions in a healthy person?

	Tone of Orad Stomach	Segmentation Contractions in Small Intestine	Tone of Pyloric Sphincter
A)	Decrease	Decrease	Decrease
B)	Decrease	Increase	Decrease
C)	Increase	Decrease	Decrease
D)	Increase	Decrease	Increase
E)	Increase	Increase	Increase

Questions 19–21

A tropical hurricane hits a Caribbean island, and the people living there are forced to drink unclean water. Within the next several days, a large number of people experience severe diarrhea, and about half of these people die. Samples of drinking water are positive for the bacterium *Vibrio cholerae*. Use this information to answer Questions 19–21.

19. A toxin from *V. cholerae* is most likely to stimulate an increase in which of the following in the epithelial cells of the crypts of Lieberkühn in these people ?

    A) Cyclic adenosine monophosphate (cAMP)
    B) Cyclic guanosine monophosphate (cGMP)

    C) Chloride absorption
    D) Sodium absorption

20. Which type of ion channel is most likely to be irreversibly opened in the intestinal epithelial cells of these people?

    A) Calcium
    B) Chloride
    C) Magnesium
    D) Potassium
    E) Sodium

21. Which range best describes the life span (in days) of an intestinal enterocyte infected with *V. cholerae* in a person who survives?

    A) 1 to 3
    B) 3 to 6
    C) 6 to 9
    D) 9 to 12
    E) 12 to 15

22. The gastrointestinal hormones have physiological effects that can be elicited at normal concentrations as well as pharmacological effects that require higher than normal concentrations. What is the physiological effect of the various hormones on gastric emptying?

	Gastrin	Secretin	Cholecysto-kinin	GLIP	Motilin
A)	Decrease	Decrease	Decrease	Decrease	Increase
B)	Increase	Decrease	None	Decrease	Increase
C)	Increase	None	None	Increase	Increase
D)	None	None	Decrease	Increase	Increase
E)	None	None	Decrease	None	None
F)	None	None	Increase	None	None

23. A healthy 12-year-old boy ingests a meal containing 20 percent fats, 50 percent carbohydrates, and 30 percent proteins. The gastric juice is most likely to have the lowest pH in this boy at which time after the meal (in hours)?

    A) 0.5
    B) 1.0
    C) 2.0
    D) 3.0
    E) 4.0

24. CCK and gastrin share multiple effects at pharmacological concentrations. Which effects do CCK and gastrin share (or not share) at physiological concentrations?

	Stimulation of Acid Secretion	Inhibition of Gastric Emptying	Stimulation of Gastric Mucosal Growth	Stimulation of Pancreatic Growth
A)	Not shared	Not shared	Not shared	Not shared
B)	Not shared	Not shared	Shared	Not shared
C)	Not shared	Shared	Not shared	Not shared
D)	Shared	Shared	Not shared	Not shared
E)	Shared	Shared	Shared	Shared

25. Swallowing is a complex process that involves signaling between the pharynx and swallowing center in the brain stem. Which structure is critical for determining whether a bolus of food is small enough to be swallowed?

    A) Epiglottis
    B) Larynx
    C) Palatopharyngeal folds
    D) Soft palate
    E) Upper esophageal sphincter

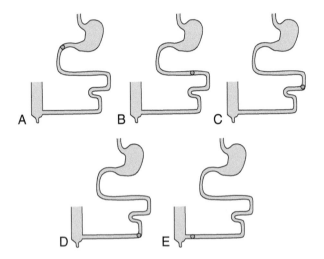

26. A 48-year-old woman consumes a healthy meal. At which location in the above figure are smooth muscle contractions most likely to have the highest frequency?

    A) A
    B) B
    C) C
    D) D
    E) E

27. The spinal cord of a 60-year-old woman is severed at T6 in an automobile accident. She devises a method to distend the rectum to initiate the rectosphincteric reflex. Rectal distention causes which of the following responses in this woman?

	Relaxation of the Internal Anal Sphincter	Contraction of the External Anal Sphincter	Contraction of the Rectum
A)	No	No	No
B)	No	No	Yes
C)	No	Yes	Yes
D)	Yes	No	Yes
E)	Yes	Yes	No
F)	Yes	Yes	Yes

28. An 82-year-old woman with upper abdominal pain and blood in the stool has been taking nonsteroidal anti-inflammatory drugs (NSAIDs) for arthritis. Endoscopy reveals patchy gastritis throughout the stomach. Biopsies were negative for *Helicobacter pylori*. Pentagastrin administered intravenously would lead to a less than normal increase in which of the following?

    A) Duodenal mucosal growth
    B) Gastric acid secretion
    C) Gastrin secretion
    D) Pancreatic enzyme secretion
    E) Pancreatic growth

29. Which substances have a physiological role in stimulating the release of hormones or stimulating nervous reflexes, which in turn can inhibit gastric acid secretion?

	Acid	Fatty Acids	Hyperosmotic Solutions	Isotonic Solutions
A)	No	No	Yes	No
B)	No	No	Yes	Yes
C)	Yes	Yes	No	Yes
D)	Yes	Yes	Yes	Yes
E)	Yes	Yes	Yes	No

30. A clinical study is conducted to determine the time course of gastric acid secretion and gastric pH in healthy volunteers after a meal consisting of 10 percent fat, 30 percent protein, and 60 percent carbohydrate. The results show an immediate increase in the pH of the gastric juice after the meal, which is followed several minutes later by a secondary increase in the rate of acid secretion. A decrease in which substance is most likely to facilitate the secondary increase in the rate of acid secretion in these volunteers?

    A) Gastrin
    B) Cholecystokinin
    C) Somatostatin
    D) Vasoactive intestinal peptide

31. Vomiting is a complex process that requires coordination of numerous components by the vomiting center located in the medulla. Which of the following occurs during the vomiting act?

	LES	Upper Esophageal Sphincter	Abdominal Muscles	Diaphragm
A)	Contract	Contract	Contract	Contract
B)	Contract	Contract	Relax	Relax
C)	Relax	Contract	Contract	Relax
D)	Relax	Relax	Contract	Contract
E)	Relax	Relax	Relax	Relax

32. A 34-year-old woman has a recurrent history of duodenal ulcers associated with diarrhea, steatorrhea, and hypokalemia. Her fasting gastrin level is 550 pg/ml, and basal acid secretion is 18 mmol/hour. Human secretin at a dose of 0.4 μg/kg of body weight is administered intravenously over 1 minute. Postinjection blood samples are collected after 1, 2, 5, 10, and 30 minutes for determination of serum gastrin concentrations. Which serum gastrin concentration is considered diagnostic for gastrinoma in this woman (in pg/ml)?

   A) 450
   B) 500
   C) 550
   D) 600
   E) 700

33. Various proteolytic enzymes are secreted in an inactive form into the lumen of the gastrointestinal tract. Which of the following substances are important for activating one or more proteolytic enzymes, converting them to an active form?

	Trypsin	Enterokinase	Pepsin
A)	No	No	No
B)	No	No	Yes
C)	No	Yes	No
D)	Yes	Yes	No
E)	Yes	Yes	Yes

34. A 71-year-old man with hematemesis and melena has a cresenteric ulcer in the duodenum. Lavage dislodged the clot, revealing an underlying raised blood vessel, which was successfully eradicated via cautery with a bipolar gold probe. Which of the following factors are diagnostic for duodenal ulcer?

	Endoscopy	Plasma Gastrin Levels	Rate of Acid Secretion
A)	No	No	No
B)	Yes	No	No
C)	Yes	No	Yes
D)	Yes	Yes	No
E)	Yes	Yes	Yes

35. A clinical study is conducted in which gastric acid secretion is stimulated using pentagastrin before and after treatment with a histamine H_2 blocker. Which rates of gastric acid secretion (in mEq/hr) are most likely to have occurred in this experiment?

	Pentagastrin Alone	Pentagastrin + H_2 Blocker
A)	15	15
B)	25	25
C)	25	15
D)	26	28
E)	40	45

36. A 23-year-old medical student consumes a cheeseburger, fries, and chocolate shake. Which of the following hormones produce physiological effects at some point during the next several hours?

	Gastrin	Secretin	Cholecystokinin	GLIP
A)	No	Yes	Yes	Yes
B)	Yes	No	Yes	Yes
C)	Yes	Yes	No	Yes
D)	Yes	Yes	Yes	Yes
E)	Yes	Yes	Yes	Yes

Questions 37 and 38

The following diagram shows manometric recordings from a patient before and after pelvic floor training. A balloon placed in the rectum was inflated (at intervals indicated by the arrows) and deflated repeatedly. Tracing Z is a manometric recording obtained from the external anal sphincter before and after pelvic floor training. Use this information and the figure below to answer Questions 37 and 38.

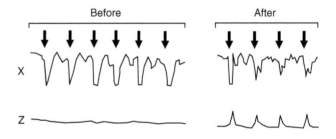

37. Which structure best describes the origin of tracing X shown in the figure?

   A) Distal rectum
   B) Ileocecal valve
   C) Internal anal sphincter
   D) LES
   E) Proximal rectum

38. Which of the following best describes the condition for which the patient received pelvic floor training?

   A) Anal fissure (i.e., a tear or superficial laceration)
   B) Chronic diarrhea
   C) Fecal incontinence (i.e., no control over defecation)
   D) Hemorrhoids
   E) Hirschsprung's disease

39. A 68-year-old woman with hematemesis has heartburn and stomach pain. An endoscopy shows inflammation involving the gastric body and antrum as well as a small gastric ulcer. Biopsies were positive for *H. pylori*. *H. pylori* damages the gastric mucosa primarily by increasing mucosal levels of which of the following?

   A) Ammonium
   B) Bile salts
   C) Gastrin
   D) NSAIDs
   E) Pepsin

40. A physiology experiment is conducted in an isolated rat small intestine. The intestine is bathed with all essential nutrients, ions, and gases in a glass dish maintained at a temperature of 37°C. The proximal jejunum is observed to contract at a frequency of five contractions per minute. A glass micropipette is then inserted into an interstitial cell of Cajal (pacemaker cell) at the same location in the jejunum, and a slow-wave frequency of 10 contractions per minute is recorded. Norepinephrine is then added to the bathing solution. Which of the following best describes the most likely slow-wave frequency and contraction frequency after treatment with norepinephrine (in occurrences per minute)?

	Slow-Wave Frequency	Contraction Frequency
A)	0	0
B)	10	0
C)	10	10
D)	10	5
E)	5	10

41. A healthy 21-year-old woman eats a big meal and then takes a 3-hour ride on a bus that does not have a bathroom. Twenty minutes after eating, the woman feels a strong urge to defecate, but manages to hold it. Which mechanisms have occurred in this woman?

	Relaxation of the Internal Anal Sphincter	Contraction of the External Anal Sphincter	Contraction of the Rectum
A)	No	No	No
B)	No	Yes	Yes
C)	Yes	No	Yes
D)	Yes	No	No
E)	Yes	Yes	Yes

42. A physiology experiment is conducted in an anesthetized rat. The distal duodenum is opened without disturbing its blood supply, and an oxygen-recording micropipette is inserted into the tip of a villus that is submerged in inert oil. An oxygen value of 10 mm Hg is recorded. The distal duodenum at the same location is then treated with the vasodilator adenosine. Which value of oxygen is most likely in the tip of the villus within 2 minutes after treatment with adenosine (in mm Hg)?

A. 0
B. 5
C. 7
D. 10
E. 12

43. One of the following hormones can stimulate growth of the intestinal mucosa, and two other hormones can stimulate pancreatic growth. Which three hormones are these?

	Gastrin	Secretin	Cholecystokinin	GLIP	Motilin
A)	No	Yes	Yes	Yes	No
B)	Yes	No	Yes	No	Yes
C)	Yes	No	Yes	Yes	No
D)	Yes	No	Yes	Yes	No
E)	Yes	Yes	Yes	No	No

44. A 65-year-old man eats a healthy meal. Approximately 40 minutes later the ileocecal sphincter relaxes and chyme moves into the cecum. Gastric distention leads to relaxation of the ileocecal sphincter by way of which reflex?

A) Enterogastric
B) Gastroileal
C) Gastrocolic
D) Intestino-intestinal
E) Rectosphincteric

45. The gastric mucosal barrier has a physiological and an anatomical basis to prevent back-leak of hydrogen ions into the mucosa. Some factors are known to strengthen the integrity of the gastric mucosal barrier, whereas other factors can weaken the barrier. Which factors strengthen or weaken the barrier?

	Bile Salts	Mucous	Aspirin	NSAIDs	Gastrin	Ethanol
A)	Strengthen	Strengthen	Weaken	Weaken	Strengthen	Strengthen
B)	Strengthen	Strengthen	Weaken	Weaken	Weaken	Strengthen
C)	Weaken	Strengthen	Strengthen	Weaken	Strengthen	Weaken
D)	Weaken	Strengthen	Weaken	Weaken	Strengthen	Weaken
E)	Weaken	Weaken	Weaken	Strengthen	Strengthen	Weaken

46. The assimilation of fats includes (1) micelle formation, (2) secretion of chylomicrons, (3) emulsification of fat, and (4) absorption of fat by enterocytes. Which sequence best describes the correct temporal order of these events?

A) 4, 3, 2, 1
B) 3, 1, 4, 2
C) 3, 4, 1, 2
D) 2, 1, 4, 3
E) 4, 2, 1, 3
F) 2, 4, 1, 3
G) 1, 2, 3, 4
H) 1, 3, 2, 4

47. A 62-year-old man with dyspepsia and a history of chronic gastric ulcer has abdominal pain. Endoscopy shows a large ulcer in the proximal gastric body. Biopsies were positive for *H. pylori*. Which substances are used clinically for treatment of gastric ulcers of various etiologies?

	Antibiotics	NSAIDs	H$_2$ Blockers	Proton Pump Inhibitors
A)	No	No	Yes	Yes
B)	Yes	No	No	Yes
C)	Yes	No	Yes	Yes
D)	Yes	Yes	Yes	Yes
E)	No	Yes	Yes	Yes

48. Cystic fibrosis (CF) is an inherited disorder of the exocrine glands affecting children and young people. Mucus in the exocrine glands becomes thick and sticky and eventually blocks the ducts of these glands (especially in the pancreas, lungs, and liver), forming cysts. A primary disruption in the transfer of which ion across cell membranes occurs in CF, leading to decreased secretion of fluid?

A) Calcium
B) Chloride
C) Phosphate
D) Potassium
E) Sodium

49. A 45-year-old man presents with abdominal pain and hematemesis. An abdominal examination was relatively benign, and abdominal radiographs were suggestive of a perforated viscus. Endoscopy revealed a chronically perforated gastric ulcer, through which the liver was visible. Which mechanism is a forerunner to gastric ulcer formation?

A) Back-leak of hydrogen ions
B) Mucus secretion
C) Proton pump inhibition
D) Tight junctions between cells
E) Vagotomy

50. A 10-year-old boy consumes a glass of milk and two cookies. His LES and fundus relax while the food is still in the esophagus. Which substance is most likely to cause relaxation of the LES and fundus in this boy?

A. Gastrin
B. Histamine
C. Motilin
D. Nitric oxide
E. Norepinephrine

51. A 19-year-old man is fed intravenously for several weeks after a severe automobile accident. The intravenous feeding leads to atrophy of the gastrointestinal mucosa, most likely because the blood level of which of the following hormones is reduced?

A) Cholecystokinin only
B) Gastrin only
C) Secretin only
D) Gastrin and cholecystokinin
E) Gastrin and secretin
F) Secretin and cholecystokinin

52. Mass movements are often stimulated after a meal by distention of the stomach (gastrocolic reflex) and distention of the duodenum (duodenocolic reflex). Mass movements often lead to which of the following?

A) Bowel movements
B) Gastric movements
C) Haustrations
D) Esophageal contractions
E) Pharyngeal peristalsis

53. A 45-year-old woman with type 1 diabetes has an early feeling of fullness when eating. She is often nauseous after a meal and vomits about once each week after eating. Glucose-induced damage to which structure is most likely to explain her gastrointestinal problem?

A) Celiac ganglia
B) Enteric nervous system
C) Esophagus
D) Stomach
E) Vagus nerve

54. Which stimulus-mediator pair normally inhibits gastrin release?

	Stimulus	Mediator
A)	Acid	CCK
B)	Acid	GLIP
C)	Acid	Somatostatin
D)	Fatty acid	Motilin
E)	Fatty acid	Somatostatin

55. A 55-year-old man consumes a meal consisting of 20 percent fat, 50 percent carbohydrate, and 30 percent protein. The following gastrointestinal hormones are released at various times during the next 6 hours: gastrin, secretin, motilin, glucose-dependent insulinotropic peptide, and cholecystokinin. Which structure is most likely to release all five hormones in this man?

    A) Antrum
    B) Colon
    C) Duodenum
    D) Esophagus
    E) Ileum

56. An 89-year-old man has a cerebrovascular accident (stroke) in the medulla and pons that completely eliminates all vagal output to the gastrointestinal tract. Which function is most likely to be totally eliminated in this man?

    A) Gastric acid secretion
    B) Gastrin release
    C) Pancreatic bicarbonate secretion
    D) Primary esophageal peristalsis
    E) Secondary esophageal peristalsis
    F) None of the above

57. An 84-year-old man with hematemesis and melena is diagnosed with a duodenal ulcer. A patient diagnosed with a duodenal ulcer is likely to exhibit which of the following?

	Parietal Cell Density	Acid Secretion	Plasma Gastrin
A)	Decreased	Decreased	Decreased
B)	Decreased	Increased	Decreased
C)	Increased	Decreased	Increased
D)	Increased	Increased	Decreased
E)	Increased	Increased	Increased

58. The gastric phase of gastric secretion accounts for about 60 percent of the acid response to a meal. Which substance can virtually eliminate the secretion of acid during the gastric phase?

    A) Antacids (e.g., Rolaids)
    B) Antigastrin antibodies
    C) Atropine
    D) Histamine H_2 blocker
    E) Proton pump inhibitor

59. A 71-year-old man with upper abdominal pain and blood in the stool takes NSAIDs for the pain and washes it down with whiskey. Pentagastrin administration produced lower than predicted levels of gastric acid secretion. Secretion of which substance is most likely to be diminished in this patient with gastritis?

    A) Intrinsic factor
    B) Ptyalin
    C) Rennin
    D) Saliva
    E) Trypsin

60. Gastric acid is secreted when a meal is consumed. Which factors have a direct action on the parietal cell to stimulate acid secretion?

	Gastrin	Somatostatin	Acetylcholine	Histamine
A)	No	No	Yes	Yes
B)	Yes	No	No	Yes
C)	Yes	No	Yes	Yes
D)	Yes	Yes	Yes	Yes
E)	Yes	Yes	No	Yes

61. A 45-year-old woman adds high-fiber wheat and bran foods to her diet to reduce her serum cholesterol levels. She had avoided eating foods containing wheat or rye since she was a child because her mother said they would make her sick. The woman loses 25 pounds on her new diet but has frequent stomach cramps, gas, and diarrhea. She has also become weaker, finding it difficult to complete her morning walks. What is most likely to be increased in this woman?

    A) Blood hemoglobin concentration
    B) Carbohydrate absorption
    C) Fecal fat
    D) Protein absorption
    E) Serum calcium

62. The control of gastric acid secretion in response to a meal involves several events that take place over a 4- or 5-hour period after the meal. These events include (1) a decrease in the pH of the gastric contents, (2) an increase in the rate of acid secretion, (3) a decrease in the rate of acid secretion, and (4) an increase in the pH of the gastric contents. Which sequence best describes the correct temporal order of events over a 4- or 5-hour period after a meal?

    A) 4, 3, 2, 1
    B) 3, 1, 4, 2
    C) 3, 4, 1, 2
    D) 2, 1, 4, 3
    E) 4, 2, 1, 3
    F) 1, 2, 3, 4
    G) 2, 3, 1, 4
    H) 1, 3, 2, 4

63. A newborn boy does not pass meconium within 48 hours of delivery. His abdomen is distended, and he begins vomiting. A suction biopsy of a distally narrowed segment of the colon shows a lack of ganglionic nerve cells. This newborn is at risk for developing which condition?

    A) Achalasia
    B) Enterocolitis
    C) Halitosis
    D) Pancreatitis
    E) Peptic ulcer

64. A 43-year-old obese woman with a history of gallstones is admitted to the emergency department because of excruciating pain in the upper right quadrant. The woman is jaundiced, and a radiograph suggests obstruction of the common bile duct. Which values of direct and indirect bilirubin are most likely to be present in the plasma of this woman (in milligrams per deciliter)?

	Direct	Indirect
A)	1.0	1.3
B)	2.3	2.4
C)	5.0	1.7
D)	1.8	6.4
E)	6.8	7.5

65. Which mechanism for transport of substances across the luminal cell membrane of an enterocyte is present in newborns and infants but not in adults?

A) Endocytosis
B) Facilitated diffusion
C) Passive diffusion
D) Primary active transport
E) Secondary active transport

66. Damage to the gastric mucosal barrier is a forerunner of a gastric ulcer. Which substance can both damage the gastric mucosal barrier and stimulate gastric acid secretion?

A) Bile salts
B) Epidermal growth factor
C) Gastrin
D) *H. pylori*
E) Mucus

67. CF is the most common cause of pancreatitis in children. Which option best explains the mechanism of CF-induced pancreatitis?

A) Activation of enterokinase
B) Activation of trypsin inhibitor
C) Autodigestion of pancreas
D) Excessive secretion of CCK
E) Gallstone obstruction

↑ direct/conjugated billy

1. B) Patients with a lactase deficiency cannot digest milk products that contain lactose (milk sugar). The operons of gut bacteria quickly switch over to lactose metabolism, which results in fermentation that produces copious amounts of gas (a mixture of hydrogen, carbon dioxide, and methane). This gas, in turn, may cause a range of abdominal symptoms including stomach cramps, bloating, and flatulence. The gas is absorbed by blood (especially in the colon) and exhaled from the lungs. Blood glucose levels do not increase because lactose is not digested to glucose and galactose in these patients.

   TMP13 pp. 833-834

2. A) The appearance of mass movements after meals is facilitated by gastrocolic and duodenocolic reflexes. These reflexes result from distention of the stomach and duodenum. They are greatly suppressed when the extrinsic autonomic nerves to the colon have been removed; therefore, the reflexes are likely transmitted by way of the autonomic nervous system. All the gut reflexes are named with the anatomical origin of the reflex as the prefix followed by the name of the gut segment in which the outcome of the reflex is observed. For example, the duodeno-colic reflex begins in the duodenum and ends in the colon. When the duodenum is distended, nervous signals are transmitted to the colon, which stimulates mass movements. The enterogastric reflex occurs when signals originating in the intestines inhibit gastric motility and gastric secretion. The intestino-intestinal reflex occurs when overdistention or injury to a bowel segment signals the bowel to relax. The rectosphincteric reflex, also called the *defecation reflex,* is initiated when feces enters the rectum and stimulates the urge to defecate.

   TMP13 pp. 815, 816, 846

3. D) About 94 percent of the bile salts are reabsorbed into the blood from the small intestine, with about half of this by diffusion through the mucosa in the early portions of the small intestine and the remainder by an active transport process through the intestinal mucosa in the distal ileum.

   TMP13 pp. 829, 830

4. E) Vitamin B_{12} is absorbed in the ileum; this absorption requires intrinsic factor, which is a glycoprotein secreted by parietal cells in the stomach. Binding of intrinsic factor to dietary vitamin B_{12} is necessary for attachment to specific receptors located in the brush border of the ileum. Atrophic gastritis is a type of autoimmune gastritis that is mainly confined to the acid-secreting corpus mucosa. The gastritis is diffuse, and severe atrophy eventually develops. Ileal resection is

likely to cause diarrhea but not constipation. A gastric ulcer is possible but relatively unlikely. GERD is caused by gastric acid and bile reflux into the esophagus; mucosal damage and epithelial cell transformation lead to Barrett esophagus, which is a forerunner to adenocarcinoma, a particularly lethal cancer.

   TMP13 pp. 822, 844

5. A) Although the potassium concentration in saliva is about seven times greater than that of plasma, and the bicarbonate concentration in saliva is only about three times greater than that of plasma, the actual concentration of bicarbonate in saliva is 50 to 70 mEq/L, whereas the concentration of potassium is about 30 mEq/L, under basal conditions.

   TMP13 p. 819

6. B) GLIP is the only gastrointestinal hormone released by all three major foodstuffs (fats, proteins, and carbohydrates). The presence of fat and protein in the small intestine stimulates the release of CCK, but carbohydrates do not stimulate its release. The presence of protein in the antrum of the stomach stimulates the release of gastrin, but fat and carbohydrates do not stimulate its release. Fat has a minor effect to stimulate the release of motilin and secretin, but neither hormone is released by the presence of protein or carbohydrate in the gastrointestinal tract.

   TMP13 p. 802

7. D) GLIP is released by the presence of fat, carbohydrate, or protein in the gastrointestinal tract. GLIP is a strong stimulator of insulin release and is responsible for the observation that an oral glucose load releases more insulin and is metabolized more rapidly than an equal amount of glucose administered intravenously. Intravenously administered glucose does not stimulate the release of GLIP. Neither CCK nor VIP stimulates the release of insulin. GLIP does not stimulate glucagon release, and glucagon has the opposite effect of insulin; that is, it would decrease the rate of glucose clearance from the blood. VIP does not stimulate GLIP release.

   TMP13 p. 802

8. C) Achlorhydria means simply that the stomach fails to secrete hydrochloric acid. This condition is diagnosed when the pH of the gastric secretions fails to decrease below 4 after stimulation by pentagastrin. When acid is not secreted, pepsin also usually is not secreted. Even when it is, the lack of acid prevents it from functioning because pepsin requires an acid medium for activity. Thus, protein digestion is impaired.

   TMP13 p. 844

9. C) Achalasia is a condition in which the LES fails to relax during swallowing. As a result, food swallowed into the esophagus fails to pass from the esophagus into the stomach. Trace C shows a high, positive pressure that fails to decrease after swallowing, which is indicative of achalasia. Trace A shows a normal pressure tracing at the level of the LES, reflecting typical receptive relaxation in response to the food bolus. Trace E is similar to trace C, but the pressures are subatmospheric. Subatmospheric pressures occur only in the esophagus where it passes through the chest cavity.
TMP13 p. 843

10. D) Pepsinogen is the precursor of the enzyme pepsin. Pepsinogen is secreted from the peptic or chief cells of the gastric gland (also called the *oxyntic gland*). To be converted from the precursor form to the active form (pepsin), pepsinogen must come in contact with hydrochloric acid or pepsin itself. Pepsin is a proteolytic enzyme that digests collagen and other types of connective tissue in meats.
TMP13 p. 821

11. A) CCK is the only gastrointestinal hormone that inhibits gastric emptying under physiological conditions. This inhibition of gastric emptying keeps the stomach full for a prolonged time, which is one reason why a breakfast containing fat and protein "sticks with you" better than breakfast meals containing mostly carbohydrates. CCK also has a direct effect on the feeding centers of the brain to reduce further eating. Although CCK is the only gastrointestinal hormone that inhibits gastric emptying, all the gastrointestinal hormones with the exception of gastrin are released to some extent by the presence of fat in the intestine.
TMP13 p. 802

12. C) Under basal conditions, saliva contains high concentrations of potassium and bicarbonate ions and low concentrations of sodium and chloride ions. The primary secretion of saliva by acini has an ionic composition similar to that of plasma. As the saliva flows through the ducts, sodium ions are actively reabsorbed and potassium ions are actively secreted in exchange for sodium. Because sodium is absorbed in excess, chloride ions follow the electrical gradient, causing chloride levels in saliva to decrease greatly. Bicarbonate ions are secreted by an active transport process causing an elevation of bicarbonate concentration in saliva. The net result is that, under basal conditions, sodium and chloride concentrations in saliva are about 10 percent to 15 percent of that of plasma, bicarbonate concentration is about threefold greater than that of plasma, and potassium concentration is about seven times greater than that of plasma.
TMP13 p. 819

13. F) All these factors can inhibit gastric acid secretion under normal physiological conditions. Gastric acid stimulates the release of somatostatin (a paracrine factor), which has a direct effect on the parietal cell to inhibit acid secretion, as well as an indirect effect mediated by suppression of gastrin secretion. Secretin and GLIP inhibit acid secretion through a direct action on parietal cells as well as indirectly through suppression of gastrin secretion. Enterogastrones are unidentified substances released from the duodenum and jejunum that directly inhibit acid secretion. When acid or hypertonic solutions enter the duodenum, a neurally mediated decrease in gastric acid secretion follows.
TMP13 pp. 802, 824

14. B) Gastrin stimulates gastric acid secretion, and secretin and GLIP inhibit gastric acid secretion under normal physiological conditions. It is important to differentiate the physiological effects of the gastrointestinal hormones from their pharmacological actions. For example, gastrin and CCK have identical actions on gastrointestinal function when large, pharmacological doses are administered, but they do not share any actions at normal physiological concentrations. Likewise, GLIP and secretin share multiple actions when pharmacological doses are administered, but only one action is shared at physiological concentrations: inhibition of gastric acid secretion.
TMP13 p. 802

15. E) The cephalic phase of gastric secretion occurs before food enters the stomach. Seeing, smelling, chewing, and anticipating food is perceived by the brain, which, in essence, tells the stomach to prepare for a meal. Stimuli for the cephalic phase thus include mechanoreceptors in the mouth, chemoreceptors (smell and taste), thought of food, and hypoglycemia. Because the cephalic phase of gastric secretion is mediated entirely by way of the vagus nerve, vagotomy can abolish the response. Antacids neutralize gastric acid, but they do not inhibit gastric secretion. An antigastrin antibody would attenuate (but not abolish) the cephalic phase because this would have no effect on histamine and acetylcholine stimulation of acid secretion. Atropine would attenuate the cephalic phase by blocking acetylcholine receptors on parietal cells; however, atropine does not abolish acetylcholine stimulation of gastrin secretion. A histamine H_2 blocker would attenuate the cephalic phase of gastric secretion but would not abolish it.
TMP13 p. 823

16. C) MMCs (sometimes called *interdigestive myoelectric complexes*) are peristaltic waves of contraction that begin in the stomach and slowly migrate in an aboral direction along the entire small intestine to the colon. By sweeping undigested food residue from the stomach, through the small intestine, and into the colon, MMCs function to maintain low bacterial counts in the upper intestine. Bacterial overgrowth syndrome can occur when the normally low bacterial colonization in the upper gastrointestinal tract increases significantly. It should be clear that an absence of MMCs would decrease duodenal motility and gastric emptying. MMCs do not have a direct effect on mass movements and swallowing.

TMP13 pp. 802-803

17. **C)** Trace C shows a basal subatmospheric pressure with a positive pressure wave caused by passage of the food bolus. Trace A does not correspond to any normal event in the esophagus. Trace B could represent the LES in a patient with achalasia. Trace D depicts normal operation of the LES. Trace E show a basal positive pressure trace, which does not occur where the esophagus passes through the chest cavity.

TMP13 p. 808

18. **C)** Gastric emptying is accomplished by coordinated activities of the stomach, pylorus, and small intestine. Conditions that favor gastric emptying include (a) increased tone of the orad stomach, which helps to push chyme toward the pylorus; (b) forceful peristaltic contractions in the stomach that move chyme toward the pylorus; (c) relaxation of the pylorus; which allows chyme to pass into the duodenum; and (d) absence of segmentation contractions in the intestine, which can otherwise impede the entry of chyme into the intestine.

TMP13 p. 812

19. **A)** The toxin from *V. cholerae* (cholera toxin) causes an irreversible increase in cAMP levels (not cGMP levels) in the enterocytes located in the crypts of Lieberkühn of the small intestine. This increase in cAMP causes an irreversible opening of chloride channels on the luminal membrane. Movement of chloride ions into the gut lumen causes a secondary movement of sodium ions to maintain electrical neutrality. Water follows the osmotic gradient created by sodium and chloride, causing a tremendous increase in fluid loss into the gut lumen. Severe diarrhea follows.

TMP13 pp. 840, 842, 846

20. **B)** Cholera toxin causes an irreversible opening of chloride channels in the enterocytes located in the crypts of Lieberkühn of the small intestine, as indicated in the explanation for the previous answer. Although sodium ions enter the gut lumen to maintain electrical neutrality after the flux of chloride ions into the gut lumen, the sodium ions move through relatively large paracellular pathways rather than through actual sodium channels. Calcium, potassium, and magnesium do not have a significant role in the course of an infection with *V. cholerae*.

TMP13 pp. 840, 842, 846

21. **B)** Enterocytes are derived from stem cells located in the crypts of Lieberkühn of the small intestine. They mature as they migrate upward toward the villus tip, where they are extruded into the gut lumen, becoming

part of the ingesta. In humans, the entire population of epithelial cells is replaced in 3 to 6 days. Cholera also usually runs its course in 3 to 6 days. Because cholera toxin causes an irreversible opening of chloride channels in the enterocytes, it is thought that the time course of cholera is dictated by the life span of the enterocytes.

TMP13 pp. 840, 842, 846

22. **E)** CCK is the only gastrointestinal hormone that inhibits gastric emptying under normal physiological conditions. CCK inhibits gastric emptying by relaxing the orad stomach, which increases its compliance. When the compliance of the stomach is increased, the stomach can hold a larger volume of food without excess buildup of pressure in the lumen. None of the gastrointestinal hormones increases gastric emptying under physiological conditions; however, gastrin, secretin, and GLIP can inhibit gastric emptying when pharmacological doses are administered experimentally.

TMP13 p. 802

23. **E)** The figure below shows the time course of gastric pH, rate of acid secretion, and stomach volume immediately before and for 4 hours after a meal. Note that the pH of the gastric juice is lowest immediately before the meal (not an answer choice) and 4 hours after consuming the meal (the correct answer). It is a common misconception that the pH of the gastric juice is lowest (most acidic) after a meal, when acid secretion is highest.

TMP13 pp. 821-822

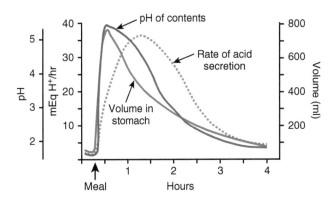

24. **A)** Gastrin and CCK do not share any effects on gastrointestinal function at normal physiological conditions; however, they have identical actions on gastrointestinal function when pharmacological doses are administered. Gastrin stimulates gastric acid secretion and mucosal growth throughout the stomach and intestines under physiological conditions. CCK stimulates growth of the exocrine pancreas and inhibits gastric emptying under normal conditions. CCK also stimulates gallbladder contraction, relaxation of the sphincter of Oddi, and secretion of bicarbonate and enzymes from the exocrine pancreas.

TMP13 p. 802

25. C) The palatopharyngeal folds located on each side of the pharynx are pulled medially, forming a sagittal slit through which the bolus of food must pass. This slit performs a selective function, allowing food that has been masticated sufficiently to pass by but impeding the passage of larger objects. The soft palate is pulled upward to close the posterior nares, which prevents food from passing into the nasal cavities. The vocal cords of the larynx are strongly approximated during swallowing, and the larynx is pulled upward and anteriorly by the neck muscles. The epiglottis then swings backward over the opening of the larynx. The upper esophageal sphincter relaxes, allowing food to move from the posterior pharynx into the upper esophagus.

TMP13 p. 808

26. A) The frequency of slow waves is fixed in various parts of the gut. The maximum frequency of smooth muscle contractions cannot exceed the slow-wave frequency. The slow-wave frequency averages about 3 per minute in the stomach, 12 per minute in the duodenum, 10 per minute in the jejunum, and 8 per minute in the ileum. Therefore, the duodenum is most likely to have the highest frequency of smooth muscle contractions.

TMP13 p. 798

27. D) When feces enters the rectum, distention of the rectal wall initiates signals that spread through the myenteric plexus to initiate peristaltic waves in the descending colon, sigmoid colon, and rectum, all of which force feces toward the anus. At the same time the internal anal sphincter relaxes, allowing the feces to pass. In people with transected spinal cords, the defecation reflexes can cause automatic emptying of the bowel because the external anal sphincter is normally controlled by the conscious brain through signals transmitted in the spinal cord.

TMP13 pp. 815-816

28. B) The use of NSAIDs may result in NSAID-associated gastritis or peptic ulceration. Chronic gastritis, by definition, is a histopathological entity characterized by chronic inflammation of the stomach mucosa. When inflammation affects the gastric corpus, parietal cells are inhibited, leading to reduced acid secretion. Although diagnosis of chronic gastritis can only be ascertained histologically, the administration of pentagastrin should produce a less than expected increase in gastric acid secretion. Pentagastrin is a synthetic gastrin composed of the terminal four amino acids of natural gastrin plus the amino acid alanine. It has all the same physiological properties of natural gastrin. Although gastrin and pentagastrin can both stimulate growth of the duodenal mucosa, it should be clear that intravenous pentagastrin would not cause substantial growth in the context of a clinical test. In any case, chronic administration of pentagastrin would not lead to a less than expected growth of the duodenal mucosa.

Pentagastrin is not expected to increase gastrin secretion, pancreatic enzyme secretion, or pancreatic growth.

TMP13 p. 844

29. E) The presence of acid, fatty acids, and hyperosmotic solutions in the duodenum and jejunum leads to suppression of acid secretion through a variety of mechanisms. Acid stimulates the secretion of secretin from the small intestine, which in turn inhibits acid secretion from parietal cells. Acidification of the antrum and oxyntic gland area of the stomach stimulates the release of somatostatin, which in turn inhibits acid secretion by a direct action on the parietal cells and an indirect action mediated by suppression of gastrin secretion. The presence of fatty acids in the small intestine stimulates the release of GLIP, which inhibits acid secretion both directly (parietal cell inhibition) and indirectly (by decreasing gastrin secretion). Hyperosmotic solutions in the small intestine cause the release of unidentified enterogastrones, which directly inhibit acid secretion from parietal cells. Isotonic solutions have no effect on acid secretion.

TMP13 pp. 802, 824

30. C) Before a meal, when the stomach is empty, the pH of the gastric juice is at its lowest point and acid secretion is suppressed. Acid secretion is suppressed in part because (a) the concentrated hydrogen ions in the gastric juice stimulate somatostatin release, which has a direct action to decrease the secretion of both gastrin and acid, and (b) the acid itself has a direct effect to suppress parietal cell secretions. When a meal is taken, the buffering effects of the food cause the gastric pH to increase, which in turn decreases somatostatin release. Cholecystokinin and vasoactive intestinal peptide do not have a role in the regulation of gastric acid secretion.

TMP13 p. 824

31. D) The act of vomiting is preceded by antiperistalsis that may begin as far down in the gastrointestinal tract as the ileum. Distention of the upper portions of the gastrointestinal tract (especially the duodenum) becomes the exciting factor that initiates the actual act of vomiting. At the onset of vomiting, strong contractions occur in the duodenum and stomach along with partial relaxation of the lower esophageal sphincter. From then on, a specific vomiting act ensues that involves (a) a deep breath, (b) relaxation of the upper esophageal sphincter, (c) closure of the glottis, and (d) strong contractions of the abdominal muscles and diaphragm.

TMP13 pp. 847-848

32. E) Secretin inhibits gastrin secretion from normal G cells in the antrum and duodenum but actually stimulates gastrin secretion in gastrinoma cells. Any increase in serum gastrin concentration greater than 110 pg/ml above baseline after administration of human secretin is diagnostic of gastrinoma (also called *Zollinger-Ellison syndrome*). The secretin test is considered the most sensitive and accurate diagnostic method for gastrinoma.

TMP13 pp. 827, 828, 844-845

33. E) Essentially all proteolytic enzymes are secreted in an inactive form, which prevents autodigestion of the secreting organ. Enterokinase is physically attached to the brush border of the enterocytes that line the inner surface of the small intestine. Enterokinase activates trypsinogen to become trypsin in the gut lumen. The trypsin then catalyzes the formation of additional trypsin from trypsinogen, as well as several other proenzymes (e.g., chymotrypsinogen, procarboxypeptidase, proelastase). Pepsin is first secreted as pepsinogen, which has no proteolytic activity. However, as soon as it comes into contact with hydrochloric acid, and especially in contact with previously formed pepsin plus hydrochloride acid, it is activated to form pepsin.

TMP13 pp. 822, 825

34. B) Neither plasma gastrin levels nor the rate of acid secretion are diagnostic for duodenal ulcer. However, when patients with a duodenal ulcer are pooled together, they exhibit a statistically significant increase in the rate of acid secretion and a statistically significant decrease in plasma gastrin levels. How is this possible? The basal and maximal acid secretion rates of normal subjects range from 1 to 5 mEq/h and from 6 to 40 mEq/h, respectively, which overlaps with the basal (2-10 mEq/h) and maximal (30-80 mEq/h) acid secretion rates of persons with a duodenal ulcer. The increase in acid secretion of the average person with a duodenal ulcer suppresses the secretion of gastrin from the antrum of the stomach. It should be obvious that endoscopy is diagnostic for duodenal ulcer.

TMP13 p. 845

35. C) The various secretagogues, which include acetylcholine, gastrin, and histamine, have a multiplicative or synergistic effect on gastric acid secretion. This means that histamine potentiates the effects of gastrin and acetylcholine and that H_2 blockers attenuate the secretory responses to both acetylcholine and gastrin. Likewise, acetylcholine potentiates the effects of gastrin and histamine and atropine attenuates the secretory effects of histamine and gastrin. Therefore, in the experiment described, the stimulation of acid secretion by pentagastrin is attenuated by the H_2 blocker because of this multiplicative effect of the secretagogues.

TMP13 pp. 824-825

36. E) All of the gastrointestinal hormones are released after a meal and all have physiological effects.

TMP13 p. 802

37. C) The internal anal sphincter relaxes when the rectum is stretched, as indicated by repeated decreases in

pressure after inflation of the rectal balloon. Pressures in the distal and proximal rectum are expected to increase after inflation of the rectal balloon. Inflation of a rectal balloon should not affect pressures at the lower esophageal sphincter or ileocecal valve.

TMP13 pp. 815-816

38. C) Before pelvic floor training, the pressure at the external anal sphincter was unchanged after inflation of the rectal balloon. This failure of the external anal sphincter to contract is expected to result in defecation. After pelvic floor training, the external anal sphincter contracts when the rectal balloon is inflated, which prevents inappropriate defecation.

TMP13 pp. 815-816

39. A) *H. pylori* is a bacterium that accounts for 95 percent of patients with a duodenal ulcer and virtually 100 percent of patients with a gastric ulcer when chronic use of aspirin or other NSAIDs are eliminated. *H. pylori* is characterized by high urease activity, which metabolizes urea to NH_3 (ammonia). Ammonia reacts with H^+ to become ammonium (NH_4^+). This reaction allows the bacterium to withstand the acid environment of the stomach. The ammonium production is believed to be the major cause of cytotoxicity because the ammonium directly damages epithelial cells, increasing the permeability of the gastric mucosal barrier. Bile salts and NSAIDs can also damage the gastric mucosal barrier, but these substances are not directly related to *H. pylori* infection. Pepsin can exacerbate the mucosal lesions cause by *H. pylori* infection, but pepsin levels are not increased by *H. pylori*. It should be clear that gastrin does not mediate the mucosal damage caused by *H. pylori*.

TMP13 p. 845

40. B) Slow-wave frequency is not affected significantly by either the autonomic nervous system or hormones; it is relatively constant at any given location in the small intestine. When a slow wave reaches a threshold value, a calcium spike potential (action potential) occurs and calcium ions enter the smooth muscle cell, which causes it to contract. Norepinephrine hyperpolarizes smooth muscle cells in the intestine and thereby decreases the likelihood that the membrane potential can reach a threshold value. Therefore, norepinephrine does not affect the basal slow-wave frequency of 10 occurrences per minute but does lower the contraction frequency of the smooth muscle cells to 0 occurrences per minute in this problem.

TMP13 pp. 797-799

41. E) The defecation reflex (also called the *rectosphincteric reflex*) occurs when a mass movement forces feces into the rectum. When the rectum is stretched, the internal anal sphincter relaxes and the rectum contracts pushing the feces toward the anus. The external anal sphincter is controlled voluntarily and can be

contracted when defecation is not possible. Therefore, when a person feels the urge to defecate, the internal anal sphincter is relaxed, the rectum contracts, and the external anal sphincter is either contracted or relaxed depending on the circumstances.
TMP13 pp. 815-816

42. E) Oxygen is shunted from the artery of a villus into its venous drainage so that by the time the arterial blood reaches the villus tip, the oxygen tension has been reduced to about 10 mm Hg. Adenosine dilates the villus artery, increasing blood flow to the villus tip. This increase in blood flow decreases the residence time for blood in the artery so that greater amounts of oxygen can reach the villus tip, thus increasing the oxygen tension at the villus tip. Factors that decrease intestinal blood flow (e.g., hemorrhagic shock and a severe degree of exercise) can lead to ischemic death of villi because of their basal low level of oxygenation.
TMP13 pp. 805-806

43. E) One of the most critical actions of gastrointestinal hormones is their trophic activity. Gastrin can stimulate mucosal growth throughout the gastrointestinal tract as well as growth of the exocrine pancreas. If most of the endogenous gastrin is removed by antrectomy, the gastrointestinal tract atrophies. Exogenous gastrin prevents the atrophy. Partial resection of the small intestine for tumor removal, morbid obesity, or other reasons results in hypertrophy of the remaining mucosa. The mechanism for this adaptive response is poorly understood. Both cholecystokinin and secretin stimulate growth of the exocrine pancreas. GLIP and motilin do not appear to have trophic actions on the gastrointestinal tract.
TMP13 p. 802

44. B) Relaxation of the ileocecal sphincter occurs with or shortly after eating. This reflex has been termed the *gastroileal reflex*. It is not clear whether the reflex is mediated by gastrointestinal hormones (gastrin and cholecystokinin) or extrinsic autonomic nerves to the intestine. Note that the gastroileal reflex is named with the origin of the reflex first (gastro) and the target of the reflex named second (ileal). This method of naming is characteristic of all the gastrointestinal reflexes. The enterogastric reflex involves signals from the colon and small intestine that inhibit gastric motility and gastric secretion. The gastrocolic reflex causes the colon to evacuate when the stomach is stretched. The intestino-intestinal reflex causes a bowel segment to relax when it is overstretched. The rectosphincteric reflex is also called the *defecation reflex*.
TMP13 pp. 813, 816

45. D) Damage to the gastric mucosal barrier allows hydrogen ions to back-leak into the mucosa in exchange for sodium ions. A low pH in the mucosa causes mast cells to leak histamine, which damages the vasculature, causing ischemia. The ischemic mucosa allows a greater leakage of hydrogen ions—leading to more cell injury and death—resulting in a vicious cycle. Factors that normally strengthen the gastric mucosal barrier include mucus (which impedes the influx of hydrogen ions), gastrin (which stimulates mucosal growth), certain prostaglandins (which can stimulate mucus secretion), and various growth factors that can stimulate growth of blood vessels, gastric mucosa, and other tissues. Factors that weaken the gastric mucosal barrier include *H. pylori* (a bacterium that produces toxic levels of ammonium), as well as aspirin, NSAIDs, ethanol, and bile salts.
TMP13 pp. 823-824

46. B) Fat entering the small intestine is first emulsified into smaller globules by bile released from the gallbladder. Pancreatic lipase in conjunction with the co-enzyme colipase then digests the fat (which is mostly triglycerides) into monoglycerides and free fatty acids; these substances then become surrounded by bile salts to form water-soluble aggregates called *micelles*. When a micelle makes contact with an enterocyte of the intestinal wall, the monoglycerides and free fatty acids diffuse directly through the cell membrane into the enterocyte; triglycerides are too large to be absorbed. Once inside the enterocyte, the monoglycerides and free fatty acids form new triglyceride molecules that are subsequently packaged by the Golgi apparatus into chylomicrons. The chylomicrons exocytose at the basolateral membrane of the enterocyte and enter a lymphatic capillary (central lacteal) in the villus.
TMP13 pp. 836-837

47. C) The medical treatment of gastric ulcers is aimed at restoring the balance between acid secretion and mucosal protective factors. Proton pump inhibitors are drugs that covalently bind and irreversibly inhibit the H^+/K^+ adenosine triphosphatase (ATPase) pump, effectively inhibiting acid release. Therapy can also be directed toward histamine release, that is, H_2 blockers, such as cimetidine (Tagamet), ranitidine (Zantac), famotidine (Pepcid), and nizatidine (Axid). These agents selectively block the H_2 receptors in the parietal cells. Antibiotic therapy is used to eradicate the *H. pylori* infection. NSAIDs can cause damage to the gastric mucosal barrier, which is a forerunner of gastric ulcer.
TMP13 p. 845

48. B) Movement of chloride ions out of cells leads to secretion of fluid by cells. CF is caused by abnormal chloride ion transport on the apical surface of epithelial cells in exocrine gland tissues. The CF transmembrane regulator (CFTR) protein functions both as a cAMP-regulated Cl^- channel and, as its name implies, a regulator of other ion channels. The fully processed form of CFTR is found in the plasma membrane of normal epithelia. Absence of CFTR at appropriate cellular sites is

often part of the pathophysiology of CF. However, other mutations in the CF gene produce CFTR proteins that are fully processed but are nonfunctional or only partially functional at the appropriate cellular sites.
TMP13 pp. 819, 831-832, 840

49. **A)** Hydrogen ions leak into the mucosa when it is damaged. As the hydrogen ions accumulate in the mucosa, the intracellular buffers become saturated, and the pH of the cells decreases, resulting in injury and cell death. The hydrogen ions also damage mast cells, causing them to secrete excess amounts of histamine. The histamine exacerbates the condition by damaging blood capillaries within the mucosa. The result is focal ischemia, hypoxia, and vascular stasis. The mucosal lesion is a forerunner of gastric ulcer. Mucus secretion helps strengthen the gastric mucosal barrier because mucus impedes the leakage of hydrogen ions into the mucosa. Various proton pump inhibitors are used as a treatment modality for gastric ulcers because these inhibitors can decrease the secretion of hydrogen ions (protons). The tight junctions between cells within the mucosa help prevent the back-leak of hydrogen ions. Vagotomy was once used to treat gastric ulcer disease because severing or crushing the vagus nerve decreases gastric acid secretion.
TMP13 pp. 823-824

50. **D)** The fundus of the stomach and lower esophageal sphincter both relax during a swallow while the bolus of food is still higher in the esophagus. This phenomenon is called *receptive relaxation*. Receptive relaxation is mediated by afferent and efferent pathways in the vagus nerves. Nitric oxide is the neurotransmitter thought to mediate receptive relaxation at the smooth muscle cell. Motilin is a gastrointestinal hormone that mediates migrating motility complexes (also called *housekeeping contractions*); these contractions occur between meals. Gastrin and histamine do not have significant effects on smooth muscle contraction or relaxation at physiological levels. Norepinephrine can decrease smooth muscle contraction in the small intestine but is not involved in receptive relaxation.
TMP13 pp. 803, 809, 843

51. **B)** Gastrin has a critical role in stimulating mucosal growth throughout the gastrointestinal system.
TMP13 p. 802

52. **A)** Mass movements force feces into the rectum. When the walls of the rectum are stretched by the feces, the defecation reflex is initiated and a bowel movement follows when this is convenient. Mass movements do not affect gastric motility. Haustrations are bulges in the large intestine caused by contraction of adjacent circular and longitudinal smooth muscle. It should be clear that mass movements in the colon do not affect esophageal contractions or pharyngeal peristalsis.
TMP13 pp. 814-815

53. **E)** This woman has gastroparesis (also called *delayed gastric emptying*). This disorder slows or at times even stops the movement of chyme from the stomach to the duodenum. Diabetes is the most common known cause of gastroparesis; it occurs in about 20 percent of persons with type 1 diabetes. The high blood glucose is thought to damage the vagus nerve and thereby delay gastric emptying.
TMP13 p. 812

54. **C)** Acid acts directly on somatostatin cells to stimulate the release of somatostatin. The somatostatin decreases acid secretion by directly inhibiting the acid-secreting parietal cells and indirectly by inhibiting gastrin secretion from G cells in the antrum. Acid is a weak stimulus for CCK release, but CCK does not inhibit (or stimulate) gastrin release. Acid does not stimulate GLIP release. Fatty acids are a weak stimulus for motilin, but motilin does not affect gastrin release. Fatty acids are not thought to stimulate somatostatin release.
TMP13 p. 824

55. **C)** All five gastrointestinal hormones are released from both the duodenum and jejunum. Only gastrin is released from the antrum. Small amounts of cholecystokinin and secretin are also released from the ileum. No gastrointestinal hormones are released from the colon or esophagus.
TMP13 p. 802, Table 63-1

56. **D)** Primary peristalsis of the esophagus is a continuation of pharyngeal peristalsis; central control originates in the swallowing center located in the medulla and pons. Visceral somatic fibers in the vagus nerves directly innervate smooth muscle fibers of the pharynx and upper esophagus, which coordinate pharyngeal peristalsis and primary peristalsis of the esophagus. Esophageal contractions can occur independently of vagal stimulation by a local stretch reflex initiated by the food bolus itself; this phenomenon is called *secondary peristalsis*. Although the vagus nerves can stimulate gastric acid secretion, gastrin release, and pancreatic bicarbonate secretion, these processes can be activated by other mechanisms. Thus, elimination of vagal stimulation does not completely eliminate them.
TMP13 p. 809

57. **D)** Persons with duodenal ulcers have about 2 billion parietal cells and can secrete about 40 mEq H$^+$ per hour. Unaffected individuals have about 50 percent of these values. Plasma gastrin levels are related inversely to acid secretory capacity because of a feedback mechanism by which antral acidification inhibits gastrin release. Thus, plasma gastrin levels are reduced in persons with duodenal ulcers. Maximal acid secretion and plasma gastrin levels are not diagnostic for duodenal ulcer disease because of significant overlap with the normal population among persons in each group.
TMP13 pp. 844-845

58. C) Gastrin, acetylcholine, and histamine can directly stimulate parietal cells to secrete acid. These three secretagogues also have a multiplicative effect on acid secretion such that inhibition of one secretagogue reduces the effectiveness of the remaining two secretagogues. Acetylcholine also has an indirect effect to increase acid secretion by stimulating gastrin secretion from G cells. Somatostatin inhibits acid secretion.
TMP13 pp. 802, 822, 824

59. A) Intrinsic factor is a glycoprotein secreted from parietal cells (i.e., acid-secreting cells in the stomach) that is necessary for absorption of vitamin B_{12}. The patient has a diminished capacity to secrete acid because of chronic gastritis. Because acid and intrinsic factor are both secreted by parietal cells, a diminished capacity to secrete acid is usually associated with diminished capacity to secrete intrinsic factor. Ptyalin, also known as *salivary amylase*, is an enzyme that begins carbohydrate digestion in the mouth. The secretion of ptyalin is not affected by gastritis. Rennin, known also as *chymosin*, is a proteolytic enzyme synthesized by chief cells in the stomach. Its role in digestion is to curdle or coagulate milk in the stomach, a process of considerable importance in very young animals. It should be clear that saliva secretion is not affected by gastritis. Trypsin is a proteolytic enzyme secreted by the pancreas.
TMP13 p. 822

60. E) A proton pump inhibitor such as omeprazole inhibits all acid secretion by directly inhibiting the H^+, K^+-ATPase (H^+ pump). The parietal cell has receptors for secretagogues such as gastrin, acetylcholine, and histamine. Therefore, antigastrin antibodies, atropine, and histamine H_2 blockers can reduce the secretion of acid, but none of these can completely eliminate acid secretion. Antacids neutralize gastric acid once it has entered the stomach, but they cannot inhibit acid secretion from parietal cells.
TMP13 pp. 823, 845

61. C) This woman has celiac disease, also called gluten-sensitive enteropathy, which is a chronic disease of the digestive tract that interferes with the absorption of nutrients from food. Mucosal lesions seen on upper gastrointestinal biopsy specimens are the result of an abnormal, genetically determined, cell-mediated immune response to gliadin, a constituent of the gluten found in wheat; a similar response occurs to comparable proteins found in rye and barley. Gluten is not found in oats, rice, or corn. When persons with celiac disease ingest gluten, the mucosa of their small intestine is damaged by an immunologically mediated inflammatory response, which results in malabsorption and maldigestion at the brush border. Digestion of fat is normal in persons with celiac disease because lipase secreted by the pancreas still functions normally. Malabsorption in celiac disease increases the stool content of carbohydrates, fat, and nitrogen. There is no cure

for celiac disease, but a strict gluten-free diet can help manage symptoms and promote intestinal healing.
TMP13 pp. 845-846

62. E) After a meal, the pH of the gastric contents increases because the food buffers the acid in the stomach. This increase in pH suppresses the release of somatostatin from delta cells in the stomach (hydrogen ions stimulate the release of somatostatin). Because somatostatin inhibits secretion of both gastrin and gastric acid, the fall in somatostatin levels leads to an increase in acid secretion. The increase in acid secretion causes the pH of the gastric contents to decrease. As the pH of the gastric contents decreases, the rate of acid secretion also decreases.
TMP13 pp. 821-822

63. B) This infant has Hirschsprung's disease, which is characterized by a congenital absence of ganglion cells in the distal colon resulting in a functional obstruction. Prolonged fecal stasis can lead to enterocolitis (i.e., inflammation of the colon); full-thickness necrosis and perforation can occur in severe cases. In achalasia, the LES fails to relax during swallowing. Halitosis (bad breath) can occur in persons with Hirschsprung's disease, but this condition is not serious. Peptic ulcer and pancreatitis (inflammation of the pancreas) are not common in persons with Hirschsprung's disease.
TMP13 p. 846

64. C) Pancreatitis is inflammation of the pancreas. The pancreas secretes digestive enzymes into the small intestine that are essential in the digestion of fats, proteins, and carbohydrates. Reduced secretion of fluid into the pancreatic ducts in CF cause these digestive enzymes to accumulate in the ducts. The digestive enzymes then become activated in the pancreatic ducts (which typically would not occur) and can begin to "digest" the pancreas, leading to inflammation and a myriad of other problems (cysts and internal bleeding). Enterokinase is located at the brush border of intestinal enterocytes where it normally activates trypsin from its precursor, trypsinogen. Trypsin inhibitor is normally present in the pancreatic ducts where it prevents trypsin from being activated, and thus prevents autodigestion of the pancreas. When the ducts are blocked in cystic fibrosis, the available trypsin inhibitor is insufficient to prevent trypsin from being activated. Excessive secretion of CCK does not occur in persons with CF. Gallstone obstruction can lead to pancreatitis (by autodigestion) when the obstruction prevents pancreatic juice from entering the intestine, but this is unrelated to CF.
TMP13 p. 845

65. A) Intestinal absorption of immunoglobulins (present in colostrum) during early infancy occurs by endocytosis. This ability to absorb large molecules by endocytosis occurs during the first several months of life but does not occur thereafter. Facilitated diffusion, passive diffusion, and primary and secondary active transport are all normal transport processes in enterocytes.

TMP13 pp. 841-842

66. **D)** The discovery of *H. pylori* and its association with peptic ulcer disease, adenocarcinoma, gastric lymphoma, and other diseases make it one of the most significant medical discoveries of this century. In the United States about 26 million people will experience ulcer disease in their lifetime, and in up to 90 percent, it will likely be due to *H. pylori*. *H. pylori* is a gram-negative bacterium with high urease activity, an enzyme that catalyzes the formation of ammonia from urea. The ammonia (NH_3) is converted to ammonium (NH_4^+) in the acid environment of the stomach. The ammonium damages the gastric mucosal barrier because it damages epithelial cells. *H. pylori* also increases gastric acid secretion, possibly by increasing parietal cell mass. This combination of increased acid secretion along

with damage to the gastric mucosal barrier promotes the development of gastric ulcer. Bile salts can damage the gastric mucosal barrier, but they do not have a clinically significant effect on acid secretion. Epidermal growth factor, gastrin, and mucus strengthen the gastric mucosal barrier.

TMP13 p. 845

67. **C)** About 20 percent of persons older than 65 years have gallstones (cholelithiasis) in the United States, and 1 million newly diagnosed cases of gallstones are reported each year. Gallstones are the most common cause of biliary obstruction. Regardless of the cause of gallstones, serum bilirubin values (especially direct or conjugated) are usually elevated. Indirect or unconjugated bilirubin values are usually normal or only slightly elevated. Only answer C shows a high level of direct bilirubin (conjugated bilirubin) compared with the level of indirect bilirubin (unconjugated bilirubin).

TMP13 p. 830

Metabolism and Temperature Regulation

1. Fatty acid degradation in mitochondria produces which two-carbon substance?

   A) Acetyl coenzyme A
   B) Carnitine
   C) Glycerol
   D) Glycerol 3-phosphate
   E) Oxaloacetic acid

2. The following events occurred during the course of a fever in a 12-year-old boy: (1) cutaneous vasodilation and sweating; (2) a return of the set-point temperature to normal; (3) an increase in the set-point temperature to 103°F; and (4) shivering, chills, and cutaneous vaso-constriction. Which of the following best describes the correct temporal order of events during the course of the fever in this boy?

   A) 4, 3, 2, 1
   B) 3, 4, 2, 1
   C) 2, 1, 4, 3
   D) 4, 2, 1, 3
   E) 3, 4, 1, 2
   F) 1, 2, 3, 4
   G) 2, 3, 1, 4
   H) 1, 3, 2, 4

3. A 72-year-old man with a 25-year history of alcoholism and liver disease visits his physician because of sudden weight gain. One year ago the man had a body mass index (BMI) of 24.9 kg/m²; today his BMI is 28.5 kg/m². Physical examination shows +3 edema in his feet and moderate ascites. Which condition is most likely to have promoted the development of both ascites and peripheral edema in this man?

   A) Decreased capillary hydrostatic pressure
   B) Decreased plasma colloid osmotic pressure
   C) Increased capillary hydrostatic pressure
   D) Increased plasma colloid osmotic pressure

4. A 24-year-old student goes hiking in the Mojave Desert during spring break. The environmental temperature is 105°F and the relative humidity is 20 percent. Which option best describes the major mechanism of heat loss in this student?

   A) Conduction to air
   B) Conduction to objects
   C) Convection
   D) Evaporation
   E) Radiation

5. A 32-year-old student consumes a meal containing 10 percent fat, 50 percent carbohydrate, and 40 percent protein. Four hours later the metabolic rate has increased by about 30 percent, even though the student is sitting at rest. Which substance is most likely to cause the greatest increase in metabolic rate in this student 4 hours after consuming the meal?

   A) Carbohydrate
   B) Fat
   C) Protein

6. A 70-year-old man is found sitting in his yard, vomiting on a hot summer day with the lawnmower running. The man is confused and dizzy. He is admitted to the hospital as an emergency patient. His body temperature is 105°F, his heart rate is 110 beats/min, and his skin turgor is poor. Which symptom is unlikely in this man?

   A) Headache
   B) Hot skin
   C) Hypotension
   D) Nausea
   E) Sweating

7. A 22-year-old woman on a camping trip has underestimated the cool evening temperatures, so she wraps herself in a thin sheet of polyester film with a reflective surface (Mylar), also known as an emergency blanket or space blanket. She feels warm immediately. Which heat loss mechanism most likely accounts for the effectiveness of this paper-thin, reflective Mylar blanket?

   A) Conduction to air
   B) Conduction to objects
   C) Convection
   D) Evaporation
   E) Radiation

Questions 8 and 9
Refer to the following figure to answer Questions 8 and 9.

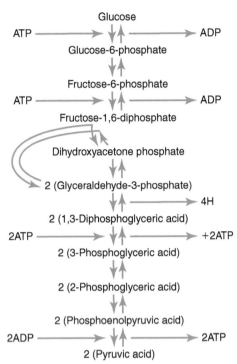

Net reaction per molecule of glucose:
Glucose + 2ADP + 2PO$_4^{\equiv}$ ⟶ 2 Pyruvic acid + 2ATP + 4H

8. Abundant amounts of adenosine triphosphate (ATP) in the cytoplasm of the cell inhibit which step in glycolysis?

 A) Conversion of glucose to glucose-6-phosphate
 B) Conversion of fructose-6-phosphate to fructose-1,6-diphosphate
 C) Conversion of 1,3-diphosphoglyceric acid to 3-phosphoglyceric acid
 D) Conversion of phosphoenolpyruvic acid to pyruvic acid

9. Abundant amounts of adenosine diphosphate (ADP) or adenosine monophosphate (AMP) stimulate which step in glycolysis?

 A) Conversion of glucose to glucose-6-phosphate
 B) Conversion of fructose-6-phosphate to fructose-1,6-diphosphate
 C) Conversion of 1,3-diphosphoglyceric acid to 3-phosphoglyceric acid
 D) Conversion of phosphoenolpyruvic acid to pyruvic acid

10. The transport of glucose through the membranes of most tissue cells occurs by what process?

 A) Facilitated diffusion
 B) Primary active transport
 C) Secondary active co-transport
 D) Secondary active countertransport
 E) Simple diffusion

11. A 65-year-old woman with hepatic cirrhosis comes to her physician for a checkup. Physical examination shows ascites. The woman's prothrombin time has doubled since her last visit 3 months ago, and her hematocrit is now 30 percent. What is the most likely cause of this low hematocrit?

 A) Colon cancer
 B) Esophageal varices
 C) Jaundice
 D) Pancreatitis
 E) Scleral icterus

12. During resting conditions, about 75 percent of the blood flowing through the liver is from the portal vein, and the remainder is from the hepatic artery. Which option best describes the liver circulation in terms of resistance, pressure, and flow?

	Resistance	Pressure	Flow
A)	High	High	High
B)	High	Low	High
C)	Low	High	Low
D)	Low	Low	High
E)	Low	Low	Low

13. A scuba diver explores an underwater lava flow where the water temperature is 102°F. Which profile best describes the mechanisms of heat loss that are effective in this man?

	Evaporation	Radiation	Convection	Conduction
A)	No	No	No	Yes
B)	No	No	No	No
C)	Yes	Yes	No	Yes
D)	No	Yes	No	Yes
E)	Yes	Yes	Yes	Yes

14. A 34-year-old black man is admitted to the hospital because of steadily increasing intense pain in the upper right side of the abdomen. He is nauseated and vomiting. His hematocrit is 30. Ultrasonography shows the presence of gallstones. Which of the following is the most likely major composition of the gallstones in this man?

 A) Bile pigments
 B) Calcium carbonate
 C) Calcium oxalate
 D) Cholesterol

15. *Deamination* means removal of the amino groups from the amino acids. Which substance is produced when deamination occurs by transamination?

 A) Acetyl coenzyme A
 B) Ammonia
 C) Citrulline
 D) Ornithine
 E) α-Ketoglutaric acid

16. Most of the energy released from a glucose molecule occurs as a result of which process?

    A) Citric acid cycle
    B) Glycogenesis
    C) Glycogenolysis
    D) Glycolysis
    E) Oxidative phosphorylation

17. A 29-year-old woman visits her physician because of loss of appetite, fatigue, nausea, and dizziness. Physical examination shows thinning hair. Blood tests show a hematocrit of 32. The woman began following a vegetarian diet suggested by a friend 1 year ago. The physician suspects a dietary deficiently of which substance?

    A) Alanine
    B) Glycine
    C) Lysine
    D) Serine
    E) Tyrosine

18. A 45-year-old man is admitted to the emergency department after he was found lying in the street in an inebriated state. He is markedly pale with icteric conjunctivae and skin. His abdomen is distended, and he has shifting dullness, indicating ascites. His liver is enlarged about 5 centimeters below the right costal margin and tender. His spleen cannot be palpated. He has bilateral edema of the legs and feet. Which values of direct and indirect bilirubin (in milligrams per deciliter) are most likely to be present in this man's plasma?

	Direct	Indirect
A)	1.1	1.2
B)	1.7	5.4
C)	2.4	2.5
D)	5.2	1.8
E)	5.8	7.2

Questions 19–21
Use the following figure to answer Questions 19–21. The diagram shows the effects of changing the set point of the hypothalamic temperature controller. The red line indicates the body temperature, and the blue line represents the hypothalamic set-point temperature.

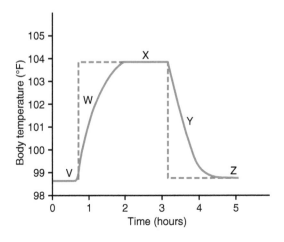

19. Which set of changes occurs at point W compared with point V?

	Shivering	Sweating	Vasoconstriction	Vasodilation
A)	No	No	No	No
B)	No	Yes	No	Yes
C)	No	Yes	Yes	No
D)	Yes	No	No	Yes
E)	Yes	No	Yes	No
F)	Yes	Yes	Yes	Yes

20. Which set of changes occurs at point Y compared with point V?

	Shivering	Sweating	Vasoconstriction	Vasodilation
A)	No	No	No	No
B)	No	Yes	No	Yes
C)	No	Yes	Yes	No
D)	Yes	No	No	Yes
E)	Yes	No	Yes	No
F)	Yes	Yes	Yes	Yes

21. Which set of changes occurs at point X compared with point V?

	Shivering	Sweating	Vasoconstriction	Vasodilation
A)	No	No	No	No
B)	No	Yes	No	Yes
C)	No	Yes	Yes	No
D)	Yes	No	No	Yes
E)	Yes	No	Yes	No
F)	Yes	Yes	Yes	Yes

22. Which of the following is the most abundant source of high-energy phosphate bonds in the cells?

    A) ATP
    B) Phosphocreatine
    C) ADP
    D) Creatine
    E) Creatinine

23. A 54-year-old man is admitted to the emergency department after being found lying in his yard near a running lawnmower on a hot summer day. His body temperature is 106°F, his blood pressure is normal, and his heart rate is 160 beats/min. Which set of changes is most likely to be present in this man?

	Sweating	Hyperventilation	Vasodilation of Skin
A)	No	No	No
B)	No	Yes	Yes
C)	Yes	No	Yes
D)	Yes	Yes	No
E)	Yes	Yes	Yes

24. What accounts for the largest component of daily energy expenditure in a sedentary person?

    A) Basal metabolic rate
    B) Maintaining body posture
    C) Nonshivering thermogenesis
    D) Thermic effect of food

25. Most of the energy for strenuous exercise that lasts for more than 5 to 10 seconds but less than 1 to 2 minutes comes from what source?

    A) ATP
    B) Anaerobic glycolysis
    C) Oxidation of carbohydrates
    D) Oxidation of lactic acid
    E) Conversion of lactic acid into pyruvic acid

26. The ammonia released during deamination of amino acids is removed from the blood almost entirely by conversion into what substance?

    A) Ammonium
    B) Carbon dioxide
    C) Citrulline
    D) Ornithine
    E) Urea

27. Erythrocytes are constantly dying and being replaced. Heme from the hemoglobin is converted to what substance before being eliminated from the body?

    A) Bilirubin
    B) Cholesterol
    C) Cholic acid
    D) Globin
    E) Glucuronic acid

28. Which of the following best describes the process by which glucose can be formed from amino acids?

    A) Gluconeogenesis
    B) Glycogenesis
    C) Glycogenolysis
    D) Glycolysis
    E) Hydrolysis

29. A 32-year-old pregnant woman in her third trimester is admitted to the emergency department because of severe upper right quadrant pain after eating a meal of chicken-fried steak. Her blood pressure is 130/84 mm Hg, her heart rate is 105 beats/min, and her respirations are 30/min. Her body mass index before pregnancy was 45 kg/m². Physical examination shows abdominal guarding and diaphoresis. Her serum bilirubin levels and white blood cell count are both normal. This patient most likely has which condition?

    A) Cholelithiasis
    B) Constipation
    C) Hepatitis
    D) Pancreatitis
    E) Peritonitis

30. An experimental device containing hepatocytes is developed to provide effective support for patients with hepatic failure pending liver regeneration or liver transplantation. Hepatocyte viability is best documented by an increase in which function?

    A) Lactate dehydrogenase uptake
    B) Ethanol output
    C) Albumin output
    D) Glucuronic acid uptake
    E) Oxygen output
    F) Carbon dioxide uptake

31. The metabolic rate of a person is typically expressed in terms of the rate of heat liberation that results from the chemical reactions of the body. Metabolic rate can be estimated with reasonable accuracy from the oxygen consumption of a person. Which factors tend to increase or decrease a person's metabolic rate?

	Growth Hormone	Fever	Sleep	Malnutrition
A)	Decrease	Decrease	Decrease	Decrease
B)	Decrease	Increase	Decrease	Increase
C)	Increase	Increase	Increase	Increase
D)	Increase	Increase	Decrease	Increase
E)	Increase	Increase	Decrease	Decrease

32. An 8-year-old girl is taken to the physician because of diarrhea and a red scaly rash. Physical examination shows mild cerebellar ataxia. She is suspected of having pellagra because of these chronic symptoms. However, she appears to be ingesting adequate amounts of niacin in her diet, which is rich in meat. A brother has a similar problem. Urine studies show large amounts of free amino acids. Which diagnosis is most likely?

    A) Alkaptonuria
    B) Beriberi
    C) Hartnup's disease
    D) Scurvy
    E) Stickler's syndrome

33. In a person with type 1 diabetes who is not receiving insulin therapy and who has a fasting blood glucose of 400 mg/100 ml, what would the respiratory quotient likely be 2 hours after eating a light meal containing 60 percent carbohydrates, 20 percent protein, and 20 percent fat?

    A) 0.5
    B) 0.7
    C) 0.9
    D) 1.0
    E) 1.2

34. A 3-year-old white boy is extremely obese (weight of 37.5 kg), and his parents report that he has a voracious appetite. What is the most likely cause of his hyperphagia and obesity?

    A) A lesion/destruction of the lateral hypothalamus
    B) Excessive stimulation of the ventromedial nuclei of the hypothalamus
    C) A mutation that produces nonfunctional melanocortin-4 receptor protein
    D) Excessive stimulation of pro-opiomelanocortin (POMC) neurons
    E) Excessive secretion of leptin
    F) A mutation that prevents neuropeptide Y (NPY) formation in hypothalamic neurons

35. Deficiency of which of the following would cause "night blindness" in humans?

    A) Vitamin A
    B) Vitamin B_1
    C) Vitamin B_6
    D) Vitamin B_{12}
    E) Vitamin C
    F) Niacin

36. Which changes would be expected to stimulate hunger in a person who has not eaten for 24 hours?

    A) Increased NPY in the hypothalamus
    B) Increased leptin secretion
    C) Increased peptide YY (PYY) secretion
    D) Decreased ghrelin secretion
    E) Activation of hypothalamic POMC neurons
    F) Increased cholecystokinin secretion

37. Which of the following would be most important in contributing to satiety after eating a large meal containing carbohydrates (50 percent), fat (40 percent), and protein (10 percent)?

    A) Release of cholecystokinin by the duodenum
    B) Decreased leptin secretion
    C) Increased release of endorphins
    D) Increased ghrelin release by the stomach
    E) Decreased release of PYY by the intestine

38. Deficiency of which vitamin is most likely to cause impaired blood clotting?

    A) Vitamin A
    B) Vitamin B_6
    C) Vitamin C
    D) Vitamin D
    E) Vitamin K

39. Deficiency of which vitamin is the main cause of beriberi?

    A) Vitamin A
    B) Thiamine (vitamin B_1)
    C) Riboflavin (vitamin B_2)
    D) Vitamin B_{12}
    E) Pyridoxine (vitamin B_6)

40. Which of the following would tend to decrease hunger?

    A) Increased release of endorphins
    B) Increased ghrelin release by the stomach
    C) Increased release of PYY by the intestine
    D) Increased release of NPY by the hypothalamus
    E) Increased release of cortisol by the adrenals

41. Which substance might be most useful in stimulating appetite in a patient with cancer who has anorexia/cachexia?

    A) Leptin
    B) α-Melanocyte-stimulating hormone
    C) PYY
    D) Melanocortin-4 receptor antagonist
    E) Ghrelin antagonist
    F) Neuropeptide YY antagonist

42. The first stage in using triglycerides for energy is hydrolysis of the triglycerides to which substances?

    A) Acetyl coenzyme A and glycerol
    B) Cholesterol and fatty acids
    C) Glycerol 3-phosphate and cholesterol
    D) Glycerol and fatty acids
    E) Phospholipids and glycerol

43. Urinary nitrogen excretion measured in a patient is 16.0 grams in 24 hours. What is the approximate amount of protein breakdown in this patient for 24 hours in grams?

    A) 16.0
    B) 17.6
    C) 100
    D) 110
    E) 120

1. A) Fatty acids are degraded in mitochondria by the progressive release of two-carbon segments in the form of acetyl coenzyme A. This process is known as the beta-oxidation process for degradation of fatty acids.

TMP13 p. 866

2. B) The typical series of events that occur during the course of a fever are shown in the below figure. When pyrogens raise the set-point temperature above its normal value, the body activates heat conservation and heat production mechanisms that include cutaneous vasoconstriction, piloerection, epinephrine secretion, and shivering. Within several minutes, the body temperature increases to the elevated set-point value of 103°F in this example. If the factor that is causing the high temperature is removed, the hypothalamic set-point temperature returns to a normal value of about 98.6°F, which leads to activation of heat-loss mechanisms such as sweating and cutaneous vasodilation. The body temperature then returns to its basal level.

TMP13 pp. 919-920

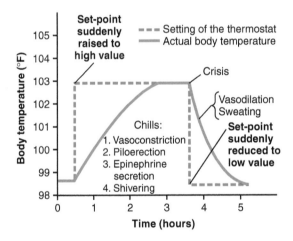

3. B) This man has cirrhosis of the liver. Fluid accumulates in the abdomen (ascites) for two main reasons: (1) decreased plasma colloid osmotic pressure (COP), and (2) increased capillary hydrostatic pressure in the splanchnic organs. The decrease in plasma COP results from decreased production of albumin by liver hepatocytes; albumin accounts for nearly 80 percent of the plasma COP. The low plasma COP also promotes edema formation in the periphery, especially the feet. Liver parenchymal cells are damaged or destroyed in persons with cirrhosis of the liver; they are replaced with fibrous tissue that eventually contracts around the blood vessels, thereby greatly impeding the flow of portal blood through the liver. This increase in vascular resistance leads to an increase in portal vein pressure,

which in turn raises the capillary hydrostatic pressure of the splanchnic organs. There is no reason to assume that capillary hydrostatic pressure is also increased above normal in the feet of this man.

TMP13 pp. 877, 881-882

4. D) Evaporation is the only mechanism of heat loss from the body when the environmental temperature is greater than the body temperature. Each gram of water that evaporates from the surface of the body causes 0.58 kilocalorie of heat to be lost from the body. Even when a person is not sweating, water still evaporates insensibly from the skin and lungs at a rate of 450 to 600 ml/day, which amounts to about 12 to 16 kilocalories of heat loss per hour. Radiation, convection, and conduction are mechanisms of heat loss when the body temperature is greater than the environmental temperature.

TMP13 pp. 912-913

5. C) The metabolic rate increases after a meal because of various chemical reactions associated with digestion, absorption, and storage of food; this phenomenon is known as the thermogenic effect of food. After a meal containing mostly carbohydrates and fats, the metabolic rate usually increases by about 4 percent. However, a high-protein meal often increases the metabolic rate by as much as 30 percent; this effect can last from 3 to 12 hours after the meal and is called the specific dynamic action of proteins. Clearly, assimilation of proteins requires far more energy expenditure compared with fats and carbohydrates.

TMP13 p. 909

6. E) This man has heatstroke. When the body temperature rises into the range of 105°F to 108°F, heatstroke is likely to develop. Heat loss mechanisms are overwhelmed by excessive metabolic production of heat and excessive environmental heat. Heatstroke is usually accompanied by dehydration (poor skin turgor is common), which can produce nausea, vomiting, hypotension, and fainting or dizziness. Interestingly, the skin is frequently dry because the anterior hypothalamic-preoptic area of the brain that normally initiates sweating is often compromised by the elevation in body temperature.

TMP13 pp. 914-915, 921

7. E) Most of the heat loss from the body occurs by radiation in the form of infrared heat waves, which is a type of electromagnetic wave. Heat waves radiate from all objects toward the body, and the body radiates heat waves to all surrounding objects. The reflective surface of the Mylar blanket prevents heat loss by reflecting

infrared heat waves from the body back to the body, which causes the body to warm. At room temperature, 60 percent of the heat loss occurs by radiation, 22 percent by evaporation, 15 percent by conduction to air, and 3 percent by conduction to objects. Convection (i.e., air currents) can increase heat loss by removing the unstirred layer of air close to the skin.
TMP13 pp. 912-913

8. B) Continual release of energy from glucose when energy is not needed by the cells would be an extremely wasteful process. Both ATP and ADP control the rate of chemical reactions in the energy metabolism sequence. When ATP is abundant within the cell, it helps control energy metabolism by inhibiting the conversion of fructose-6-phosphate to fructose-1,6-diphosphate. It does so by inhibiting the enzyme phosphofructokinase.
TMP13 p. 859

9. B) Both ADP and AMP increase the activity of the enzyme phosphofructokinase and increase the conversion of fructose-6-phosphate to fructose-1,6-diphosphate.
TMP13 p. 856

10. A) The transport of glucose through the membranes of most cells is different from that which occurs through the gastrointestinal membrane or through the epithelium of the renal tubules. In both these latter cases, the glucose is transported by the mechanism of secondary active co-transport, in which active transport of sodium provides energy for absorbing glucose against a concentration difference. This sodium co-transport mechanism functions only in certain special epithelial cells that are specifically adapted for active absorption of glucose. At all other cell membranes, glucose is transported only from higher concentrations toward lower concentrations by facilitated diffusion made possible by the special binding properties of membrane glucose carrier protein.
TMP13 pp. 854-855

11. B) Esophageal varices are extremely dilated submucosal veins in the lower third of the esophagus. The submucosal veins have a normal diameter of about 1 millimeter and can enlarge to 1 to 2 centimeters with prolonged portal hypertension, which is common in persons with cirrhosis of the liver. The presence of ascites indicates that the patient has portal hypertension. The dilated esophageal veins often bleed and thus lower the hematocrit. Although colon cancers can also bleed, there is no reason to assume colon cancer in this woman. Pancreatitis can occur in persons with chronic alcoholism, but there is no evidence for this condition, and substantial bleeding is not common in persons with pancreatitis. Jaundice and scleral icterus (i.e., yellowing of the sclera) are common in persons with cirrhosis, but these conditions are unlikely to cause significant bleeding.
TMP13 pp. 881-882

12. D) The liver has a high blood flow, low vascular resistance, and low blood pressure. During resting conditions, about 27 percent of the cardiac output flows through the liver, yet the pressure in the portal vein leading into the liver averages only 9 mm Hg. This high flow and low pressure indicate that the resistance to blood flow through the hepatic sinusoids is normally very low.
TMP13 pp. 881-882

13. B) None of the mechanisms of heat loss is effective when a person is placed in water that has a temperature greater than body temperature. Instead, the body will continue to gain heat until the body temperature becomes equal to the water temperature.
TMP13 pp. 912-913

14. A) This man has sickle cell disease, which is a hemolytic disease that results in the premature destruction of red blood cells. Release of hemoglobin from damaged red blood cells leads to high levels of bilirubin in the blood plasma. This increase in bilirubin can lead to the development of pigment stones in the gallbladder that are composed primarily of bilirubin. Cholesterol stones are very common, but pigment stones are more likely in this patient because of the decrease in hematocrit, which is indicative of hemolysis. Pigment stones may contain small amounts of calcium carbonate. Kidney stones are often composed of calcium oxalate.
TMP13 pp. 830, 885-886

15. B) The degradation of amino acids occurs almost entirely in the liver, and it begins with deamination, which occurs mainly by the following transamination schema: The amino group from the amino acid is transferred to α-ketoglutaric acid, which then becomes glutamic acid. The glutamic acid then transfers the amino group to still other substances or releases it in the form of ammonia. In the process of losing the amino group, the glutamic acid once again becomes α-ketoglutaric acid, so that the cycle can repeat again and again.
TMP13 p. 878

16. E) About 90 percent of the total ATP produced by glucose metabolism is formed during oxidation of the hydrogen atoms released during the early stages of glucose degradation. This process is called *oxidative phosphorylation.* Only two ATP molecules are formed by glycolysis, and another two are formed in the citric acid cycle. ATP is not formed by glycogenesis or glycogenolysis.
TMP13 p. 858

17. C) Lysine is an essential amino acid, which means that it must be included in the diet because the body cannot synthesize it. Alanine, glycine, serine, and tyrosine can be synthesized by the body and are therefore considered nonessential amino acids. This woman has a lysine deficiency, which is common in poorly designed vegetarian

diets; symptoms include nausea, fatigue, dizziness, anemia, loss of appetite, and thinning hair. Good dietary sources of lysine include eggs, meat, beans, legumes, soy, dairy products, and certain fish (such as cod and sardines). L-lysine is a building block for all proteins in the body.
TMP13 pp. 876, 878

18. **D)** This man has cirrhosis of the liver. In this condition, the rate of bilirubin production is normal, and the free bilirubin still enters the liver cells and becomes conjugated in the usual way. The conjugated bilirubin (direct) is mostly returned to the blood, probably by rupture of congested bile canaliculi, so that only small amounts enter the bile. The result is elevated levels of conjugated (direct) bilirubin in the plasma, with normal or near-normal levels of unconjugated (indirect) bilirubin.
TMP13 pp. 884-885

19. **E)** When the hypothalamic set-point temperature is greater than the body temperature, the person feels cold and exhibits responses that lead to an elevation of body temperature. These responses include shivering and vasoconstriction, as well as piloerection and epinephrine secretion. Shivering increases heat production. The increase in epinephrine secretion causes an immediate increase in the rate of cellular metabolism, which is an effect called *chemical thermogenesis.* Vasoconstriction of the skin blood vessels decreases heat loss through the skin.
TMP13 p. 920

20. **B)** When the hypothalamic set-point temperature is lower than the body temperature, the person feels hot and exhibits responses that cause body temperature to decrease. These responses include sweating and vasodilation. Sweating increases heat loss from the body by evaporation. Vasodilation of skin blood vessels facilitates heat loss from the body by increasing the skin blood flow.
TMP13 p. 920

21. **A)** When the hypothalamic set-point temperature is equal to the body temperature, the body exhibits neither heat loss nor heat conservation mechanisms, even when the body temperature is far above normal. Therefore, the person does not feel hot even when the body temperature is 104°F.
TMP13 p. 920

22. **B)** Phosphocreatine contains high-energy phosphate bonds and is three to eight times as abundant as ATP or ADP in a cell. Creatine does not contain high-energy phosphate bonds. Creatinine is a breakdown product of creatine phosphate in muscle.
TMP13 p. 904

23. **B)** This patient has heatstroke. Patients with heatstroke commonly exhibit tachypnea and hyperventilation caused by direct central nervous system stimulation, acidosis, or hypoxia. The blood vessels in the skin are vasodilated, and the skin is warm. Sweating ceases in patients with true heatstroke, most likely because the high temperature itself causes damage to the anterior hypothalamic-preoptic area. The nerve impulses from this area are transmitted in the autonomic pathways to the spinal cord and then through sympathetic outflow to the skin to cause sweating.
TMP13 pp. 913, 920

24. **A)** Basal metabolic rate counts for about 50 percent to 70 percent of the daily energy expenditure in most sedentary persons. Nonexercise activity, such as fidgeting or maintaining posture, accounts for approximately 7 percent of daily energy expenditure, and the thermic effect of food accounts for about 8 percent. Nonshivering thermogenesis can occur in response to cold stress, but the maximal response in adults is less than 15 percent of the total metabolic rate.
TMP13 p. 907

25. **B)** Most of the extra energy required for strenuous activity that lasts for more than 5 to 10 seconds but less than 1 to 2 minutes is derived from anaerobic glycolysis. Release of energy by glycolysis occurs much more rapidly than oxidative release of energy, which is much too slow to supply the needs of the muscle in the first few minutes of exercise. ATP and phosphocreatine already present in the cells are rapidly depleted in less than 5 to 10 seconds. After the muscle contraction is over, oxidative metabolism is used to reconvert much of the accumulated lactic acid into glucose; the remainder becomes pyruvic acid, which is degraded and oxidized in the citric acid cycle.
TMP13 pp. 904-905

26. **E)** Two molecules of ammonia and one molecule of carbon dioxide combine to form one molecule of urea and one molecule of water. Essentially all urea formed in the human body is synthesized in the liver. In the absence of the liver or in serious liver disease, ammonia accumulates in the blood. The ammonia is toxic to the brain, often leading to a state called *hepatic coma.*
TMP13 p. 879

27. **A)** Hemoglobin is metabolized by tissue macrophages (also called the *reticuloendothelial system*). The hemoglobin is first split into globin and heme, and the heme ring is opened to produce free iron and a straight chain of four pyrrole nuclei, from which bilirubin will eventually be formed. The free bilirubin is taken up by hepatic cells, and most of it is conjugated with glucuronic acid; the conjugated bilirubin passes into the bile canaliculi and then into the intestines.
TMP13 p. 884

28. A) When the body's stores of carbohydrates decrease below normal, moderate quantities of glucose can be formed from amino acids and the glycerol portion of fat. This process is called *gluconeogenesis.* Glycogenesis is the formation of glycogen. Glycogenolysis means the breakdown of the cell's stored glycogen to re-form glucose in the cells. Glycolysis means splitting of the glucose molecule to form two molecules of pyruvic acid. Hydrolysis is a process in which a molecule is split into two parts by the addition of a water molecule.
 TMP13 pp. 861-862

29. A) Cholelithiasis is the presence of gallstones (choleliths) in the gallbladder or bile ducts. This patient exhibits typical symptoms caused by gallstones.
 TMP13 pp. 830, 886

30. C) Hepatocytes produce essentially all the albumin normally present in blood. Viable hepatocytes use oxygen and produce carbon dioxide. Glucuronic acid produced by hepatocytes is used to conjugate bilirubin, forming bilirubin glucuronide. Lactate dehydrogenase is an enzyme that converts pyruvic acid to lactic acid under anaerobic conditions.
 TMP13 p. 877

31. E) Growth hormone can increase the metabolic rate 15 percent to 20 percent as a result of direct stimulation of cellular metabolism. Fever, regardless of its cause, increases the chemical reactions of the body by an average of about 120 percent for every 10°C rise in temperature. The metabolic rate decreases 10 percent to 15 percent below normal during sleep. Prolonged malnutrition can decrease the metabolic rate 20 percent to 30 percent, presumably because of the paucity of food substances in the cells.
 TMP13 pp 907-908

32. C) This child has Hartnup's disease. This condition resembles pellagra (because of the symptoms of diarrhea, dementia, and dermatitis) and may be misdiagnosed as a nutritional deficiency of niacin. Hartnup's disease is an autosomal-recessive trait caused by a defective gene that codes for a sodium-dependent and chloride-independent neutral amino acid transporter expressed mainly in kidney and intestinal epithelium. Poor epithelial transport of neutral amino acids (such as tryptophan) leads to poor absorption of dietary amino acids, as well as excess amino acid excretion in the urine. Tryptophan is a precursor of niacin; it is an essential amino acid that must be included in the diet. Alkaptonuria, also called "black urine disease," is a genetic disorder of phenylalanine and tyrosine metabolism. Beriberi is caused by a nutritional deficit in thiamine. Scurvy results from a deficiency of vitamin C, which is required for collagen synthesis. Stickler's syndrome is a group of genetic disorders that affect connective tissues; it is characterized by eye problems, hearing loss, joint problems, and facial abnormalities.
 TMP13 p. 899

33. B) Type 1 diabetes is characterized by a lack of insulin. In the absence of adequate insulin, little carbohydrate can be used by the body's cells, and the respiratory quotient remains near that for fat metabolism (0.70).
 TMP13 p. 889

34. C) Mutations that produce a nonfunctional melanocortin-4 receptor cause extreme obesity and may account for as much as 5 percent to 6 percent of early onset, morbid obesity in children. All the other changes would tend to reduce food intake and/or increase energy expenditure and thus cause weight loss rather than obesity.
 TMP13 pp. 889-902

35. A) One of the basic functions of vitamin A is in the formation of retinal pigments and therefore the prevention of night blindness.
 TMP13 p. 898

36. A) NPY is an orexigenic neurotransmitter that stimulates feeding and is increased during food deprivation. Leptin, PYY, cholecystokinin, and activation of POMC neurons are all reduced by fasting. Ghrelin is increased, not decreased, by fasting.
 TMP13 pp. 890-893

37. A) Cholecystokinin is released mainly in response to fats and proteins entering the duodenum and activates sensory receptors in the duodenum, sending messages to the brain stem via vagal afferents that contribute to satiation and meal cessation. All the other changes would tend to increase rather than decrease food intake.
 TMP13 p. 892

38. E) Vitamin K is an essential co-factor to a liver enzyme that adds a carboxyl group to factors II (prothrombin), VII (proconvertin), IX, and X, all of which are important to blood coagulation. The other vitamins listed are not directly involved in coagulation.
 TMP13 p. 900

39. B) Thiamine is needed for the final metabolism of carbohydrates and amino acids. Decreased utilization of these nutrients secondary to thiamine deficiency is responsible for many of the characteristics of beriberi, including peripheral vasodilation and edema, lesions of the central and peripheral nervous system, and gastrointestinal tract disturbances.
 TMP13 pp. 919-920

40. C) PYY is released from most parts of the intestinal tract, but especially from the ileum and colon, in response to food intake. Increased levels of PYY have been shown to decrease food intake. All the other changes tend to increase food intake.
 TMP13 pp. 891-892

41. D) Antagonists of melanocortin-4 receptors have been shown to markedly attenuate anorexia (i.e., reduced food intake due to decreased appetite) and cachexia (i.e., increased energy expenditure as well as decreased food intake) by blocking hypothalamic melanocortin-4 receptors. All the others choices would tend to decrease appetite and/or increase energy expenditure, exacerbating the anorexia/cachexia of a patient with cancer.

    TMP13 pp. 891, 897

42. D) Triglycerides are hydrolyzed to glycerol and fatty acids, which, in turn, are oxidized to provide energy. Almost all cells, with the exception of some brain tissue, can use fatty acids almost interchangeably with glucose for energy.

    TMP13 pp. 863-864

43. D) The rate of protein metabolism can be estimated by measuring the nitrogen in the urine, then adding 10 percent (about 90 percent of the nitrogen in proteins is excreted in the urine) and multiplying by 6.25 (100/16) because the average protein contains about 16 percent nitrogen.

    TMP13 p. 889

Endocrinology and Reproduction

1. Which receptor controls nitric oxide (NO) release to cause vasodilation during penile erection?

   A) Leptin receptor

   B) Angiotensin AT1 receptor

   C) Endothelin ETA receptor

   D) Muscarinic receptor — *parasympathetic postganglionic*

2. Which statement about antidiuretic hormone (ADH) is true?

   A) It is synthesized in the posterior pituitary gland

   B) It increases salt and water reabsorption in the collecting tubules and ducts

   C) It stimulates thirst

   D) It has opposite effects on urine and plasma osmolality

3. After menopause, hormone replacement therapy with estrogen-like compounds is effective in preventing the progression of osteoporosis. What is the mechanism of their protective effect?

   A) They stimulate the activity of osteoblasts

   B) They increase absorption of calcium from the gastrointestinal tract

   C) They stimulate calcium reabsorption by the renal tubules

   D) They stimulate parathyroid hormone (PTH) secretion by the parathyroid gland

4. A patient has nephrogenic diabetes insipidus. Of the following options, which outcome would be expected or which intervention would be suggested?

   A) Expected outcome: decreased plasma sodium concentration

   B) Expected outcome: increased secretion of ADH from the supraoptic and paraventricular nuclei

   C) Expected outcome: high urine osmolality

   D) Suggested intervention: water restriction

   E) Suggested intervention: ADH antagonists (vaptans)

5. Within minutes after a normal delivery, flow through the foramen ovale decreases dramatically. What is the cause of this change?

   A) Increased formation of prostaglandin E_2 (PGE_2) in the endocardium

   B) Increased rate of flow through the pulmonary artery

   C) Increased left atrial pressure

   D) Increased right atrial pressure

   E) Increased partial pressure of oxygen (P_{O_2})

6. Which hormones antagonize the effect of NO and cause the penis to become flaccid after orgasm?

   A) Endothelin and norepinephrine

   B) Estrogen and progesterone

   C) Luteinizing hormone (LH) and follicle-stimulating hormone (FSH)

   D) Progesterone and LH

Questions 7–9

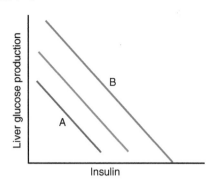

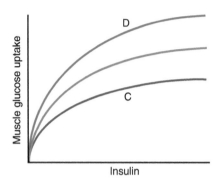

The red lines in the above figure illustrate the normal relationships between plasma insulin concentration and glucose production in the liver and between plasma insulin concentration and glucose uptake in muscle. Use this figure to answer Questions 7–9.

7. Which lines most likely illustrate these relationships in a patient with type 2 diabetes?
   A) A and C
   B) A and D
   C) B and C
   D) B and D

8. Which lines most likely illustrate these relationships in a patient with acromegaly?
   A) A and C
   B) A and D
   C) B and C
   D) B and D

   ↳high levels of
   GH = insulin
   resistance.

9. Line D most likely illustrates the influence of which of the following?
   A) Exercise
   B) Obesity
   C) Growth hormone (GH)
   D) Cortisol
   E) Glucagon

10. Thecal cells in the follicle are not able to produce what sex steroid?
    A) Estradiol
    B) Testosterone
    C) Progesterone
    D) Dihydrotestosterone

11. A baby is born with a penis, a scrotum with no testes, no vagina, and XX chromosomes. This condition is referred to as hermaphroditism. What could cause this abnormality?
    A) Abnormally high levels of human chorionic gonadotropin (HCG) production by the trophoblast cells
    B) The presence of a testosterone-secreting tumor in the mother's right adrenal gland
    C) Abnormally high levels of LH in the maternal blood
    D) Abnormally low levels of testosterone in the maternal blood
    E) Abnormally low rates of estrogen production by the placenta

12. A young woman is given daily injections of a substance beginning on the sixteenth day of her normal menstrual cycle and continuing for 3 weeks. As long as the injections continue, she does not menstruate. The injected substance could be which of the following?
    A) Testosterone
    B) FSH
    C) An inhibitor of progesterone's actions
    D) A PGE$_2$ inhibitor
    E) HCG

13. Which of the following increases secretion of GH?
    A) Senescence
    B) Insulin-like growth factor-1 (IGF-1)
    C) Somatostatin
    D) Hypoglycemia
    E) Exogenous GH administration

14. Which of the following could inhibit the initiation of labor?
    A) Administration of an antagonist of the actions of progesterone ~inhale
    B) Administration of LH ~ no offect.
    C) Administration of an antagonist of PGE$_2$ effects
    D) Mechanically dilating and stimulating the cervix~initiate
    E) Administration of oxytocin ~initiate.

15. Exposure to ultraviolet light directly facilitates which of the following?
    A) Conversion of cholesterol to 25-hydroxycholicalciferol
    B) Conversion of 25-hydroxycholicalciferol to 1,25-dihydroxycholicalciferol
    C) Transport of calcium into the extracellular fluid
    D) Formation of calcium-binding protein
    E) Storage of vitamin D$_3$ in the liver

16. Which of the following decreases the pressure in the pulmonary artery after birth?

    A) An increase in systemic arterial pressure
    B) Closure of ductus arteriosus
    C) An increase in left ventricular pressure
    D) A decrease in pulmonary vascular resistance

17. Which of the following is both synthesized and stored in the hypothalamus?

    A) ADH
    B) Thyroid-stimulating hormone (TSH)
    C) LH
    D) Somatostatin
    E) Somatomedin ~synthesized in liver (IGF+1)

18. If a radioimmunoassay is properly conducted and the amount of radioactive hormone bound to antibody is low, what would this result indicate?

    A) Plasma levels of endogenous hormone are high
    B) Plasma levels of endogenous hormone are low
    C) More antibody is needed
    D) Less radioactive hormone is needed

19. By which mechanism do LH and FSH return to baseline levels?

    A) LH surge
    B) Negative feedback on gonadotropin-releasing hormone (GnRH) by progesterone
    C) Negative feedback on GnRH by estradiol
    D) Negative feedback on GnRH from testosterone

20. Spermatogenesis is regulated by a negative feedback control system in which FSH stimulates the steps in sperm cell formation. Which negative feedback signal associated with sperm cell production inhibits pituitary formation of FSH?

    A) Testosterone
    B) Inhibin
    C) Estrogen
    D) LH

21. Which of the following is true during the 12-hour period preceding ovulation?

    A) A surge of LH is secreted from the pituitary
    B) The surge occurs immediately after the formation of the corpus luteum
    C) The surge is followed immediately by a fall in the plasma concentration of progesterone
    D) The number of developing follicles is increasing

22. When do progesterone levels rise to their highest point during the female hormonal cycle?

    A) Between ovulation and the beginning of menstruation
    B) Immediately before ovulation
    C) When the blood concentration of LH is at its highest point
    D) When 12 primary follicles are developing to the antral stage

23. What accompanies sloughing of the endometrium during the endometrial cycle in a normal woman?

    A) An increase in progesterone
    B) The LH "surge"
    C) A decrease in both progesterone and estrogen
    D) An increase in estradiol

24. Some cells secrete chemicals into the extracellular fluid that act on cells in the same tissue. Which of the following refers to this type of regulation?

    A) Neural
    B) Endocrine
    C) Neuroendocrine
    D) Paracrine
    E) Autocrine

25. Which of the following pairs is an example of the type of regulation referred to in Question 24?

    A) Somatostatin—GH secretion
    B) Somatostatin—insulin secretion
    C) Dopamine—prolactin secretion
    D) Norepinephrine—corticotropin-releasing hormone (CRH) secretion
    E) CRH—adrenocorticotropic hormone (ACTH) secretion

26. A professional athlete in her mid-20s has not had a menstrual cycle for 5 years, although a bone density scan revealed normal skeletal mineralization. Which fact may explain these observations?

    A) She consumes a high-carbohydrate diet
    B) Her grandmother sustained a hip fracture at age 79 years
    C) Her blood pressure is higher than normal
    D) Her plasma estrogen concentration is very low
    E) She has been taking anabolic steroid supplements for 5 years

27. What is the nongenomic effect of testosterone on vascular smooth muscle?

    A) Vasodilation
    B) Vasoconstriction
    C) Increase in prostaglandins
    D) Increase in estrogen receptors

28. In the circulatory system of a fetus, which of the following is greater before birth than after birth?

    A) Arterial P_{O_2}
    B) Right atrial pressure
    C) Aortic pressure
    D) Left ventricular pressure

Questions 29 and 30

Match each of the patients described in Questions 29 and 30 with the correct set of plasma values listed in the table below. Normal values are as follows: plasma aldosterone concentration, 10 ng/dl; plasma cortisol concentration, 10 mg/dl; and plasma potassium concentration, 4.5 mEq/L.

	Aldosterone Concentration	Cortisol Concentration	Potassium Concentration
A)	10.0	2.0	4.5
B)	2.0	2.0	6.0
C)	40.0	30.0	2.0
D)	40.0	10.0	4.5
E)	40.0	10.0	2.0

29. A patient with Conn's syndrome. E. ↑Aldosterone: ↓K hypokalemia

30. A patient consuming a low-sodium diet. D

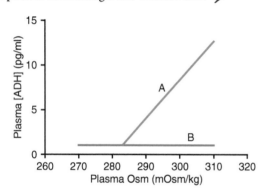

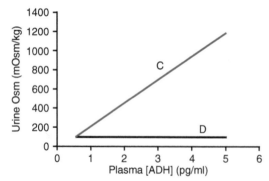

31. In the above figure, which lines most likely reflect the responses in a patient with nephrogenic diabetes insipidus?
    A) A and C
    B) A and D ✓
    C) B and C
    D) B and D

32. Which enzyme in the cytochrome P450 steroid synthesis cascade is directly responsible for estradiol synthesis?
    A) 17-beta-hydroxysteroid dehydrogenase
    B) 5-alpha reductase
    C) Aromatase
    D) Side chain cleavage enzyme

33. Which of the following is greater after birth than before birth?
    A) Flow through the foramen ovale
    B) Pressure in the right atrium
    C) Flow through the ductus arteriosus
    D) Aortic pressure

34. PTH does what directly?
    A) Controls the rate of 25-hydroxycholicalciferol formation
    B) Controls the rate of calcium transport in the mucosa of the small intestine
    C) Controls the rate of formation of calcium-binding protein
    D) Controls the rate of formation of 1,25-dihydroxycholicalciferol
    E) Stimulates renal tubular phosphate reabsorption

35. Which substances are most likely to produce the greatest increase in insulin secretion?
    A) Amino acids
    B) Amino acids and glucose
    C) Amino acids and somatostatin
    D) Glucose and somatostatin

36. Which of the following would be expected in a child with dwarfism due to pituitary dysfunction?

	Plasma [IGF-1]	Growth-Hormone-Releasing Hormone Secretion	Fasting Plasma [Glucose]
A)	↑	↑	↓
B)	↑	↑	↑
C)	↑	↓	↓
D)	↓	↓	↑
E)	↓	↓	↓
F)	↓	↑	↓

37. For male differentiation to occur during embryonic development, testosterone must be secreted from the testes. What stimulates the secretion of testosterone during embryonic development?
    A) LH from the maternal pituitary gland
    B) HCG
    C) Inhibin from the corpus luteum
    D) GnRH from the embryo's hypothalamus

38. A patient has an elevated plasma thyroxine (T_4) concentration, a low plasma TSH concentration, and her thyroid gland is smaller than normal. What is the most likely explanation for these findings?
    A) A lesion in the anterior pituitary that prevents TSH secretion
    B) The patient is taking propylthiouracil
    C) The patient is taking thyroid extract
    D) The patient is consuming large amounts of iodine
    E) Graves' disease

39. Extracellular ionic calcium activity will be decreased within 1 minute by which of the following?

    A) An increase in extracellular phosphate ion activity
    B) An increase in extracellular pH
    C) A decrease in extracellular partial pressure of carbon dioxide (P_{CO_2})
    D) All the above
    E) None of the above

40. As menstruation ends, estrogen levels in the blood rise rapidly. What is the source of the estrogen?

    A) Corpus luteum
    B) Developing follicles
    C) Endometrium
    D) Stromal cells of the ovaries
    E) Anterior pituitary gland

41. A 30-year-old woman reports to the clinic for a routine physical examination. The examination reveals she is pregnant. Her plasma levels of TSH are high, but her total thyroid hormone concentration is normal. Which of the following best reflects the patient's clinical state?

    A) Graves' disease
    B) Hashimoto's disease
    C) A pituitary tumor secreting TSH
    D) A hypothalamic tumor secreting thyrotropin-releasing hormone (TRH)
    E) The patient is taking thyroid extract

42. Which anterior pituitary hormone plays a major role in the regulation of a nonendocrine target gland?

    A) ACTH
    B) TSH
    C) Prolactin
    D) FSH
    E) LH

43. A female athlete who took testosterone-like steroids for several months stopped having normal menstrual cycles. What is the best explanation for this observation?

    A) Testosterone stimulates inhibin production from the corpus luteum
    B) Testosterone binds to receptors in the endometrium, resulting in the failure of the endometrium to develop during the normal cycle
    C) Testosterone binds to receptors in the anterior pituitary that stimulate the secretion of FSH and LH
    D) Testosterone inhibits the hypothalamic secretion of GnRH and the pituitary secretion of LH and FSH

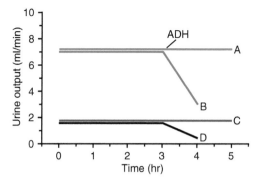

44. An experiment is conducted in which ADH is administered at hour 3 to four subjects (A to D). In the above figure, which lines most likely reflect the response to ADH administration in a normal patient and in a patient with central diabetes insipidus?

	Normal	Central Diabetes Insipidus
A)	B	A
B)	B	D
C)	D	A
D)	D	B

45. Which of the following decreases the resistance in the arteries leading to the sinuses of the penis?

    A) Stimulation of the sympathetic nerves innervating the arteries
    B) NO
    C) Inhibition of activity of the parasympathetic nerves leading to the arteries
    D) All the above

46. A patient has a goiter associated with high plasma levels of both TRH and TSH. Her heart rate is elevated. This patient most likely has which condition?

    A) An endemic goiter
    B) A hypothalamic tumor secreting large amounts of TRH
    C) A pituitary tumor secreting large amounts of TSH
    D) Graves' disease

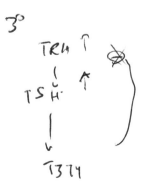

47. A man eats a low-carbohydrate meal that is rich in proteins containing the amino acids that stimulate insulin secretion. Which response accounts for the absence of hypoglycemia?

    A) Suppression of GH
    B) Suppression of somatomedin C secretion
    C) Stimulation of cortisol secretion
    D) Stimulation of glucagon secretion
    E) Stimulation of epinephrine secretion

48. A 46-year-old man has "puffy" skin and is lethargic. His plasma TSH concentration is low and increases markedly when he is given TRH. What is the most likely diagnosis?

    A) Hyperthyroidism due to a thyroid tumor
    B) Hyperthyroidism due to an abnormality in the hypothalamus
    C) Hypothyroidism due to an abnormality in the thyroid
    D) Hypothyroidism due to an abnormality in the hypothalamus
    E) Hypothyroidism due to an abnormality in the pituitary

49. Negative feedback on FSH release from the anterior pituitary in men that results in a reduction in estradiol production is due to which hormone?

    A) Progesterone
    B) Estradiol
    C) Testosterone
    D) Inhibin

50. During the first few years after menopause, FSH levels are normally extremely high. A 56-year-old woman completed menopause 3 years ago. However, she is found to have low levels of FSH in her blood. What is the best explanation for this finding?

    A) She has been receiving hormone replacement therapy with estrogen and progesterone since she completed menopause
    B) Her adrenal glands continue to produce estrogen
    C) Her ovaries continue to secrete estrogen
    D) She took birth control pills for 20 years before menopause

51. Blockade of what receptors will prolong erection in the male?

    A) Estrogen receptors
    B) Cholesterol receptors
    C) Muscarinic receptors
    D) Phosphodiesterase-5 receptors

52. Which of the following pairs of hormones and the corresponding action is incorrect?

    A) Glucagon—increased glycogenolysis in liver
    B) Glucagon—increased glycogenolysis in skeletal muscle

    C) Glucagon—increased gluconeogenesis
    D) Cortisol—increased gluconeogenesis
    E) Cortisol—decreased glucose uptake in muscle

53. A large dose of insulin is administered intravenously to a patient. Which set of hormonal changes is most likely to occur in the plasma in response to the insulin injection?

	Growth Hormone	Glucagon	Epinephrine
A)	↑	↓	↔
B)	↔	↑	↑
C)	↑	↑	↑
D)	↓	↑	↑
E)	↓	↓	↔

54. What is a frequent cause of delayed breathing at birth?

    A) Fetal hypoxia during the birth process
    B) Maternal hypoxia during the birth process
    C) Fetal hypercapnia
    D) Maternal hypercapnia

55. Which hormone is largely unbound to plasma proteins?

    A) Cortisol
    B) T$_4$
    C) ADH – largely unbound.
    D) Estradiol
    E) Progesterone

56. What is the mechanism by which the zona pellucida becomes "hardened" after penetration of a sperm cell to prevent a second sperm from penetrating?

    A) A reduction in estradiol
    B) The proteins released from the acrosome of the sperm
    C) An increase in intracellular calcium in the oocyte
    D) An increase in testosterone that affects the sperm

57. Why is milk produced by a woman only after delivery, not before?

    A) Levels of LH and FSH are too low during pregnancy to support milk production
    B) High levels of progesterone and estrogen during pregnancy suppress milk production
    C) The alveolar cells of the breast do not reach maturity until after delivery
    D) High levels of oxytocin are required for milk production to begin, and oxytocin is not secreted until the baby stimulates the nipple

58. Which of the following increases the rate of excretion of calcium ions by the kidney?

    A) A decrease in calcitonin concentration in the plasma
    B) An increase in phosphate ion concentration in the plasma
    C) A decrease in the plasma level of PTH
    D) Metabolic alkalosis

↓ PTH. ↑ calcium excretion

59. A patient has hyperthyroidism due to a pituitary tumor. Which set of physiological changes would be expected?

	Thyroglobulin Synthesis	Heart Rate	Exophthalmos
A)	↑	↑	+
B)	↑	↑	−
C)	↑	↓	+
D)	↓	↓	+
E)	↓	↓	−
F)	↓	↑	−

60. A 25-year-old man is severely injured when hit by a speeding vehicle and loses 20 percent of his blood volume. Which set of physiological changes would be expected to occur in response to the hemorrhage?

	Atrial Stretch Receptor Activity	Arterial Baroreceptor Activity	ADH Secretion
A)	↓	↓	↑
B)	↓	↓	↓
C)	↔	↑	↑
D)	↑	↑	↑
E)	↑	↑	↓

61. If a woman has a tumor that is secreting large amounts of estrogen from the adrenal gland, which of the following will occur?

A) Progesterone levels in the blood will be very low
B) Her LH secretion rate will be totally suppressed
C) She will not have normal menstrual cycles
D) Her bones will be normally calcified
E) All the above

62. When compared with the postabsorptive state, which set of metabolic changes would most likely occur during the postprandial state?

	Hepatic Glucose Uptake	Muscle Glucose Uptake	Hormone-Sensitive Lipase Activity
A)	↑	↑	↑
B)	↑	↓	↑
C)	↓	↑	↓
D)	↑	↑	↓
E)	↓	↑	↑

63. Very early in embryonic development, testosterone is formed within the male embryo. What is the function of this hormone at this stage of development?

A) Stimulation of bone growth
B) Stimulation of development of male sex organs
C) Stimulation of development of skeletal muscle
D) Inhibition of LH secretion

64. Which change would be expected to occur with increased binding of a hormone to plasma proteins?

A) Increase in plasma clearance of the hormone
B) Decrease in half-life of the hormone
C) Increase in hormone activity
D) Increase in degree of negative feedback exerted by the hormone
E) Increase in plasma reservoir for rapid replenishment of free hormone

65. A patient arrives in the emergency department apparently in cardiogenic shock due to a massive heart attack. His initial arterial blood sample reveals the following concentrations of ions and pH level:

Sodium	137 mmol/L
Bicarbonate	14 mmol/L
Free calcium	2.8 mmol/L
Potassium	4.8 mmol/L
pH	7.16

To correct the acidosis, the attending physician begins an infusion of sodium bicarbonate and after 1 hour obtains another blood sample, which reveals the following values:

Sodium	138 mmol/L
Bicarbonate	22 mmol/L
Free calcium	2.3 mmol/L
Potassium	4.5 mmol/L
pH	7.34

What is the cause of the decrease in calcium ion concentration?

A) The increase in arterial pH resulting from the sodium bicarbonate infusion inhibited PTH secretion
B) The increase in pH resulted in the stimulation of osteoblasts, which removed calcium from the circulation
C) The increase in pH resulted in an elevation in the concentration of HPO_4^-, which shifted the equilibrium between HPO_4^- and Ca^{++} toward $CaHPO_4$
D) The increase in arterial pH stimulated the formation of 1,25-dihydroxycholecalciferol, which resulted in an increased rate of absorption of calcium from the gastrointestinal tract

↑ pH · ↓ free calcium

66. A patient presents with tachycardia and heat intolerance. You suspect Graves' disease. Which of the following is not consistent with your diagnosis?

    A) Increased total and free T_4
    B) Suppressed plasma [TSH]
    C) Exophthalmos
    D) Goiter
    E) Decreased thyroid radioactive iodine uptake

67. A 30-year-old woman is breastfeeding her infant. During suckling, which hormonal response is expected in the woman?

    A) Increased secretion of ADH from the supraoptic nuclei
    B) Increased secretion of ADH from the paraventricular nuclei
    C) Increased secretion of oxytocin from the paraventricular nuclei
    D) Decreased secretion of neurophysin
    E) Increased plasma levels of both oxytocin and ADH

68. A 30-year-old man has Conn's syndrome. Which set of physiological changes is most likely to occur in this patient compared with a healthy person?

	Arterial Pressure	Extracellular Fluid Volume	Sodium Excretion
A)	↔	↔	↔
B)	↑	↔	↔
C)	↑	↑	↔
D)	↔	↑	↓
E)	↑	↑	↓

69. Why is it important to feed newborn infants every few hours?

    A) The hepatic capacity to store and synthesize glycogen and glucose is not adequate to maintain the plasma glucose concentration in a normal range for more than a few hours after feeding
    B) If adequate fluid is not ingested frequently, the plasma protein concentration will rise to greater than normal levels within a few hours
    C) The function of the gastrointestinal system is poorly developed and can be improved by keeping food in the stomach at all times
    D) The hepatic capacity to form plasma proteins is minimal and requires the constant availability of amino acids from food to avoid hypoproteinemic edema

70. Dehydroepiandrosterone sulfate (DHEAS), the precursor for the high levels of estradiol that occur in pregnancy, is made in what tissue?

    A) Fetal adrenal gland
    B) Ovary of the mother
    C) Placenta
    D) Adrenal gland of the mother

71. What is the consequence of sporadic nursing of the neonate by the mother?

    A) An increase in prolactin-releasing hormone
    B) An increase in oxytocin
    C) Lack of birth control
    D) Lack of prolactin surge

72. Which of the following would be associated with parallel changes in aldosterone and cortisol secretion?

    A) Addison's disease
    B) Cushing's disease
    C) Cushing's syndrome (adrenal tumor)
    D) A low-sodium diet
    E) Administration of a converting enzyme inhibitor

73. A chronic increase in the plasma concentration of thyroxine-binding globulin (TBG) would result in which of the following?

    A) An increased delivery of T_4 to target cells
    B) A decrease in plasma free $[T_4]$
    C) An increase in the conversion of T_4 to triiodothyronine (T_3) in peripheral tissues
    D) An increase in TSH secretion
    E) No change in metabolic rate

74. RU486 causes abortion if it is administered before or soon after implantation. What is the specific effect of RU486?

    A) It binds to LH receptors, stimulating the secretion of progesterone from the corpus luteum
    B) It blocks progesterone receptors so that progesterone has no effect within the body
    C) It blocks the secretion of FSH by the pituitary
    D) It blocks the effects of oxytocin receptors in the uterine muscle

75. A 55-year-old man has developed the syndrome of inappropriate antidiuretic hormone secretion due to carcinoma of the lung. Which physiological response would be expected?

    A) Increased plasma osmolality
    B) Inappropriately low urine osmolality (relative to plasma osmolality)
    C) Increased thirst
    D) Decreased secretion of ADH from the pituitary gland

76. During pregnancy, the uterine smooth muscle is quiescent. During the ninth month of gestation, the uterine muscle becomes progressively more excitable. What factor contributes to the increase in excitability?

    A) Placental estrogen synthesis rises to high rates
    B) Progesterone synthesis by the placenta decreases
    C) Uterine blood flow reaches its highest rate
    D) PGE_2 synthesis by the placenta decreases
    E) Activity of the fetus falls to low levels

77. A 20-year-old woman is not having menstrual cycles. Her plasma progesterone concentration is found to be minimal. What is the explanation for the low level of progesterone?

    A) LH secretion rate is elevated
    B) LH secretion rate is suppressed
    C) FSH secretion rate is suppressed
    D) No corpus luteum is present
    E) High inhibin concentration in the plasma has suppressed progesterone synthesis

78. Before the preovulatory surge in LH, granulosa cells of the follicle secrete which hormone?

    A) Testosterone
    B) Progesterone
    C) Estrogen
    D) Inhibin

Questions 79 and 80

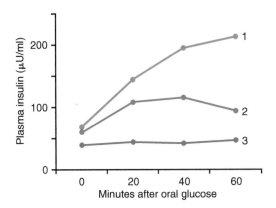

79. Based on the above figure, which set of curves most likely reflects the responses in a healthy individual and in patients with type 1 or type 2 diabetes mellitus (DM)?

	Healthy	Type 1 DM	Type 2 DM
A)	3	2	1
B)	1	2	3
C)	1	3	2
D)	2	1	3
E)	2	3	1

80. Based on the above figure, which set of curves most likely reflects the responses in a healthy person and in a patient in the early stages of Cushing's syndrome?

	Healthy	Cushing's Syndrome
A)	3	2
B)	1	2
C)	1	3
D)	2	1
E)	2	3

81. Which hormone activates enzyme-linked receptors?

    A) ADH
    B) Insulin
    C) ACTH
    D) PTH
    E) Aldosterone

82. Which of the following is produced by the trophoblast cells during the first 3 weeks of pregnancy?

    A) Estrogen
    B) LH
    C) Oxytocin
    D) HCG
    E) None of the above

83. Which of the following is higher in the neonate than in the fetus?

    A) Flow through the foramen ovale
    B) Right atrial pressure
    C) Flow through the ductus arteriosus
    D) Aortic pressure

84. Which finding is most likely in a patient who has myxedema?

    A) Somnolence
    B) Palpitations
    C) Increased respiratory rate
    D) Increased cardiac output
    E) Weight loss

85. At birth, a large, well-nourished baby is found to have a plasma glucose concentration of 17 mg/dl (normal is 80 to 100 mg/dl) and a plasma insulin concentration twice the normal value. What is the explanation for these findings?

    A) The neonate experienced in utero malnutrition
    B) The mother was malnourished during pregnancy
    C) The mother is diabetic, with poorly controlled hyperglycemia
    D) The mother is obese

86. In the fetus, why can normal growth occur despite low P_{O_2} levels?

    A) The concentration of hemoglobin A is increased in the fetus
    B) The hemoglobin of the fetus can carry more oxygen at lower P_{CO_2} levels
    C) The oxyhemoglobin curve in the fetus is shifted to the left
    D) The mother has increased blood volume during pregnancy

87. Which of the following stimulates the secretion of PTH?

    A) An increase in extracellular calcium ion activity above the normal value
    B) An increase in calcitonin concentration
    C) Respiratory acidosis
    D) Increased secretion of PTH-releasing hormone from the hypothalamus
    E) None of the above

88. A 40-year-old woman consumes a high-potassium diet for several weeks. Which hormonal change is most likely to occur?

    A) Increased secretion of DHEA
    B) Increased secretion of cortisol
    C) Increased secretion of aldosterone
    D) Increased secretion of ACTH
    E) Decreased secretion of CRH

89. After implantation into the uterus, nutrition of the blastocyst comes from which structure?

    A) Placenta
    B) Decidua
    C) Glomerulosa cells
    D) Corpus luteum

90. Which hormone is not stored in its endocrine-producing gland?

    A) T_4
    B) PTH
    C) Aldosterone — K^+ secretion.
    D) ACTH
    E) Insulin

91. A young woman comes to the emergency department with a vertebral compression fracture. Radiographs of the spine indicate generalized demineralization. She is vegetarian, does not smoke or drink alcohol, and has a normal plasma potassium concentration of 5.4 mEq/L, a sodium concentration of 136 mEq/L, and a plasma calcium concentration of 7.0 mg/dl. Her vitamin D_3 value is several times greater than normal, although her 1,25-dihydroxycholecalciferol concentration is at the lower limit of detectability. She has been in renal failure for the past 5 years and undergoes hemodialysis three times each week. What is the cause of her low 1,25-dihydroxycholecalciferol level?

    A) Metabolic acidosis
    B) Metabolic alkalosis
    C) She is unable to form 1,25-dihydroxycholecalciferol because of her extensive kidney disease
    D) She is undergoing dialysis with a dialysis fluid that does not contain calcium
    E) She is taking receiving calcium supplements

92. The placenta is incapable of synthesizing which hormones?

    A) Estrogen
    B) Progesterone
    C) Androgens
    D) Estriol

93. A neonate develops jaundice and has a bilirubin concentration of 10 mg/dl on day 2 (normal is 3 mg/dl at 2 days old). The neonatologist can be confident that the condition is not erythroblastosis fetalis if which of the following is true?

    A) The bilirubin concentration rises no further
    B) Hematocrit falls only slightly
    C) The mother, father, and neonate are all Rh-negative
    D) The mother has no history of hepatic dysfunction

94. Which finding would likely be reported in a patient with a deficiency in iodine intake? Hypothyroidism

    A) Weight loss
    B) Nervousness
    C) Increased sweating
    D) Increased synthesis of thyroglobulin
    E) Tachycardia

95. A 37-year-old woman presents to her physician with an enlarged thyroid gland and high plasma levels of T_4 and T_3. Which of the following is likely to be decreased?

    A) Heart rate
    B) Cardiac output
    C) Peripheral vascular resistance
    D) Ventilation rate
    E) Metabolic rate

96. Before intercourse, a woman irrigates her vagina with a solution that lowers the pH of the vaginal fluid to 4.5. What will be the effect on sperm cells in the vagina?

    A) The metabolic rate will increase
    B) The rate of movement will decrease
    C) The formation of PGE_2 will increase
    D) The rate of oxygen consumption will increase

97. Which hormonal responses would be expected after a meal high in protein?

	Insulin	Glucagon	Growth Hormone
A)	↑	↑	↓
B)	↑	↑	↑
C)	↑	↓	↓
D)	↓	↓	↑
E)	↓	↑	↑

98. Men who take large doses of testosterone-like androgenic steroids for long periods are sterile in the reproductive sense of the word. What is the explanation for this finding?

    A) High levels of androgens bind to testosterone receptors in the Sertoli cells, resulting in overstimulation of inhibin formation
    B) Overstimulation of sperm cell production results in the formation of defective sperm cells
    C) High levels of androgen compounds inhibit the secretion of GnRH by the hypothalamus, resulting in the inhibition of LH and FSH release by the anterior pituitary
    D) High levels of androgen compounds produce hypertrophic dysfunction of the prostate gland

99. Cortisone is administered to a 30-year-old woman for the treatment of an autoimmune disease. Which of the following is most likely to occur?

    A) Increased ACTH secretion
    B) Increased cortisol secretion
    C) Increased insulin secretion
    D) Increased muscle mass
    E) Hypoglycemia between meals

100. In the hypothalamic-pituitary-gonadal axis of the female, what is the follicular cell type that produces inhibin?

    A) Cytotrophoblasts
    B) Synthiotrophoblasts
    C) Granulosa
    D) Thecal

101. The function of which of the following is increased by an elevated parathyroid hormone concentration?

    A) Osteoclasts
    B) Hepatic formation of 25-hydroxycholecalciferol
    C) Phosphate reabsorptive pathways in the renal tubules
    D) All the above

102. Which statement about peptide or protein hormones is usually true?

    A) They have longer half-lives than steroid hormones
    B) They have receptors on the cell membrane
    C) They have a slower onset of action than both steroid and thyroid hormones
    D) They are not stored in endocrine-producing glands

103. Which set of physiological changes would be most likely to occur in a patient with acromegaly?

	Pituitary Mass	Kidney Mass	Femur Length
A)	↓	↓	↑
B)	↓	↑	↑
C)	↑	↔	↔
D)	↑	↑	↔
E)	↑	↑	↑

104. Cortisol and GH are most dissimilar in their metabolic effects on which of the following?

    A) Protein synthesis in muscle
    B) Glucose uptake in peripheral tissues
    C) Plasma glucose concentration
    D) Mobilization of triglycerides

105. Why do infants of mothers who had adequate nutrition during pregnancy not require iron supplements or a diet rich in iron until about 3 months of age?

    A) Growth of the infant does not require iron until after the third month
    B) The fetal liver stores enough iron to meet the infant's needs until the third month
    C) Synthesis of new red blood cells begins after 3 months
    D) Muscle cells that develop before the third month do not contain myoglobin

106. Cortisone is administered to a patient for the treatment of an autoimmune disease. Which of the following would least likely occur in response to the cortisone treatment?

    A) Hypertrophy of the adrenal glands
    B) Increased plasma levels of C-peptide
    C) Decreased CRH secretion
    D) Increased blood pressure
    E) Hyperglycemia

107. Which symptom would least likely be associated with thyrotoxicosis?

    A) Tachycardia
    B) Increased appetite
    C) Somnolence
    D) Increased sweating
    E) Muscle tremor

108. If a male is born without a penis and testes, a defect is likely in which gene on the Y chromosome?

    A) ERE—estrogen response element
    B) ARE—androgen response element
    C) SRY—affecting Sertoli cells
    D) ERG—early response genes

109. Where does fertilization normally take place?

    A) Uterus
    B) Cervix
    C) Ovary
    D) Ampulla of the fallopian tubes

110. Which finding is most likely to occur in a patient who has uncontrolled type 1 DM?

    A) Decreased plasma osmolality
    B) Increased plasma volume
    C) Increased plasma pH
    D) Increased release of glucose from the liver
    E) Decreased rate of lipolysis

111. GH secretion would most likely be suppressed under which condition?

    A) Acromegaly
    B) Gigantism
    C) Deep sleep
    D) Exercise
    E) Acute hyperglycemia

112. Pregnenolone is not in the biosynthetic pathway of which substance?

    A) Cortisol
    B) Estrogen
    C) Aldosterone
    D) 1,25(OH)2D
    E) DHEA

113. Two days before the onset of menstruation, secretions of FSH and LH reach their lowest levels. What is the cause of this low level of secretion?

    A) The anterior pituitary gland becomes unresponsive to the stimulatory effect of GnRH
    B) Estrogen from the developing follicles exerts a feedback inhibition on the hypothalamus
    C) The rise in body temperature inhibits hypothalamic release of GnRH
    D) Secretion of estrogen, progesterone, and inhibin by the corpus luteum suppresses hypothalamic secretion of GnRH and pituitary secretion of FSH

114. Which condition contributes to "sodium escape" in persons with Conn's syndrome?

    A) Decreased plasma levels of atrial natriuretic peptide
    B) Increased plasma levels of angiotensin II
    C) Decreased sodium reabsorption in the collecting tubules
    D) Increased arterial pressure

115. An experiment is conducted in which patients in group 1 are given compound X and patients in group 2 are given compound Y. After 3 weeks, studies show that patients in group 1 have a higher rate of ACTH secretion and a lower blood glucose concentration than those in group 2. Identify compounds X and Y.

	Compound X	Compound Y
A)	Cortisone	Placebo
B)	Cortisol	Placebo
C)	Placebo	Cortisol
D)	ACTH	Placebo
E)	Placebo	ACTH

116. A 30-year-old woman reports to the clinic for a routine physical examination, which reveals she is pregnant. Her plasma levels of TSH are high, but her total T_4 concentration (protein bound and free) is normal. Which of the following best reflects this patient's clinical state?

    A) Graves' disease
    B) Hashimoto's disease
    C) A pituitary tumor that is secreting TSH
    D) A hypothalamic tumor that is secreting TRH
    E) The patient is taking thyroid extract

117. A man has a disease that destroyed only the motor neurons of the spinal cord below the thoracic region. Which aspect of sexual function would not be possible?

    A) Arousal
    B) Erection
    C) Lubrication
    D) Ejaculation

118. Which component of the reproductive system has the most far-reaching effects on the physiology of the organism?

    A) /Y chromosomal effects
    B) X dose—one X chromosome versus two X chromosomes
    C) Gonadal steroid hormones
    D) Prenatal testosterone levels

119. A sustained program of lifting heavy weights will increase bone mass. What is the mechanism of this effect of weightlifting?

    A) Elevated metabolic activity stimulates parathyroid hormone secretion
    B) Mechanical stress on the bones increases the activity of osteoblasts
    C) Elevated metabolic activity results in an increase in dietary calcium intake
    D) Elevated metabolic activity results in stimulation of calcitonin secretion

120. Birth control pills containing combinations of synthetic estrogen and progesterone compounds that are given for the first 21 days of the menstrual cycle are effective in preventing pregnancy. What is the explanation for their efficacy?

    A) Prevention of the preovulatory surge of LH secretion from the pituitary gland
    B) Prevention of development of the ovarian follicles
    C) Suppression of the function of the corpus luteum soon after it forms
    D) Prevention of normal development of the endometrium

121. Which of the following would be expected in a patient with a genetic deficiency of 11-β-hydroxysteroid dehydrogenase type II?
    A) Hyperkalemia
    B) Hypertension
    C) Increased plasma renin activity
    D) Increased plasma [aldosterone]
    E) Hyperglycemia

122. Which physiological response is greater for T₃ than for T₄?
    A) Secretion rate from the thyroid
    B) Plasma concentration
    C) Plasma half-life
    D) Affinity for nuclear receptors in target tissues
    E) Latent period for the onset of action in target tissues

123. A "birth control" compound for men has been sought for several decades. Which substance would provide effective sterility?
    A) A substance that mimics the actions of LH
    B) A substance that blocks the actions of inhibin
    C) A substance that blocks the actions of FSH
    D) A substance that mimics the actions of GnRH

124. For milk to flow from the nipple of the mother into the mouth of the nursing infant, what must occur?
    A) Myoepithelial cells must relax
    B) Prolactin levels must fall
    C) Oxytocin secretion from the posterior pituitary must take place
    D) The baby's mouth must develop a strong negative pressure over the nipple
    E) All the above

125. Failure of the ductus arteriosus to close is a common developmental defect. Which condition would likely be present in a 12-month-old infant with patent ductus arteriosus?
    A) Below normal arterial P_{O_2}
    B) Below normal arterial P_{CO_2}
    C) Greater than normal arterial blood pressure
    D) Lower than normal pulmonary arterial pressure

126. Which set of physiological changes would be expected in a nondiabetic patient with Cushing's disease?

	Plasma Aldosterone	Plasma Cortisol	Plasma Insulin
A)	↑	↑	↑
B)	↑	↑	↔
C)	↑	↔	↔
D)	↔	↔	↑
E)	↔	↑	↔
F)	↔	↑	↑

127. When compared with the late-evening values typically observed in normal subjects, plasma levels of both ACTH and cortisol would be expected to be higher in which persons?
    A) Normal subjects after waking in the morning
    B) Normal subjects who have taken dexamethasone
    C) Patients with Cushing's syndrome (adrenal adenoma)
    D) Patients with Addison's disease
    E) Patients with Conn's syndrome

128. Which of the following conditions or hormones would most likely increase GH secretion?
    A) Hyperglycemia
    B) Exercise
    C) Somatomedin
    D) Somatostatin
    E) Aging

129. Which set of findings would be expected in a person maintained on a long-term low-sodium diet?

	Plasma [Aldosterone]	Plasma [Atrial Natriuretic Peptide]	Plasma [Cortisol]
A)	↑	↑	↔
B)	↑	↓	↓
C)	↑	↓	↔
D)	↔	↔	↔
E)	↓	↓	↓
F)	↓	↑	↓

130. What would be associated with parallel changes in aldosterone and cortisol secretion?
    A) Addison's disease
    B) Cushing's disease
    C) Cushing's syndrome (ectopic ACTH-producing tumor)
    D) A high-sodium diet
    E) Administration of a converting enzyme inhibitor

131. Which blood vessel in the fetus has the highest P_{O_2}?
    A) Ductus arteriosus
    B) Ductus venosus
    C) Ascending aorta
    D) Left atrium

132. A 59-year-old woman has osteoporosis, hypertension, hirsutism, and hyperpigmentation. Magnetic resonance imaging indicates that the pituitary gland is not enlarged. Which condition is most consistent with these findings?
    A) Pituitary ACTH-secreting tumor
    B) Ectopic ACTH-secreting tumor
    C) Inappropriately high secretion rate of CRH
    D) Adrenal adenoma
    E) Addison's disease

133. Which set of findings is an inappropriate hypophysial hormone response to the hypothalamic hormone listed?

	Hypothalamic Hormone Secretion	Hypophysial Hormone
A)	Somatostatin	↓ GH
B)	Dopamine	↑ Prolactin
C)	GnRH	↑ LH
D)	TRH	↑ TSH
E)	CRH	↑ ACTH

134. A patient is administered sufficient T_4 to increase plasma levels of the hormone severalfold. Which set of changes is most likely in this patient after several weeks of T_4 administration?

	Respiratory Rate	Heart Rate	Plasma Cholesterol Concentration
A)	↑	↑	↑
B)	↑	↑	↓
C)	↑	↓	↑
D)	↓	↓	↑
E)	↓	↑	↓

135. During the latter stages of pregnancy, many women experience an increase in body hair growth in a masculine pattern. What is the explanation for this phenomenon?

A) The ovaries secrete some testosterone along with the large amounts of estrogen produced late in pregnancy

B) The fetal ovaries and testes secrete androgenic steroids

C) The maternal and fetal adrenal glands secrete large amounts of androgenic steroids that are used by the placenta to form estrogen

D) The placenta secretes large amounts of estrogen, some of which is metabolized to testosterone

136. What causes menopause?

A) Reduced levels of gonadotropic hormones secreted from the anterior pituitary gland

B) Reduced responsiveness of the follicles to the stimulatory effects of gonadotropic hormones

C) Reduced rate of secretion of progesterone from the corpus luteum

D) Reduced numbers of follicles available in the ovary for stimulation by gonadotropic hormones

137. What does not increase when insulin binds to its receptor?

A) Fat synthesis in adipose tissue
B) Protein synthesis in muscle
C) Glycogen synthesis
D) Gluconeogenesis in the liver
E) Intracellular tyrosine kinase activity

138. Release of which hormone is an example of neuroendocrine secretion?

A) GH
B) Cortisol
C) Oxytocin
D) Prolactin
E) ACTH

139. During the week after ovulation, the endometrium increases in thickness to 5 to 6 millimeters. What stimulates this increase in thickness?

A) LH
B) Estrogen from the corpus luteum
C) Progesterone from the corpus luteum
D) FSH

140. Inhibition of the iodide pump would be expected to cause which change?

A) Increased synthesis of T_4
B) Increased synthesis of thyroglobulin
C) Increased metabolic rate
D) Decreased TSH secretion
E) Extreme nervousness

141. Before implantation, the blastocyst obtains its nutrition from uterine endometrial secretions. How does the blastocyst obtain nutrition during the first week after implantation?

A) It continues to derive nutrition from endometrial secretions

B) The cells of the blastocyst contain stored nutrients that are metabolized for nutritional support

C) The placenta provides nutrition derived from maternal blood

D) The trophoblast cells digest the nutrient-rich endometrial cells and then absorb their contents for use by the blastocyst

142. Which pituitary hormone has a chemical structure most similar to that of ADH?

A) Oxytocin
B) ACTH
C) TSH
D) FSH
E) Prolactin

143. Which option would not be efficacious in the treatment of patients with type 2 diabetes?

A) Glucocorticoids
B) Insulin injections
C) Thiazolidinediones
D) Sulfonylureas
E) Weight loss

144. Which of the following is most likely to occur in the early stages of type 2 diabetes?

    A) Increased insulin sensitivity
    B) Decreased hepatic glucose output
    C) Increased plasma levels of C-peptide
    D) Increased plasma [β-hydroxybutyric acid]
    E) Hypovolemia

145. What is the most common cause of respiratory distress syndrome in neonates born at 7 months' gestation?

    A) Pulmonary edema due to pulmonary arterial hypertension
    B) Formation of a hyaline membrane over the alveolar surface
    C) Failure of the alveolar lining to form adequate amounts of surfactant
    D) Excessive permeability of the alveolar membrane to water

146. Which of the following would be expected to occur during the postprandial period?

	Adipocyte α-Glycerol Phosphate	Plasma [Insulin]	Glycogen Phosphorylase
A)	↑	↑	↓
B)	↑	↑	↑
C)	↑	↓	↑
D)	↓	↓	↑
E)	↓	↓	↓
F)	↓	↑	↓

147. A 45-year-old woman has a mass in the sella turcica that compresses the portal vessels, disrupting pituitary access to hypothalamic secretions. The secretion rate of which hormone would most likely increase in this patient?

    A) ACTH
    B) GH
    C) Prolactin
    D) LH
    E) TSH

148. Which of the following is not produced by osteoblasts?

    A) Alkaline phosphatase
    B) RANK ligand
    C) Collagen
    D) Pyrophosphate
    E) Osteoprotegerin

149. Which set of findings would be expected in a patient with primary hyperparathyroidism?

	Plasma [1,25-(OH)2D3]	Plasma [Phosphate]	Urinary Ca++ Excretion
A)	↑	↑	↑
B)	↑	↓	↑
C)	↑	↓	↓
D)	↓	↓	↑
E)	↓	↑	↓
F)	↓	↑	↑

150. A man who has been exposed to high levels of gamma radiation is sterile due to destruction of the germinal epithelium of the seminiferous tubules, although he has normal levels of testosterone. Which of the following would be found in this patient?

    A) A normal secretory pattern of GnRH
    B) Normal levels of inhibin
    C) Suppressed levels of FSH
    D) Absence of Leydig cells

Questions 151 and 152

An experiment was conducted in which rats were injected with one of two hormones or saline solution (control) for 2 weeks. Autopsies were then performed, and organ weights were measured (in milligrams). Use this information to answer Questions 151 and 152.

	Control	Hormone 1	Hormone 2
Pituitary	12.9	8.0	14.5
Thyroid	250	500	245
Adrenal glands	40	37	85
Body weight	300	152	175

151. What is hormone 1?

    A) TRH
    B) TSH
    C) T_4
    D) ACTH
    E) Cortisol

152. What is hormone 2?

    A) TSH
    B) T_4
    C) CRH
    D) ACTH
    E) Cortisol

153. Which of the following would be expected in a patient with vitamin D deficiency?

	Plasma [1,25-(OH)2D3]	Bone Resorption	Intestinal Calbindin
A)	↑	↑	↑
B)	↑	↓	↑
C)	↑	↓	↓
D)	↓	↓	↑
E)	↓	↑	↓
F)	↓	↑	↑

1. D) Parasympathetic postganglionic fibers release acetylcholine that activates muscarinic receptors on endothelium to produce NO and increases cyclic guanosine monophosphate, which activates protein kinase G, causing a reduction in intracellular calcium (also increasing NO by positive feedback) and causing vasodilation.
TMP13 p. 1027

2. D) ADH increases the permeability of the collecting tubules and ducts to water, but not to sodium, which in turn increases water reabsorption and decreases water excretion. As a result, urine concentration increases and the retained water dilutes the plasma. ADH is synthesized in the supraoptic and paraventricular nuclei of the hypothalamus and has no direct effect on the thirst center.
TMP13 pp. 949-364, 404, 949

3. A) Estrogen compounds are believed to have an osteoblast-stimulating effect. When the amount of estrogen in the blood falls to very low levels after menopause, the balance between the bone-building activity of the osteoblasts and the bone-degrading activity of the osteoclasts is tipped toward bone degradation. When estrogen compounds are added as part of hormone replacement therapy, the bone-building activity of the osteoblasts is increased to balance the osteoclastic activity.
TMP13 pp. 949, 1045

4. B) In nephrogenic diabetes insipidus, the kidneys cannot respond to ADH. Consequently, dilute urine and loss of water from the extracellular fluid occurs, resulting in hypernatremia. Hypernatremia stimulates thirst, which attenuates the severity of hypernatremia, whereas water restriction exacerbates hypernatremia. Hypernatremia also stimulates ADH secretion from the magnocellular neurons in the hypothalamus.
TMP13 p. 949

5. C) After birth, systemic arterial resistance increases dramatically due to loss of the placental vasculature. Consequently, arterial pressure, left ventricular pressure, and left atrial pressure all increase. At the same time, pulmonary vascular resistance decreases due to expansion of the lungs, and pulmonary artery pressure, right ventricular pressure, and right atrial pressure all fall. Blood flow through the foramen is a function of the pressure gradient, which after birth favors flow from the left to the right atrium, but most of the flow is blocked by the septal flap on the septal wall of the left atrium.
TMP13 pp. 1073-1075

6. A) Norepinephrine is released from the nerve terminals and endothelin is released from endothelial cells in the vasculature, causing vasoconstriction of the vasculature.
TMP13 p. 1027

7. C) Type 2 DM is characterized by diminished sensitivity of target tissues to the metabolic effects of insulin—that is, there is insulin resistance. As a result, hepatic uptake of glucose is impaired and glucose release is enhanced. In muscle, the uptake of glucose is impaired.
TMP13 pp. 985-986, 995

8. C) In acromegaly, high plasma levels of GH cause insulin resistance. Consequently, glucose production by the liver is increased and glucose uptake by peripheral tissues is impaired.
TMP13 pp. 943-944, 996-997

9. A) During exercise, glucose utilization by muscle is increased, which is largely independent of insulin.
TMP13 p. 985

10. A) Thecal cells do not have the capacity to produce estradiol because they lack aromatase.
TMP13 pp. 1040, 1043, 1044

11. B) A very high concentration of testosterone in a female embryo will induce formation of male genitalia. An adrenal tumor in the mother that synthesizes testosterone at a high, uncontrolled rate could produce the masculinizing effect.
TMP13 pp. 1043, 1044

12. E) HCG has the same stimulatory effect as LH on the corpus luteum. Administration of HCG would cause the corpus luteum to continue to secrete estrogen and progesterone, preventing degradation of the endometrium and the onset of menstruation.
TMP13 p. 1059

13. D) Hypoglycemia is a potent stimulus for GH. GH decreases with aging and in response to the hypothalamic inhibitory hormone somatostatin. GH secretion would decrease in response to both exogenous GH administration and IGF-1 as a result of negative feedback inhibition.
TMP13 p. 945

14. C) Antagonism of progesterone's effects, dilation of the cervix, and oxytocin all increase uterine smooth muscle excitability and facilitate contractions and the onset of labor. LH would have no effect. Prostaglandin

E₂ strongly stimulates uterine smooth muscle contraction and is formed at an increasing rate by the placenta late in gestation.
    TMP13 p. 1064, 1066

15. **A)** Ultraviolet light absorbed by the skin directly facilitates conversion of cholesterol to 25-hydroxycholesterol.
    TMP13 p. 1007

16. **D)** Pulmonary vascular resistance greatly decreases as a result of expansion of the lungs. In the unexpanded fetal lungs, the blood vessels are compressed because of the small volume of the lungs. Immediately upon expansion, these vessels are no longer compressed, and the resistance to blood flow decreases severalfold.
    TMP13 pp. 1073, 1074

17. **D)** The inhibitory hormone somatostatin is both synthesized and stored in the hypothalamus. Both TSH and LH are synthesized and stored in the anterior pituitary gland. ADH is synthesized in the hypothalamus but is stored in the posterior pituitary gland. Somatomedin (IGF-1) is synthesized in the liver.
    TMP13 p. 946

18. **A)** In a radioimmunoassay, there is too little antibody to completely bind the radioactively tagged hormone and the hormone in the fluid (plasma) to be assayed. Thus, there is competition between the labeled and endogenous hormone for binding sites on the antibody. Consequently, if the amount of radioactive hormone bound to antibody is low, this finding would indicate that plasma levels of endogenous hormone are high.
    TMP13 p. 936

19. **C)** Just before the LH surge, estradiol levels increase, which causes negative feedback on GnRH to stop producing LH and FSH, resulting in the decrease in their levels.
    TMP13 p. 1039

20. **B)** The Sertoli cells of the seminiferous tubules secrete inhibin at a rate proportional to the rate of production of sperm cells. Inhibin has a direct inhibitory effect on anterior pituitary secretion of FSH. FSH binds to specific receptors on the Sertoli cells, causing the cells to grow and secrete substances that stimulate sperm cell production. The secretion of inhibin thereby provides the negative feedback control signal from the seminiferous tubules to the pituitary gland.
    TMP13 p. 1033

21. **B)** Ovulation will not take place unless a surge of LH precedes it. Immediately prior to ovulation, the number of follicles is decreasing due to normal attrition of all but one follicle, and consequently estrogen synthesis by the ovary is decreasing. Progesterone synthesis is stimulated by the LH surge.
    TMP13 pp. 1039, 1040

22. **A)** The corpus luteum is the only source of progesterone production, except for minute quantities secreted from the follicle before ovulation. The corpus luteum is functional between ovulation and the beginning of menstruation, during which time the concentration of LH is suppressed below the level achieved during the preovulatory LH surge.
    TMP13 pp. 1046-1047

23. **C)** At the end of the luteal phase, the corpus luteum is resorbed and fails to produce progesterone and estradiol, making levels fall precipitously and causing the endometrium to slough.
    TMP13 p. 1039

24. **D)** Paracrine communication refers to cell secretions that diffuse into the extracellular fluid to affect neighboring cells.
    TMP13 p. 925

25. **B)** The delta cells of the pancreas secrete somatostatin, which inhibits the secretion of insulin and glucagon from the pancreatic beta and alpha cells, respectively. Choice D is an example of neural communication, and the remaining choices are examples of neuroendocrine communication.
    TMP13 pp. 925, 993

26. **E)** Anabolic steroids bind to testosterone receptors in the hypothalamus, providing feedback inhibition of normal ovarian cycling and preventing menstrual cycling as well as stimulation of osteoblastic activity in the bones.
    TMP13 pp. 1028, 1031

27. **A)** Testosterone causes vasodilation by inhibiting L-type calcium channels to inhibit calcium influx into the cells, thus causing vasodilation.
    TMP13 p. 1026

28. **B)** Right atrial pressure falls dramatically after the onset of breathing because of a reduction in pulmonary vascular resistance, pulmonary arterial pressure, and right ventricular pressure.
    TMP13 pp. 1073-1075

29. **E)** Patients with Conn's syndrome have tumors of the zona glomerulosa that secrete large amounts of aldosterone. Consequently, plasma levels of aldosterone are elevated, causing hypokalemia. The secretion of cortisol from the zona fasciculata is normal.
    TMP13 p. 981

30. **D)** Aldosterone secretion is elevated when dietary sodium intake is low, but cortisol secretion is normal. Although aldosterone increases the rate of potassium secretion by the principal cells of the collecting tubules, this effect is offset by a low distal tubular flow rate. Consequently, there is little change in either potassium excretion or plasma potassium concentration.
    TMP13 pp. 971-972

31. B) In patients with nephrogenic diabetes insipidus, the kidneys do not respond appropriately to ADH, and the ability to form concentrated urine is impaired. In contrast, there is a normal ADH secretory response to changes in plasma osmolality.
    TMP13 pp. 380-381, 949

32. C) Aromatase causes conversion of testosterone to estradiol.
    TMP13 p. 1043

33. D) Because of the loss of blood flow through the placenta, systemic vascular resistance doubles at birth, which increases the aortic pressure as well as the pressure in the left ventricle and left atrium.
    TMP13 pp. 1073, 1074

34. D) Parathyroid hormone acts in the renal cortex to stimulate the reaction forming 1,25-dihydroxycholicalciferol from 25-hydroxycholicalciferol. It has no effects on other the other reactions.
    TMP13 pp. 1007-1008

35. B) Both amino acids and glucose stimulate insulin secretion. Furthermore, amino acids strongly potentiate the glucose stimulus for insulin secretion. Somatostatin inhibits insulin secretion.
    TMP13 pp. 990-991, 993

36. F) In this form of dwarfism, there is decreased synthesis and secretion of GH into the circulation. As a result, stimulation of hepatic IGF-1 secretion is decreased and secretion of hypothalamic GnRH is increased due to diminished negative feedback. GH has several actions to increase blood levels of glucose, and when blood levels of GH are inappropriately low, fasting blood glucose concentration tends to fall.
    TMP13 pp. 943-947

37. B) HCG also binds to LH receptors on the interstitial cells of the testes of the male fetus, resulting in the production of testosterone in male fetuses up to the time of birth. This small secretion of testosterone is what causes the fetus to develop male sex organs instead of female sex organs.
    TMP13 pp. 1033, 1060-1061

38. C) If a subject took sufficient amounts of exogenous thyroid extract to increase plasma levels of T_4 above normal, feedback would cause the secretion of TSH to decrease. Low plasma levels of TSH would result in atrophy of the thyroid gland. In a person with Graves' disease, the same changes in plasma levels of T_4 and TSH would be present, but the thyroid gland would not be atrophied. In fact, goiter is often present in patients with Graves' disease. A lesion in the anterior pituitary that prevents TSH secretion or the taking of propylthiouracil or large amounts of iodine would be associated with low plasma levels of T_4.
    TMP13 pp. 959-960

39. D) Choices A to C would all shift the mass action balance toward the side favoring association of ionic calcium with phosphate compounds or other anionic compounds, resulting in reduced levels of free ionic calcium.
    TMP13 p. 1001

40. B) In the nonpregnant female, the only significant source of estrogen is ovarian follicles or corpus luteae. Menstruation begins when the corpus luteum degenerates. Menstruation ends when developing follicles secrete estrogen sufficiently to raise circulating concentration to a level that stimulates regrowth of the endometrium.
    TMP13 pp. 1039, 1042, 1046-1047

41. B) As a result of negative feedback, plasma levels of TSH are a sensitive index of circulating levels of unbound (free) thyroid hormones. High plasma levels of TSH indicate inappropriately low levels of free thyroid hormones in the circulation, such as are present with autoimmune destruction of the thyroid gland in persons with Hashimoto's disease. However, because elevated plasma levels of estrogen in pregnancy increase hepatic production of TBG, the total amount (bound + free) of thyroid hormones in the circulation is elevated. Plasma levels of thyroid hormones are elevated in persons with Graves' disease and in patients with a pituitary TSH-secreting tumor, as well in patients given thyroid extract for therapy.
    TMP13 pp. 954, 958-962

42. C) The major target tissue for prolactin is the breast, where it stimulates the secretion of milk. The other anterior pituitary hormones (ACTH, TSH, FSH, and LH) stimulate hormones from endocrine glands.
    TMP13 p. 927

43. D) The cells of the anterior pituitary that secrete LH and FSH, along with the cells of the hypothalamus that secrete GnRH, are inhibited by both estrogen and testosterone. The steroids taken by the woman caused sufficient inhibition to result in cessation of the monthly menstrual cycle.
    TMP13 pp. 1033, 1047-1048

44. D) Patients with central diabetes insipidus have an inappropriately low secretion rate of ADH in response to changes in plasma osmolality, but their renal response to ADH is not impaired. Because plasma levels of ADH are depressed, the ability to concentrate urine is impaired, and a large volume of dilute urine is excreted. Loss of water tends to increase plasma osmolality, which stimulates the thirst center and leads to a very high rate of water turnover.
    TMP13 p. 949

45. B) NO is the vasodilator that is normally released, causing vasodilation in these arteries.
    TMP13 pp. 1027, 1034

46. B) A hypothalamic tumor secreting large amounts of TRH would stimulate the pituitary gland to secrete increased amounts of TSH. As a result, the secretion of thyroid hormones would increase, which would result in an elevated heart rate. In comparison, a patient with either a pituitary tumor secreting large amounts of TSH or Graves' disease would have low plasma levels of TRH because of feedback. Both TRH and TSH levels would be elevated in an endemic goiter, but the heart rate would be depressed because of the low rate of T_4 secretion.

TMP13 pp. 957-962

47. D) Consumption of amino acids stimulates both GH and glucagon secretion. Increased glucagon secretion tends to increase blood glucose concentration and thus opposes the effects of insulin to cause hypoglycemia.

TMP13 pp. 992-993

48. D) Lethargy and myxedema are signs of hypothyroidism. Low plasma levels of TSH indicate that the abnormality is in either the hypothalamus or the pituitary gland. The responsiveness of the pituitary to the administration of TRH suggests that pituitary function is normal and that the hypothalamus is producing insufficient amounts of TRH.

TMP13 pp. 958-962

49. D) Inhibin prevents FSH release from the anterior pituitary, preventing Sertoli cells from causing aromatization to produce estradiol.

TMP13 p. 1032

50. A) After menopause, the absence of feedback inhibition by estrogen and progesterone results in extremely high rates of FSH secretion. Women taking estrogen as part of hormone replacement therapy for symptoms associated with postmenopausal conditions have suppressed levels of FSH as a result of the inhibitory effect of estrogen.

TMP13 pp. 1050, 1051

51. D) Phosphodiesterase-5 receptors prevent hydrolysis of cyclic guanosine monophosphate, thus keeping the levels high and maintaining vasodilation.

TMP13 p. 1034

52. B) Glucagon stimulates glycogenolysis in the liver, but it has no physiological effects in muscle. Both glucagon and cortisol increase gluconeogenesis, and cortisol impairs glucose uptake by muscle.

TMP13 pp. 972-973, 992

53. C) Injection of insulin leads to a decrease in blood glucose concentration. Hypoglycemia stimulates the secretion of GH, glucagon, and epinephrine, all of which have counter-regulatory effects to increase glucose levels in the blood.

TMP13 p. 945, 993-994

54. A) Prolonged fetal hypoxia during delivery can cause serious depression of the respiratory center. Hypoxia may occur during delivery because of compression of the umbilical cord, premature separation of the placenta, excessive contraction of the uterus, or excessive anesthesia of the mother.

TMP13 p. 1073

55. C) In general, peptide hormones are water soluble and are not highly bound by plasma proteins. ADH, a neurohypophysial peptide hormone, is virtually unbound by plasma proteins. In contrast, steroid and thyroid hormones are highly bound to plasma proteins.

TMP13 p. 929-930

56. C) The rise in intracellular calcium in the oocyte triggers the cortical reaction in which granules that previously lay at the base of the plasma membrane undergo exocytosis. That process leads to the release of enzymes that "harden" the zona pellucida and prevent other sperm from penetrating.

TMP13 p. 1025

57. B) Although estrogen and progesterone are essential for the physical development of the breast during pregnancy, a specific effect of both these hormones is to inhibit the actual secretion of milk. Even though prolactin levels are increased 10- to 20-fold at the end of pregnancy, the suppressive effects of estrogen and progesterone prevent milk production until after the baby is born. Immediately after birth, the sudden loss of both estrogen and progesterone secretion from the placenta allows the lactogenic effect of prolactin to promote milk production.

TMP13 pp. 1066-1067

58. C) The concentration of PTH strongly regulates the absorption of calcium ion from the renal tubular fluid. A reduction in hormone concentration reduces calcium reabsorption and increases the rate of calcium excretion in the urine. The other choices either have little effect on or decrease calcium excretion.

TMP13 pp. 1011-1012

59. B) A pituitary tumor secreting increased amounts of TSH would be expected to stimulate the thyroid gland to secrete increased amounts of thyroid hormones. TSH stimulates several steps in the synthesis of thyroid hormones, including the synthesis of thyroglobulin. Increased heart rate is among the many physiological responses to high plasma levels of thyroid hormones. However, high plasma levels of thyroid hormones do not cause exophthalmos. Immunoglobulins cause exophthalmos in Graves' disease, the most common form of hyperthyroidism.

TMP13 pp. 952, 957, 961

60. A) Hemorrhage decreases the activation of stretch receptors in the atria and arterial baroreceptors. Decreased activation of these receptors increases ADH secretion.
> TMP13 p. 949

61. E) Choices A to D are true: LH secretion will be suppressed (B) by the negative feedback effect of the estrogen from the tumor; consequently, she will not have menstrual cycles (C), and because she will not have normal cycles, no corpus luteae will develop, so no progesterone will be formed (A). The high levels of estrogen produced by the tumor will provide stimulation of osteoblastic activity to maintain normal bone activity (D).
> TMP13 pp. 1044, 1045

62. D) After eating a meal, insulin secretion is increased. As a result, there is an increased rate of glucose uptake by both the liver and muscle. Insulin also inhibits hormone-sensitive lipase, which decreases hydrolysis of triglycerides in fat cells.
> TMP13 pp. 985-987, 992

63. B) The primary function of testosterone in the embryonic development of males is to stimulate formation of the male sex organs.
> TMP13 pp. 219-220, 364, 383, 405, 949-950

64. E) Protein-bound hormones are biologically inactive and cannot be metabolized. Thus, an increase in protein binding would tend to decrease hormone activity and plasma clearance and increase the half-life of the hormone. Free hormone is also responsible for negative feedback inhibition of hormone secretion. Therefore, a sudden increase in hormone binding to plasma proteins would decrease negative feedback. Protein binding of hormones does, however, provide a reservoir for the rapid replacement of free hormone.
> TMP13 pp. 929-930

65. C) The reduction in hydrogen ion indicated by the elevation in pH increases the concentration of negatively charged phosphate ion species available for ionic combination with calcium ions. Consequently, the free calcium ion concentration is reduced.
> TMP13 pp. 1011-1012

66. E) In Graves' disease, antibodies against the TSH receptor in the thyroid gland stimulate many of the steps in the synthesis of thyroid hormones, including increased iodine uptake. Due to excessive stimulation of the gland, the thyroid gland hypertrophies and secretes increased amounts of thyroid hormones. High circulating levels of thyroid hormones inhibit TSH secretion due to negative feedback inhibition. The antibodies present in Graves' disease also cause pathological changes in the tissue surrounding the eyes, leading to protrusion of the eyeballs.
> TMP13 pp. 960-961

67. C) During suckling, stimulation of receptors on the nipples increases neural input to both the supraoptic and paraventricular nuclei. Activation of these nuclei leads to the release of oxytocin and neurophysin from secretion granules in the posterior pituitary gland. Suckling does not stimulate the secretion of appreciable amounts of ADH.
> TMP13 pp. 1066, 1067

68. C) In Conn's syndrome, large amounts of aldosterone are secreted. Because aldosterone causes sodium retention, hypertension is a common finding in patients with this condition. However, the degree of sodium retention is modest, as is the resultant increase in extracellular fluid volume. This occurs because the rise in arterial pressure offsets the sodium-retaining effects of aldosterone, limiting sodium retention and permitting daily sodium balance to be achieved.
> TMP13 pp. 970, 981

69. A) Because the liver functions imperfectly during the first weeks of life, the glucose concentration in the blood is unstable and falls to very low levels within a few hours after feeding.
> TMP13 pp. 1075, 1076

70. D) DHEA sulfate produced by the fetal adrenal gland diffuses to the placenta and is converted to DHEA and then to estradiol and provides estradiol to the mother.
> TMP13 pp. 1060, 1061

71. D) Sporadic nursing of the mother results in a lack of prolactin surge because mechanosensors in the nipple cause prolactin release. Without prolactin release, there is a lack of milk production, and the mother eventually will not be able to provide milk for the baby.
> TMP13 pp. 1066, 1067

72. A) Persons with Addison's disease have diminished secretion of both glucocorticoids (cortisol) and mineralocorticoids (aldosterone). In persons with Cushing's disease or Cushing's syndrome, cortisol secretion is elevated but aldosterone secretion is normal. A low-sodium diet is associated with a high rate of aldosterone secretion but a secretion rate of cortisol that is normal. By inhibiting the generation of angiotensin II and thus the stimulatory effects of angiotensin II on the zona glomerulosa, administration of a converting enzyme inhibitor would decrease aldosterone secretion without altering the rate of cortisol secretion.
> TMP13 pp. 971-972, 979-980

73. E) In the steady state, high plasma levels of TBG would simply increase the reservoir for hormone and, therefore, the total amount of thyroid hormone in the circulation. However, protein-bound hormone is inactive. The metabolic effects of thyroid hormones and their feedback inhibition on TSH secretion are determined

by the free thyroid hormone and not the total amount of thyroid hormone in the circulation. Both the plasma levels of free thyroid hormone and TSH would be expected to be normal in the steady state. Consequently, the metabolic rate would be unchanged.
TMP13 pp. 929-930, 955-960

74. **B)** Progesterone is required to maintain the decidual cells of the endometrium. If progesterone levels fall, as they do during the last days of a nonpregnant menstrual cycle, menstruation will follow within a few days, with loss of pregnancy. Administration of a compound that blocks the progesterone receptor during the first few days after conception will terminate the pregnancy.
TMP13 pp. 1060-1061

75. **D)** An inappropriately high rate of ADH secretion from the lung promotes excess water reabsorption, which tends to produce concentrated urine and a decrease in plasma osmolality. Low plasma osmolality suppresses both thirst and ADH secretion from the pituitary gland.
TMP13 pp. 404, 949

76. **B)** A very high plasma concentration of progesterone maintains the uterine muscle in a quiescent state during pregnancy. In the final month of gestation the concentration of progesterone begins to decline, increasing the excitability of the muscle.
TMP13 pp. 1027, 971-972

77. **D)** The corpus luteum is the only source of progesterone. If she is not having menstrual cycles, no corpus luteum is present.
TMP13 p. 1048

78. **C)** FSH stimulates the granulosa cells of the follicle to secrete estrogen.
TMP13 pp. 1040, 1048

79. **E)** In response to increased blood levels of glucose, plasma insulin concentration normally increases during the 60-minute period following oral intake of glucose. In type 1 DM, insulin secretion is depressed. In contrast, in type 2 DM, insulin resistance is a common finding and, at least in the early stages of the disease, there is an abnormally high rate of insulin secretion.
TMP13 pp. 995-998

80. **D)** In Cushing's syndrome, high plasma levels of cortisol impair glucose uptake in peripheral tissues, which tends to increase plasma levels of glucose. As a result, the insulin response to oral intake of glucose is enhanced.
TMP13 pp. 996-998

81. **B)** In general, protein hormones cause physiological effects by binding to receptors on the cell membrane.

However, of the four protein hormones indicated, only insulin activates an enzyme-linked receptor. Aldosterone is a steroid hormone and enters the cytoplasm of the cell before binding to its receptor.
TMP13 p. 932

82. **D)** HCG is secreted from the trophoblast cells beginning shortly after the blastocyst implants in the endometrium.
TMP13 pp. 1060-1061

83. **B)** Aortic pressure increases due to the increase in left ventricular pressure. The increase in left atrial pressure causes the foramen ovale to close. The ductus arteriosus also closes within a short time after birth.
TMP13 pp. 1073-1075

84. **A)** Somnolence is a common feature of hypothyroidism. Palpitations, increased respiratory rate, increased cardiac output, and weight loss are all associated with hyperthyroidism.
TMP13 pp. 957, 962-963

85. **C)** An infant born of an untreated diabetic mother will have considerable hypertrophy and hyperfunction of the islets of Langerhans in the pancreas. As a consequence, the infant's blood glucose concentration may fall to lower than 20 mg/dl shortly after birth.
TMP13 pp. 1078-1079

86. **C)** Hemoglobin F levels are higher in the fetus than in the mother, and hemoglobin F in the fetus can carry more oxygen than can hemoglobin in the mother.
TMP13 p. 1058

87. **E)** Choices A to D would not stimulate PTH secretion. An increase in calcium concentration (A) suppresses PTH secretion; calcitonin has little to no effect on PTH secretion (B); acidosis would increase free calcium in the extracellular fluid, thereby inhibiting PTH secretion (C); and PTH-releasing hormone does not exist (D).
TMP13 pp. 1001, 1011

88. **C)** Potassium is a potent stimulus for aldosterone secretion, as is angiotensin II. Therefore, a patient consuming a high-potassium diet would exhibit high circulating levels of aldosterone.
TMP13 p. 971

89. **B)** The decidua and trophoblasts provide the nutrition needed to provide nourishment of the blastocyst.
TMP13 pp. 1057, 1060-1062

90. **C)** Steroid hormones are not stored to any appreciable extent in their endocrine producing glands. This is true for aldosterone, which is produced in the adrenal cortex. In contrast, there are appreciable stores of thyroid hormones and peptide hormones in their endocrine-producing glands.
TMP13 p. 928

91. **C)** 1,25-dihydroxycholecalciferol is formed only in the renal cortex. Extensive renal disease reduces the amount of cortical tissue, eliminating the source of this active calcium regulating hormone.
TMP13 p. 1015

92. **C)** The placenta cannot produce androgens but can only produce DHEA by removal of the sulfate from DHEAS produced in the fetal adrenal glands.
TMP13 p. 1060

93. **C)** For erythroblastosis fetalis to occur, the baby must inherit Rh-positive red blood cells from the father. If the mother is Rh-negative, she then becomes immunized against the Rh-positive antigen in the red blood cells of the fetus, and her antibodies destroy fetal red blood cells, releasing large quantities of bilirubin into the plasma of the fetus.
TMP13 p. 1076

94. **D)** Because iodine is needed to synthesize thyroid hormones, the production of thyroid hormones is impaired if iodine is deficient. As a result of feedback, plasma levels of TSH increase and stimulate the follicular cells to increase the synthesis of thyroglobulin, which results in a goiter. Increased metabolic rate, sweating, nervousness, and tachycardia are all common features of hyperthyroidism, not hypothyroidism, due to iodine deficiency.
TMP13 pp. 960-963

95. **C)** Because of the effects of thyroid hormones to increase metabolism in tissues, tissues vasodilate, thus increasing blood flow and cardiac output. All the other choices increase in response to high plasma levels of thyroid hormones.
TMP13 pp. 956-957

96. **B)** Sperm cell motility decreases as pH is reduced below 6.8. At a pH of 4.5, sperm cell motility is significantly reduced. However, the buffering effect of sodium bicarbonate in the prostatic fluid raises the pH somewhat, allowing the sperm cells to regain some mobility.
TMP13 p. 1024

97. **B)** A protein meal stimulates all three hormones indicated.
TMP13 pp. 945, 991, 993

98. **C)** Testosterone secreted by the testes in response to LH inhibits hypothalamic secretion of GnRH, thereby inhibiting anterior pituitary secretion of LH and FSH. Taking large doses of testosterone-like steroids also suppresses the secretion of GnRH and the pituitary gonadotropic hormones, resulting in sterility.
TMP13 p. 1033

99. **C)** Steroids with potent glucocorticoid activity tend to increase plasma glucose concentration. As a result,

insulin secretion is stimulated. Increased glucocorticoid activity also diminishes muscle protein. Because of feedback, cortisone administration leads to a decrease in adrenocorticotropic hormone secretion and, therefore, a decrease in plasma cortisol concentration.
TMP13 pp. 972-973

100. **C)** Inhibin is the hormone that has a negative feedback on the anterior pituitary to prevent FSH from being released. Inhibin is produced by the granulosa cells in the ovary.
TMP13 pp. 1040-1041

101. **A)** An increase in the concentration of PTH results in the stimulation of existing osteoclasts and, over longer periods, increases the number of osteoclasts present in the bone.
TMP13 pp. 1010-1011

102. **B)** In general, peptide hormones produce biological effects by binding to receptors on the cell membrane. Peptide hormones are stored in secretion granules in their endocrine-producing cells and have relatively short half-lives because they are not highly bound to plasma proteins. Protein hormones often have a rapid onset of action because, unlike steroid and thyroid hormones, protein synthesis is usually not a prerequisite to produce biological effects.
TMP13 pp. 926, 929-932

103. **D)** A pituitary tumor secreting GH is likely to present as an increase in pituitary gland size. The anabolic effects of excess GH secretion lead to enlargement of the internal organs, including the kidneys. Because acromegaly is the state of excess GH secretion after epiphyseal closure, increased femur length does not occur.
TMP13 p. 947

104. **A)** GH and cortisol have opposite effects on protein synthesis in muscle. GH is anabolic and promotes protein synthesis in most cells of the body, whereas cortisol decreases protein synthesis in extrahepatic cells, including muscle. Both hormones impair glucose uptake in peripheral tissues and, therefore, tend to increase plasma glucose concentration. Both hormones also mobilize triglycerides from fat stores.
TMP13 pp. 943-944, 972-973

105. **B)** If the mother has had adequate amounts of iron in her diet, the infant's liver usually has enough stored iron to form blood cells for 4 to 6 months after birth. However, if the mother had insufficient iron levels, severe anemia may develop in the infant after about 3 months of life.
TMP13 pp. 1072, 1077

106. **A)** High plasma levels of steroids with glucocorticoid activity suppress CRH and, consequently, ACTH secretion. Therefore, the adrenal glands would actually

atrophy with chronic cortisone treatment. Increased plasma levels of glucocorticoids tend to cause sodium retention and increase blood pressure. They also tend to increase plasma levels of glucose and, consequently, stimulate insulin secretion and C-peptide, which is part of the insulin prohormone.

TMP13 pp. 972-973, 976-977, 979-980

107. **C)** Thyrotoxicosis indicates the effects of thyroid hormone excess. Thyroid hormone excites synapses. In contrast, somnolence is characteristic of hypothyroidism. Tachycardia, increased appetite, increased sweating, and muscle tremor are all signs of hyperthyroidism.

TMP13 pp. 956-958, 961

108. **C)** SRY is the region on the Y chromosome that encodes a transcription factor that causes differentiation of Sertoli cells from precursors in testis. If SRY is not present, granulosa cells in the ovary are produced.

TMP13 p. 1029

109. **D)** Fertilization of the ovum normally takes place in the ampulla of one of the fallopian tubes.

TMP13 p. 1055

110. **D)** Because insulin secretion is deficient in persons with type 1 DM, there is increased (not decreased) release of glucose from the liver. Low plasma levels of insulin also lead to a high rate of lipolysis; increased plasma osmolality, hypovolemia, and acidosis are all symptoms of uncontrolled type 1 DM.

TMP13 pp. 995-996

111. **E)** Under acute conditions, an increase in blood glucose concentration will decrease GH secretion. GH secretion is characteristically elevated in the chronic pathophysiological states of acromegaly and gigantism. Deep sleep and exercise are stimuli that increase GH secretion.

TMP13 pp. 945-946

112. **D)** All the steroids listed include pregnenolone early in their biosynthetic pathway. 1,25(OH)2D is derived from vitamin D and does not include pregnenolone in its biosynthetic pathway.

TMP13 pp. 965-967, 1007-1008

113. **D)** Estrogen and, to a lesser extent, progesterone secreted by the corpus luteum during the luteal phase have strong feedback effects on the anterior pituitary gland to maintain low secretory rates of both FSH and LH. In addition, the corpus luteum secretes inhibin, which inhibits the secretion of FSH.

TMP13 p. 1042

114. **D)** Under chronic conditions, the effects of high plasma levels of aldosterone to promote sodium reabsorption in the collecting tubules are sustained. However, persistent sodium retention does not occur because of concomitant changes that promote sodium excretion. These changes include increased arterial pressure, increased plasma levels of atrial natriuretic peptide, and decreased plasma angiotensin II concentration.

TMP13 pp. 961, 981

115. **C)** Increased plasma levels of cortisol tend to increase plasma glucose concentration and inhibit ACTH secretion. Therefore, if cortisol were administered to patients in group 2, the patients in group 1 would have lower plasma glucose concentrations and higher plasma levels of ACTH.

TMP13 pp. 972-973, 976-977

116. **B)** Circulating levels of free T_4 exert biological effects and are regulated by feedback inhibition of TSH secretion from the anterior pituitary gland. Protein-bound T_4 is biologically inactive. Circulating T_4 is highly bound to plasma proteins, especially to TBG, which increases during pregnancy. An increase in TBG tends to decrease free T_4, which then leads to an increase in TSH secretion, causing the thyroid to increase thyroid hormone secretion. Increased secretion of thyroid hormones persists until free T_4 returns to normal levels, at which time there is no longer a stimulus for increased TSH secretion. Therefore, in a chronic steady-state condition associated with elevated TBG, high plasma total T_4 (bound and free) and normal plasma TSH levels would be expected. In this pregnant patient, the normal levels of total T_4, along with high plasma levels of TSH, would indicate an inappropriately low plasma level of free T_4. Deficient thyroid hormone secretion in this patient would be consistent with Hashimoto's disease, the most common form of hypothyroidism.

TMP13 pp. 954, 958-962

117. **D)** The motor neurons of the spinal cord of the thoracic and lumbar regions are the sources of innervation for the skeletal muscles of the perineum involved in ejaculation.

TMP13 pp. 1026, 1027

118. **C)** The gonadal steroids, in addition to controlling reproductive function, also control nonreproductive organ function via their estrogen and androgen receptors. For example, estrogens control vascular function due to their ability to increase intracellular calcium in vascular smooth cells causing vasodilation. In addition, estradiol upregulates synthesis of endothelial NO synthase, leading to vasodilation.

TMP13 p. 1034

119. **B)** Bone is deposited in proportion to the compressional load that the bone must carry. Continual mechanical stress stimulates osteoblastic deposition and calcification of bone.

TMP13 pp. 1006-1007

120. **A)** Administration of either estrogen or progesterone in appropriate quantities during the first half of the menstrual cycle can inhibit ovulation by preventing the preovulatory surge of LH secretion by the anterior pituitary gland, which is essential for ovulation.
TMP13 pp. 1040, 1041

121. **B)** In the absence of 11-β-hydroxysteroid dehydrogenase, renal epithelial cells cannot convert cortisol to cortisone and, therefore, cortisol will bind to the mineralocorticoid receptor and mimic the actions of excess aldosterone. Consequently, this would result in hypertension associated with suppression of the renin-angiotensin-aldosterone system, along with hypokalemia.
TMP13 pp. 968-970, 980-981

122. **D)** In target tissues, nuclear receptors for thyroid hormones have a greater affinity for T_3 than for T_4. The secretion rate, plasma concentration, half-life, and onset of action are all greater for T_4 than for T_3.
TMP13 pp. 953-955

123. **C)** Blocking the action of FSH on the Sertoli cells of the seminiferous tubules interrupts the production of sperm. Choice C is the only option that is certain to provide sterility.
TMP13 p. 1033

124. **C)** Oxytocin is secreted from the posterior pituitary gland and carried in the blood to the breast, where it causes the cells that surround the outer walls of the alveoli and ductile system to contract. Contraction of these cells raises the hydrostatic pressure of the milk in the ducts to 10 to 20 mm Hg. Consequently, milk flows from the nipple into the baby's mouth.
TMP13 pp. 1068-1069

125. **A)** If the ductus arteriosus remains patent, poorly oxygenated blood from the pulmonary artery flows into the aorta, giving the arterial blood an oxygen level that is below normal.
TMP13 p. 1075

126. **F)** Persons with Cushing's disease have a high rate of cortisol secretion, but aldosterone secretion is normal. High plasma levels of cortisol tend to increase plasma glucose concentration by impairing glucose uptake in peripheral tissues and by promoting gluconeogenesis. However, at least in the early stages of Cushing's disease, the tendency for glucose concentration to increase appreciably is counteracted by increased insulin secretion.
TMP13 pp. 972-973, 979-980

127. **A)** In healthy patients, the secretory rates of ACTH and cortisol are low in the late evening but high in the early morning. In patients with Cushing's syndrome (adrenal adenoma) or in patients taking dexamethasone, plasma levels of ACTH are very low and are certainly not higher than normal early morning values. In patients with Addison's disease, plasma levels of ACTH are elevated as a result of deficient adrenal secretion of cortisol. The secretion of ACTH and cortisol would be expected to be normal in Conn's syndrome.
TMP13 pp. 977-980

128. **B)** Exercise stimulates GH secretion. Hyperglycemia, somatomedin, and the hypothalamic inhibitory hormone somatostatin all inhibit GH secretion. GH secretion also decreases as persons age.
TMP13 p. 945

129. **C)** A low-sodium diet would stimulate aldosterone but not cortisol secretion. Increased atrial stretch associated with volume expansion would stimulate atrial natriuretic peptide secretion but would not be expected during a low-sodium diet.
TMP13 pp. 364, 405, 971-972

130. **A)** Adrenal gland hypofunction with Addison's disease is associated with decreased secretion of both aldosterone and cortisol. In Cushing's disease and Cushing's syndrome associated with an ectopic tumor, the mineralocorticoid-hypertension induced by high plasma levels of cortisol would suppress aldosterone secretion. Neither a high-sodium diet nor administration of a converting enzyme inhibitor would affect cortisol secretion.
TMP13 pp. 971-972, 979-980

131. **B)** Blood returning from the placenta through the umbilical vein passes through the ductus venosus. The blood coming from the placenta has the highest concentration of oxygen found in the fetus.
TMP13 p. 1074

132. **B)** Osteoporosis, hypertension, hirsutism, and hyperpigmentation are all symptoms of Cushing's syndrome associated with high plasma levels of ACTH. If the high plasma ACTH levels were the result of either a pituitary adenoma or an abnormally high rate of corticotropin-releasing hormone secretion from the hypothalamus, the patient would likely have an enlarged pituitary gland. In contrast, the pituitary gland would not be enlarged if an ectopic tumor were secreting high levels of ACTH.
TMP13 pp. 979-980

133. **B)** Prolactin secretion is inhibited, not stimulated, by the hypothalamic release of dopamine into the median eminence. GH is inhibited by the hypothalamic-inhibiting hormone somatostatin. The secretion of LH, TSH, and ACTH are all under the control of the releasing hormones indicated.
TMP13 p. 942

134. B) Increased heart rate, increased respiratory rate, and decreased cholesterol concentration are all responses to excess thyroid hormone.
TMP13 pp. 956-958

135. C) Estrogen secreted by the placenta is not synthesized from basic substrates in the placenta. Instead, it is formed almost entirely from androgenic steroid compounds that are formed in the adrenal glands of both the mother and the fetus. These androgenic compounds are transported by the blood to the placenta and converted by the trophoblast cells to estrogen compounds. Their concentration in the maternal blood may also stimulate hair growth on the body.
TMP13 pp. 1060-1061

136. D) By age 45 years, only a few primordial follicles remain in the ovaries to be stimulated by gonadotropic hormones, and the production of estrogen decreases as the number of follicles approaches zero. When estrogen production falls below a critical value, it can no longer inhibit the production of gonadotropic hormones from the anterior pituitary. FSH and LH are produced in large quantities, but as the remaining follicles become atretic, production by the ovaries falls to zero.
TMP13 pp. 1050, 1051

137. D) The binding of insulin to its receptor activates tyrosine kinase, resulting in metabolic events leading to increased synthesis of fats, proteins, and glycogen. In contrast, gluconeogenesis is inhibited.
TMP13 pp. 984-989

138. C) The secretion of chemical messengers (neurohormones) from neurons into the blood is referred to as neuroendocrine secretion. Thus, in contrast to the local actions of neurotransmitters at nerve endings, neurohormones circulate in the blood before producing biological effects at target tissues. Oxytocin is synthesized from magnocellular neurons whose cell bodies are located in the paraventricular and supraoptic nuclei and whose nerve terminals terminate in the posterior pituitary gland. Target tissues for circulating oxytocin are the breast and uterus, where the hormone plays a role in lactation and parturition, respectively.
TMP13 pp. 925, 948-950

139. C) Progesterone secreted in large quantities from the corpus luteum causes marked swelling and secretory development of the endometrium.
TMP13 pp. 1046-1047

140. B) Inhibition of the iodide pump decreases the synthesis of thyroid hormones but does not impair the production of thyroglobulin by follicular cells. Decreased plasma levels of thyroid hormones result in a low metabolic rate and lead to an increase in TSH secretion. Increased plasma levels of TSH stimulate the follicular cells to synthesize more thyroglobulin.

Nervousness is a symptom of hyperthyroidism and is not caused by thyroid hormone deficiency.
TMP13 pp. 951-952, 956-960

141. D) As the blastocyst implants, the trophoblast cells invade the decidua, digesting and imbibing it. The stored nutrients in the decidual cells are used by the embryo for growth and development. During the first week after implantation, this is the only means by which the embryo can obtain nutrients. The embryo continues to obtain at least some of its nutrition in this way for up to 8 weeks, although the placenta begins to provide nutrition after about the 16th day beyond fertilization (a little more than 1 week after implantation).
TMP13 p. 1056

142. A) Both ADH and oxytocin are peptides containing nine amino acids. Their chemical structures differ in only two amino acids.
TMP13 p. 949

143. A) Because glucocorticoids decrease the sensitivity of tissues to the metabolic effects insulin, they would exacerbate diabetes. Thiazolidinediones and weight loss increase insulin sensitivity. Sulfonylureas increase insulin secretion. If weight loss and the aforementioned drugs are ineffective, exogenous insulin may be used to regulate blood glucose concentration.
TMP13 pp. 991, 996-997

144. C) In the early stages of type 2 diabetes, the tissues have a decreased sensitivity to insulin. As a result, there is a tendency for plasma glucose to increase, in part because decreased hepatic insulin sensitivity leads to increased hepatic glucose output. Because of the tendency for plasma glucose to increase, there is a compensatory increase in insulin secretion, including C-peptide, which is part of the insulin prohormone. Hypovolemia and increased production of ketone bodies, although commonly associated with uncontrolled type 1 diabetes, are not typically present in the early stages of type 2 diabetes.
TMP13 pp. 984, 994-998

145. C) One of the most characteristic findings in respiratory distress syndrome is failure of the respiratory epithelium to secrete adequate quantities of surfactant into the alveoli. Surfactant decreases the surface tension of the alveolar fluid, allowing the alveoli to open easily during inspiration. Without sufficient surfactant, the alveoli tend to collapse, and there is a tendency to develop pulmonary edema.
TMP13 p. 1074

146. A) After eating a meal, insulin secretion increases. Increased plasma levels of insulin inhibit glycogen phosphorylase, the enzyme that causes glycogen to split into glucose. In addition, insulin promotes glucose uptake in adipose tissue, providing α-glycerol

phosphate, which is needed to combine fatty acids with triglycerides, the storage form of fat.
TMP13 pp. 985-990

147. **C)** The primary controllers of ACTH, GH, LH, and TSH secretion from the pituitary gland are hypothalamic-releasing hormones. They are secreted into the median eminence and subsequently flow into the hypothalamic-hypophysial portal vessels before bathing the cells of the anterior pituitary gland. Conversely, prolactin secretion from the pituitary gland is influenced primarily by the hypothalamic inhibiting hormone dopamine. Consequently, obstruction of blood flow through the portal vessels would lead to reduced secretion of ACTH, GH, LH, and TSH, but increased secretion of prolactin.
TMP13 p. 942

148. **D)** Osteoblasts secrete all of the above except pyrophosphate. Secretions (alkaline phosphatase) from osteoblasts neutralize pyrophosphate, an inhibitor of hydroxyapatite crystallization. Neutralization of pyrophosphate permits the precipitation of calcium salts into collagen fibers.
TMP13 pp. 1004-1006

149. **B)** In primary hyperparathyroidism, high plasma levels of PTH increase the formation of 1,25-(OH)2D3, which increases intestinal absorption of calcium. This action of PTH, along with its effects to increase bone resorption and renal calcium reabsorption, leads to hypercalcemia. However, because of the high filtered load of calcium, calcium is excreted in the urine. High plasma levels of PTH also decrease phosphate reabsorption and increase urinary excretion, leading to a fall in plasma phosphate concentration.
TMP13 pp. 1009-1012, 1014-1015

150. **A)** Gamma radiation destroys the cells undergoing the most rapid rates of mitosis and meiosis, the germinal epithelium of the testes. The man described is said to have normal testosterone levels, suggesting that the secretory patterns of GnRH and LH are normal and that his interstitial cells are functional. Because he is not producing sperm, the levels of inhibin secreted by the Sertoli cells would be maximally suppressed, and his levels of FSH would be strongly elevated.
TMP13 p. 1033

151. **B)** In this experiment, the size of the thyroid gland increased because TSH causes hypertrophy and hyperplasia of its target gland and increased secretion of thyroid hormones. Increased plasma levels of thyroid hormones inhibit the secretion of TRH, which decreases stimulation of the pituitary thyrotropes, resulting in a decrease in the size of the pituitary gland. Higher plasma levels of thyroid hormones also increase metabolic rate and decrease body weight.
TMP13 pp. 955-957, 960

152. **C)** In this experiment, the size of the pituitary and adrenal glands increased because CRH stimulates the pituitary corticotropes to secrete ACTH, which in turn stimulates the adrenals to secrete corticosterone and cortisol. Higher plasma levels of cortisol increase protein degradation and lipolysis and therefore decrease body weight.
TMP13 pp. 972-974, 976-977

153. **E)** Vitamin D deficiency leads to rickets in children and osteomalacia in adults. A deficiency in vitamin D leads to reduced synthesis of the active form of the vitamin 1,25-(OH)2D3. In turn, in the presence of low plasma levels of 1,25-(OH)2D3, the synthesis of calbindin in the intestine is reduced, resulting in impaired intestinal absorption of calcium. Impaired intestinal absorption of calcium tends to cause hypocalcemia, which stimulates PTH secretion. Increased PTH secretion contributes to the maintenance of plasma calcium concentration, in part, by increasing bone resorption.
TMP13 pp. 1010-1011, 1015

Sports Physiology

1. A Tour de France rider has the following values under resting conditions:

   > Oxygen consumption = 250 ml O_2/min
   > Hemoglobin concentration = 15 gm Hg/dl
   > Arterial partial pressure of oxygen (Po_2) = 100 mm Hg
   > Mixed venous saturation = 75 percent

   When exercising, he has the following values:

   > Oxygen consumption = 3000 ml O_2/min
   > Hemoglobin concentration = 15 gm Hg/dl
   > Arterial Po_2 = 100 mm Hg
   > Mixed venous saturation = 25 percent

   What is the absolute increase in cardiac output with exercise?

   A) 5 L/min
   B) 15 L/min
   C) 25 L/min
   D) 30 L/min

2. Which athlete is able to exercise the longest before exhaustion occurs?

   A) One on a high-fat diet
   B) One on a high-carbohydrate diet
   C) One on a mixed carbohydrate–fat diet
   D) One on a high-protein diet
   E) One on a mixed protein–fat diet

3. A female university student is comfortably running a 10K race. At 5 miles, which set of values would best describe her blood composition?

	Arterial Po_2	Arterial Pco_2	Mixed Venous Po_2
A)	↑	↑	↓
B)	↑	↑	↔
C)	↑	↓	↔
D)	↑	↔	↓
E)	↑	↔	↑
F)	↔	↔	↔
G)	↓	↑	↓
H)	↓	↓	↓
I)	↓	↑	↔

4. Which statement about respiration in exercise is most accurate?

   A) Maximum oxygen consumption of a male marathon runner is less than that of an untrained average male
   B) Maximum oxygen consumption can be increased about 100% by training
   C) Maximum oxygen diffusing capacity of a male marathon runner is much greater than that of an untrained average male
   D) Blood levels of oxygen and carbon dioxide are abnormal during exercise

5. Olympic athletes who run marathons or cross-country ski have much higher maximum cardiac outputs than nonathletes. Which statement about the hearts of these athletes compared with nonathletes is most accurate?

   A) Stroke volume in the Olympic athletes is about 5% greater at rest
   B) The percentage increase in heart rate during maximal exercise is much greater in the Olympic athletes
   C) Maximum cardiac output is only 3 percent to 4 percent greater in the Olympic athletes
   D) Resting heart rate in the Olympic athletes is significantly higher

6. Which statement comparing slow-twitch and fast-twitch muscle fibers is most accurate?

   A) Fast-twitch fibers are less dependent on the phosphagen and glycogen–lactic acid systems
   B) Slow-twitch fibers are surrounded by more mitochondria
   C) Slow-twitch fibers have less myoglobin
   D) Fewer capillaries surround slow-twitch fibers
   E) Fast-twitch fibers are smaller in diameter

7. What causes the excess muscle mass in the average male compared with a female?

   A) Increased testosterone secreted in the male
   B) Increased estrogen secreted by the female
   C) Higher exercise levels in the male
   D) Greater glycogen deposition by males

8. In athletes who use androgens to increase performance experience, which of the following would most likely occur?

   A) Decreased high-density blood lipoproteins
   B) Decreased low-density blood lipoproteins
   C) Increased testicular function
   D) Decreased incidence of hypertension

9. A person living in Maine trains regularly to run 10K races and continually finishes in the middle of the pack. What is the physiological limitation that prevents this person from improving?

   A) Lack of ability to increase pulmonary ventilation
   B) Lack of ability to use the oxygen delivered to the tissue
   C) Lack of an ability to increase cardiac output
   D) Lack of ability to dissipate the heat generated with exercise
   E) Lack of ability to convert glucose to adenosine triphosphate (ATP)

10. If muscle strength is increased with resistive training, which condition will most likely occur?

    A) A decrease in the number of myofibrils
    B) An increase in mitochondrial enzymes
    C) A decrease in the components of the phosphagen energy system
    D) A decrease in stored triglycerides

ANSWERS

1. B)

At rest:
Arterial content (Ca) = 15 × 1.34 = 20 ml O_2/100 ml blood at 100% saturation
Venous content (Cv) = 20 × 0.75 = 15 ml O_2/100 ml blood
Arteriovenous O_2 difference = 5 ml O_2/100 ml blood

Answer:
Vo_2 = Q (ml/min) (Ca – Cv)
250 ml O_2/min = Q (5 ml O_2/100 ml blood)
Q = 250 ml O_2/min ÷ 5 ml O_2/100 ml blood
Q = 5.0 L/min

Exercising:
Arterial content (Ca) = 15 × 1.34 = 20 ml O_2/100 ml blood
Venous content (Cv) = 20 × 0.25 = 5 ml O_2/100 ml blood
Arteriovenous O_2 difference = 15 ml O_2/100 ml blood

Answer:
Vo_2 = Q (ml/min) (Ca – Cv)
3000 ml O_2/min = Q (15 ml O_2/100 ml blood)
Q = 3000 ml O_2/min ÷ 15 ml O_2/100 ml blood
Q = 20 L/min

The increase in Vo_2 is 20 L/min – 5 L/min = 15 L/min.

TMP13 pp. 257, 530-531

2. B) An athlete consuming a high-carbohydrate diet will store nearly twice as much glycogen in the muscles compared with an athlete consuming a mixed carbohydrate–fat diet. This glycogen is converted to lactic acid and supplies four ATP molecules for each molecule of glucose. It also forms ATP 2.5 times as fast as oxidative metabolism in the mitochondria. This extra energy from glycogen significantly increases the time an athlete can exercise.

TMP13 p. 1089

3. D) With exercise an increase in arterial Po_2 occurs as a result of better ventilation/perfusion. Arterial Pco_2 may be normal or slightly decreased. Because of the increased metabolic rate, the venous Po_2 will decrease.

TMP13 pp. 1091-1092

4. C) During exercise the maximum oxygen consumption of a male marathon runner is much greater than that of an untrained average male. However, athletic training increases the maximum oxygen consumption by only about 10%. Therefore, the maximum oxygen consumption in marathon runners is probably partly genetically determined. These runners also have a large increase in maximum oxygen diffusing capacity, and their blood levels of oxygen and carbon dioxide remain relatively normal during exercise.

TMP13 pp. 1090-1091

5. B) When comparing Olympic athletes and nonathletes, there are several differences in the responses of the heart. Stroke volume is much higher at rest in the Olympic athlete, and heart rate is much lower. The heart rate can increase approximately 270 percent in the Olympic athlete during maximal exercise, which is a much greater percentage than occurs in a nonathlete. In addition, the maximal increase in cardiac output is approximately 30 percent greater in the Olympic athlete.

TMP13 p. 1093

6. B) The basic differences between the fast-twitch and slow-twitch fibers are the following: Fast-twitch fibers are more dependent on anaerobic metabolism, and slow-twitch fibers are more dependent on aerobic metabolism. In fast-twitch fibers, the dependence on phosphagen and glycogen–lactic acid systems is much greater than in the fast-twitch fibers. The slow-twitch fibers are organized for endurance and are dependent upon aerobic metabolism; therefore, they have many more mitochondria and myoglobin, which combines with oxygen in the muscle fiber. The number of capillaries that supply the oxygen is much greater in the vicinity of slow-twitch fibers than in the vicinity of fast-twitch fibers.

TMP13 p. 1090

7. A) The increased muscle mass in a male is caused by testosterone, which is secreted by the male testes. Testosterone has a powerful anabolic effect, causing greatly increased deposition of protein everywhere in the body, but especially in the muscles. Estrogen in the female causes a greater deposition of fat but not protein.

TMP13 p. 1085

8. A) Use of male sex hormones (androgens) or other anabolic steroids to increase muscle strength increases athletic performances under some conditions but can have adverse effects on the body. Anabolic steroids increase the risk of cardiovascular damage because they increase the instance of hypertension, decrease high-density blood lipoproteins, and increase low-density blood lipoproteins. These factors all promote heart attacks and strokes. These androgenic substances also decrease testicular function, which decreases the formation of sperm and the body's own production of natural testosterone.

TMP13 p. 1095

9. C) Pulmonary ventilation is not a limitation because people normally overventilate during exercise, and there are minimal to no changes in arterial blood gases. The muscles will use the oxygen delivered to them. The limitation is the delivery of oxygen and nutrients to muscle based on the limitation of an increase in cardiac output. Increasing cardiac output will increase exercise performance. Under hot conditions, heat dissipation can limit exercise performance. Muscles have minimal to no limitation in converting glucose to ATP.

TMP13 pp. 1090-1094

10. B) During resistive training, the muscles that are contracted with at least a 50 percent maximal force for at least three times a week experience an optimal increase in muscle strength. This increase in strength causes muscle hypertrophy, and several changes occur. There will be an increase in the number of myofibrils and up to a 120 percent increase in mitochondrial enzymes. As much as a 60 percent to 80 percent increase in the components of the phosphagen energy system can occur, and up to a 50 percent increase in stored glycogen can occur. Also, as much as a 75 percent to 100 percent increase in stored triglycerides can occur.

TMP13 pp. 1089-1090